Common ENT Disorders in Children

Editors

CHARLES M. BOWER
GRESHAM T. RICHTER

OTOLARYNGOLOGIC CLINICS OF NORTH AMERICA

www.oto.theclinics.com

October 2014 • Volume 47 • Number 5

ELSEVIER

1600 John F. Kennedy Boulevard • Suite 1800 • Philadelphia, Pennsylvania, 19103-2899

http://www.oto.theclinics.com

OTOLARYNGOLOGIC CLINICS OF NORTH AMERICA Volume 47, Number 5
October 2014 ISSN 0030-6665, ISBN-13: 978-0-323-32622-3

Editor: Joanne Husovski
Developmental Editor: Susan Showalter

Otolaryngologic Clinics of North America (ISSN 0030-6665) is published bimonthly by Elsevier, Inc., 360 Park Avenue South, New York, NY 10010-1710. Months of issue are February, April, June, August, October, and December. Business and Editorial Offices: 1600 John F. Kennedy Blvd., Suite 1800, Philadelphia, PA 19103-2899. Customer Service Office: 6277 Sea Harbor Drive, Orlando, FL 32887-4800. Periodicals postage paid at New York, NY and additional mailing offices. Subscription prices is $365.00 per year (US individuals), $692.00 per year (US institutions), $175.00 per year (US student/resident), $485.00 per year (Canadian individuals), $876.00 per year (Canadian institutions), $540.00 per year (international individuals), $876.00 per year (international institutions), $270.00 per year (international & Canadian student/resident). Foreign air speed delivery is included in all *Clinics'* subscription prices. All prices are subject to change without notice. **POSTMASTER:** Send address changes to *Otolaryngologic Clinics of North America,* Elsevier Health Sciences Division, Subscription Customer Service, 3251 Riverport Lane, Maryland Heights, MO 63043. **Telephone: 1-800-654-2452 (U.S. and Canada); 314-447-8871 (outside U.S. and Canada). Fax: 314-447-8029. E-mail: journalscustomerservice-usa@elsevier.com (for print support); journalsonlinesupport-usa@elsevier.com (for online support).**

Reprints. For copies of 100 or more of articles in this publication, please contact the Commercial Reprints Department, Elsevier Inc., 360 Park Avenue South, New York, NY 10010-1710. Tel.: 212-633-3874; Fax: 212-633-3820; E-mail: reprints@elsevier.com.

Otolaryngologic Clinics of North America is also published in Spanish by McGraw-Hill Interamericana Editores S.A., P.O. Box 5-237, 06500 Mexico D.F., Mexico.

Otolaryngologic Clinics of North America is covered in *MEDLINE/PubMed (Index Medicus), Current Contents/Clinical Medicine, Excerpta Medica, BIOSIS, Science Citation Index,* and *ISI/BIOMED.*

PROGRAM OBJECTIVE
The goal of the *Otolaryngologic Clinics of North America* is to provide information on the latest trends in patient management, the newest advances; and provide a sound basis for choosing treatment options in the field of otolaryngology.

TARGET AUDIENCE
All practicing physicians and healthcare professionals who provide patient care to *otolaryngologic* patients.

LEARNING OBJECTIVES
Upon completion of this activity, participants will be able to:
1. Review pediatric rhinosinusitis, pediatric stridor, pediatric sialadenitis, pediatric tonsillectomy, and pediatric cervical lymphadenopathy.
2. Discuss the diagnosis and management of patients with clefts.
3. Recognize the management of oropharyngeal dysphagia and the management of acute otitis media in children.

ACCREDITATION
The Elsevier Office of Continuing Medical Education (EOCME) is accredited by the Accreditation Council for Continuing Medical Education (ACCME) to provide continuing medical education for physicians.

The EOCME designates this enduring material for a maximum of 15 *AMA PRA Category 1 Credit*(s)™. Physicians should claim only the credit commensurate with the extent of their participation in the activity.

All other health care professionals requesting continuing education credit for this enduring material will be issued a certificate of participation.

DISCLOSURE OF CONFLICTS OF INTEREST
The EOCME assesses conflict of interest with its instructors, faculty, planners, and other individuals who are in a position to control the content of CME activities. All relevant conflicts of interest that are identified are thoroughly vetted by EOCME for fair balance, scientific objectivity, and patient care recommendations. EOCME is committed to providing its learners with CME activities that promote improvements or quality in healthcare and not a specific proprietary business or a commercial interest.

The planning committee, staff, authors and editors listed below have identified no financial relationships or relationships to products or devices they or their spouse/life partner have with commercial interest related to the content of this CME activity:
Charles M. Bower, MD; Jennings R. Boyette, MD; Brooke H. Davis; Venkata SPB Durvasula, MD; Carrie L. Francis, MD; Larry D. Hartzell, MD, FAAP; Kristen Helm; Christen M. Holder, PhD; Brynne Hunter; Joanne Husovski; Jonathan B. Ida, MD, MA, FAAP; Glenn Isaacson, MD, FAAP; Lauren A. Kilpatrick, MD; Christopher G. Larsen, MD; Sandy Lavery; Anthony Magit, MD, MPH; Jill McNair; Abby R. Nolder, MD; Ashley C. O'Neill, MS, CCC-SLP; Santha Priya; Eleni B. Rettig, MD; Gresham Thomas Richter, MD, FACS; Tara L. Rosenberg, MD; Rachel St. John, MD, NCC, NIC-A; Susan Showalter; Dana Mara Thompson, MD, MS, FACS; David E. Tunkel, MD; Wendy L. Ward, PhD.

The planning committee, staff, authors and editors listed below have identified financial relationships or relationships to products or devices they or their spouse/life partner have with commercial interest related to the content of this CME activity:

UNAPPROVED/OFF-LABEL USE DISCLOSURE
The EOCME requires CME faculty to disclose to the participants:
1. When products or procedures being discussed are off-label, unlabelled, experimental, and/or investigational (not US Food and Drug Administration (FDA) approved); and
2. Any limitations on the information presented, such as data that are preliminary or that represent ongoing research, interim analyses, and/or unsupported opinions. Faculty may discuss information about pharmaceutical agents that is outside of FDA-approved labelling. This information is intended solely for CME and is not intended to promote off-label use of these medications. If you have any questions, contact the medical affairs department of the manufacturer for the most recent prescribing information.

TO ENROLL
To enroll in the *Otolaryngologic Clinics of North America* Continuing Medical Education program, call customer service at 1-800-654-2452 or sign up online at http://www.theclinics.com/home/cme. The CME program is available to subscribers for an additional annual fee of USD 260.

METHOD OF PARTICIPATION

In order to claim credit, participants must complete the following:

1. Complete enrolment as indicated above.
2. Read the activity.
3. Complete the CME Test and Evaluation. Participants must achieve a score of 70% on the test. All CME Tests and Evaluations must be completed online.

CME INQUIRIES/SPECIAL NEEDS

For all CME inquiries or special needs, please contact elsevierCME@elsevier.com.

Contributors

EDITORS

CHARLES M. BOWER, MD
Pediatric Otolaryngology, Professor Otolaryngology – Head and Neck Surgery, Arkansas Children's Hospital, University of Arkansas for Medical Sciences, Little Rock, Arkansas

GRESHAM T. RICHTER, MD
Associate Professor, Department of Pediatric Otolaryngology and Head and Neck Surgery, Arkansas Children's Hospital, Little Rock, Arkansas

AUTHORS

CHARLES M. BOWER, MD
Pediatric Otolaryngology, Professor Otolaryngology – Head and Neck Surgery, Arkansas Children's Hospital, University of Arkansas for Medical Sciences, Little Rock, Arkansas

JENNINGS R. BOYETTE, MD
Assistant Professor, Department of Otolaryngology – Head and Neck Surgery, Arkansas Children's Hospital, University of Arkansas for Medical Sciences, Little Rock, Arkansas

BROOKE H. DAVIS
Student, Episcopal Collegiate School, Little Rock, Arkansas

VENKATA S.P.B. DURVASULA, MD, FRCS ENT
Clinical Fellow, Departments of Pediatric Otolaryngology and Head and Neck Surgery, Arkansas Children's Hospital, Little Rock, Arkansas

CARRIE L. FRANCIS, MD
Assistant Professor, Department of Otolaryngology – Head and Neck Surgery, University of Kansas Medical Center, Kansas City, Kansas; Division of Pediatric Otolaryngology, Children's Mercy Hospitals and Clinics, Kansas City, Missouri

LARRY D. HARTZELL, MD, FAAP
Assistant Professor, Pediatric Otolaryngology, Arkansas Children's Hospital, University of Arkansas for Medical Sciences, Little Rock, Arkansas

CHRISTEN M. HOLDER, PhD
Postdoctoral Fellow, Department of Pediatrics, Arkansas Children's Hospital, University of Arkansas for Medical Sciences, Little Rock, Arkansas

JONATHAN B. IDA, MD, MA, FAAP
Assistant Professor, Pediatric Otolaryngology – Head and Neck Surgery, Ann & Robert H. Lurie Children's Hospital of Chicago, Northwestern University Feinberg School of Medicine, Chicago, Illinois

GLENN ISAACSON, MD, FAAP
Departments of Otolaryngology – Head and Neck Surgery and Pediatrics, Temple University School of Medicine, Rydal, Pennsylvania

LAUREN A. KILPATRICK, MD
Assistant Professor, Department of Pediatric Otolaryngology, University of North Carolina School of Medicine, Chapel Hill, North Carolina

CHRISTOPHER G. LARSEN, MD
Department of Otolaryngology – Head and Neck Surgery, University of Kansas Medical Center, Kansas City, Kansas; Division of Pediatric Otolaryngology, Children's Mercy Hospitals and Clinics, Kansas City, Missouri

ANTHONY MAGIT, MD, MPH
Clinical Professor, Department of Surgery, Rady Children's Hospital, University of California San Diego School of Medicine, San Diego, California

ABBY R. NOLDER, MD
Department of Otolaryngology – Head and Neck Surgery, Arkansas Children's Hospital, University of Arkansas for Medical Sciences, Little Rock, Arkansas

ASHLEY C. O'NEILL, MS
Speech-Language Pathologist, Departments of Audiology and Speech Pathology, Arkansas Children's Hospital, Little Rock, Arkansas

ELENI RETTIG, MD
Department of Otolaryngology – Head and Neck Surgery, Johns Hopkins University School of Medicine, Baltimore, Maryland

GRESHAM T. RICHTER, MD
Associate Professor, Department of Pediatric Otolaryngology and Head and Neck Surgery, Arkansas Children's Hospital, Little Rock, Arkansas

TARA L. ROSENBERG, MD
Department of Otolaryngology – Head and Neck Surgery, Arkansas Children's Hospital, University of Arkansas for Medical Sciences, Little Rock, Arkansas

RACHEL ST. JOHN, MD, NCC, NIC-A
Director, Family Focused Center for Deaf and Hard of Hearing Children, Department of Otolaryngology, Dallas Children's Medical Center, UT Southwestern Medical Center, Dallas, Texas

DANA MARA THOMPSON, MD, MS, FACS
Professor and Division Chair, Pediatric Otolaryngology – Head and Neck Surgery, Ann & Robert H. Lurie Children's Hospital of Chicago, Northwestern University Feinberg School of Medicine, Chicago, Illinois

DAVID E. TUNKEL, MD
Director, Division of Pediatric Otolaryngology, Department of Otolaryngology – Head and Neck Surgery, Johns Hopkins University School of Medicine, Baltimore, Maryland

WENDY L. WARD, PhD
Professor, Department of Pediatrics, Arkansas Children's Hospital, University of Arkansas for Medical Sciences, Little Rock, Arkansas

Contents

> Infant hearing loss is common. Screening is performed in more than 98% of US infants. Otolaryngologists play an important role in identification and management of infants and children who are deaf and hard of hearing. Otolaryngologists should routinely assess for hearing screening results and intervene for screens not passed. Long-term follow-up and reassessment of patients with hearing loss is an ongoing component of otolaryngology practice. This article reviews the otolaryngologist's role in the management of infants and children who are deaf or hard of hearing from screening to intervention and management.

> Acute otitis media (AOM) is a common disease of childhood. AOM is most appropriately diagnosed by careful otoscopy with an understanding of clinical signs and symptoms. The distinction between AOM and chronic otitis media with effusion should be emphasized. Treatment should include pain management, and initial antibiotic treatment should be given to those most likely to benefit, including young children, children with severe symptoms, and those with otorrhea and/or bilateral AOM. Tympanostomy tube placement may be helpful for those who experience frequent episodes of AOM or fail medical therapy. Recent practice guidelines may assist the clinician with such decisions.

> This article reviews current knowledge of the science of pediatric tonsillectomy—developmental anatomy of the tonsil, physiology of the operation, and wound healing after surgery. It outlines indication for surgery and best practices for intraoperative and postoperative care as described in the American Academy of Otolaryngology—Head and Neck Surgery Foundation clinical practice guideline: Tonsillectomy in Children. Finally, it discusses areas of uncertainty in the field and opportunity for future improvement.

> Oropharyngeal dysphagia (OPD) is a challenging and relatively common condition in children. Both developmentally normal and delayed children

may be affected. The etiology of OPD is frequently multifactorial with neurologic, inflammatory, and anatomic conditions contributing to discoordination of the pharyngeal phase of swallowing. Depending on the severity and source, OPD may persist for several years with significant burden to a patient's health and family. This article details current understanding of the mechanism and potential sources of OPD in children while providing an algorithm for managing it in the acute and chronic setting.

Tara L. Rosenberg and Abby R. Nolder

This article provides an overview for evaluation and management of the pediatric patient with cervical lymphadenopathy. A thorough history and physical examination are crucial in developing a differential diagnosis for these patients. Although infectious causes of lymphadenopathy are more prevalent in the pediatric population compared with adults, neoplasms should also be considered. Judicious use of imaging studies, namely ultrasound, can provide valuable information for accurate diagnosis. Common and uncommon infectious causes of cervical lymphadenopathy are reviewed. Surgical intervention is occasionally necessary for diagnosis and treatment of infections, and rarely indicated for the possibility of malignancy. Indications for surgery are discussed.

Anthony Magit

This review addresses the diagnosis and treatment of acute and chronic rhinosinusitis. Antimicrobial and adjuvant therapies, including topical treatments, are discussed. Surgical intervention is included in the treatment options. Clinical characteristics of rhinosinusitis are presented with an emphasis on history and physical examination. The use of imaging is described with regard to the indications for imaging and selection of imaging modalities. Complications of rhinosinusitis, with management recommendations based on recent data, are described. The evaluation and management of patients with cystic fibrosis and allergic fungal sinusitis is part of the discussion of less common scenarios of patients with sinus disease.

Jennings R. Boyette

Facial trauma in children differs from adults. The growing facial skeleton presents several challenges to the reconstructive surgeon. A thorough understanding of the patterns of facial growth and development is needed to form an individualized treatment strategy. A proper diagnosis must be made and treatment options weighed against the risk of causing further harm to facial development. This article focuses on the management of facial fractures in children. Discussed are common fracture patterns based on the development of the facial structure, initial management, diagnostic strategies, new concepts and old controversies regarding radiologic examinations, conservative versus operative intervention, risks of growth impairment, and resorbable fixation.

OTOLARYNGOLOGIC CLINICS
OF NORTH AMERICA

RELATED INTEREST

Pediatric Clinics, October 2013
Pediatric Emergencies
Richard Lichenstein and Getachew Teshome, *Editors*

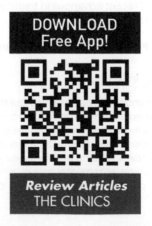

DOWNLOAD
Free App!

Review Articles
THE CLINICS

NOW AVAILABLE FOR YOUR iPhone and iPad

Preface

Common ENT Disorders in Pediatrics

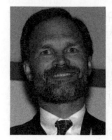 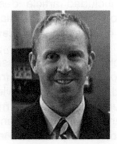

Charles M. Bower, MD   Gresham T. Richter, MD
Editors

The practice of pediatric otolaryngology includes management of a variety of disorders of the head and neck that affect a large portion of the general population and may be managed by several specialties. This issue is designed to provide the general and pediatric otolaryngologist the most up-to-date information for management of common otolaryngology disorders in children. It should also prove to be a valuable resource for pediatricians, family practice physicians, and other primary care physicians encountering ear, nose, and throat conditions.

Although rare, hearing loss is the most commonly encountered congenital malady. As a result, many states now require that one hundred percent of babies be screened for hearing loss before leaving the newborn nursery. Once identified, management of early detected hearing loss can be complicated by lack of follow-up, inconsistent and incomplete referrals, and slow progression to early intervention or amplification. The article on hearing screening will help define the role of otolaryngologists and pediatricians in terms of appropriate referrals and interventions for neonatal hearing loss. Similarly, otitis media afflicts many children and requires a systematic approach. Herein, Dr Benson and Tunkel provide comprehensive evidence-based data on the best management of acute otitis media for single episodes and recurrent disease.

Pediatric rhinosinusitis is ubiquitous and encountered by all pediatricians and otolaryngologists. The diagnosis is predominately clinical but might require imaging to help define the extent of disease for complications or perioperative planning. Management options for sinonasal disease range from observation to invasive surgery. The article by Dr Magit describes common medical strategies and options for surgical management, including endoscopic approaches, while examining uncommon causes or manifestations of pediatric sinusitis related to cystic fibrosis, immunodeficiency, and fungal allergy. The article by Dr Nolder emphasizes general medical management of infectious lymphadenopathy, but also reviews the indications for open biopsy to rule out

---

Otolaryngol Clin N Am 47 (2014) xi–xii
http://dx.doi.org/10.1016/j.otc.2014.07.002
0030-6665/14/$ – see front matter © 2014 Elsevier Inc. All rights reserved.

more serious, but fortunately much less common malignant diseases. The articles on stridor and dysphagia in this issue both provide an algorithm for diagnosis and management of these frequently related conditions in the child. Both endoscopic surgical techniques and medical management are required for these disorders. A team of physicians and ancillary services may be required for more complicated cases of stridor and dysphagia. Similarly, management of cleft lip and palate remains strongly benefited by team management. The included article describes a team-based approach to cleft lip and palate as a model for pediatric diagnoses and treatment and demonstrates how enhanced quality of care can be achieved through multidisciplinary action.

Fortunately the majority of pediatric facial trauma is soft tissue injury and managed in the emergency room or primary practitioner's office. Facial fractures in children may be more complicated and are addressed in an excellent review by Dr Boyette. The article emphasizes the variance in trauma patterns and management strategies between infants, children, and adults. An article on sialadenitis is also included in this issue to emphasize the importance of primary care management of sialadenitis through preventive immunization and conservative management strategies. Indications for referral for surgical options, including noninvasive endoscopic procedures and open surgery, are reviewed for children with more chronic disease. We complete this issue with a final article on the identification and management of behavioral problems as they relate to common otolaryngology problems, including sleep apnea, cleft lip and palate, and hearing loss. Behavioral problems are surprisingly common in these patients, but may not be adequately addressed by the otolaryngologist. A short guideline is provided to assist in appropriate referral and management strategies for behavior problems in children.

We certainly would like to thank the many authors for their excellent contributions to this special issue of *Otolaryngologic Clinics of North America*. We hope that this will be a highly beneficial resource for general as well as pediatric otolaryngologists that has great practical value for pediatricians, family practitioners, and others managing children.

Charles M. Bower, MD
Department of Pediatric Otolaryngology
Arkansas Children's Hospital
1 Children's Way, Slot #836
Little Rock, AR 72202, USA

Gresham T. Richter, MD
Department of Pediatric Otolaryngology
Arkansas Children's Hospital
1 Children's Way, Slot #836
Little Rock, AR 72202, USA

E-mail addresses:
bowercharlesm@uams.edu (C.M. Bower)
GTRichter@uams.edu (G.T. Richter)

The Otolaryngologist's Role in Newborn Hearing Screening and Early Intervention

CrossMark

Charles M. Bower, MD[a],*, Rachel St. John, MD, NCC, NIC-A[b]

KEYWORDS

- Hearing screening • Hearing loss • Newborn • Auditory evoked response
- Otoacoustic emissions • Early intervention

KEY POINTS

- All infants should complete hearing screening by 1 month of age, diagnostic testing by 3 months of age, and intervention by 6 months of age (1-3-6 guidelines).
- Otolaryngologists should routinely assess hearing status, including ascertaining the results of infant hearing screening and diagnostic tests.
- Otolaryngologists should complete an appropriate diagnostic testing algorithm in patients identified as deaf or hard of hearing.
- Otolaryngologists should monitor hearing, external and middle ear status, and speech and language development in children with hearing loss.
- Otolaryngologists should recommend referral to pediatric audiologists, speech/language pathologists, ophthalmologists, geneticists, and other indicated specialists for infants and children with hearing loss.

Author's Note: *For the purposes of this article, the terms "hearing loss" and "hearing impairment" apply to newborns and infants who are deaf or hard of hearing at birth as well as those who lose hearing at a later date. Persons with hearing loss generally prefer the terms "deaf" or "hard of hearing," and those terms are recommended when communicating with families and caregivers.*

INTRODUCTION

The main premise behind infant hearing screening is that early detection and provision of intervention is beneficial to the development of speech, language, reading, and cognition for those identified early with hearing loss.[1] The potential detrimental effects

Conflicts of Interest: None.
[a] Pediatric Otolaryngology, Arkansas Children's Hospital, University of Arkansas for Medical Sciences, 1 Children's Way, Little Rock, AR 72202, USA; [b] Family Focused Center for Deaf and Hard of Hearing Children, Department of Otolaryngology, Dallas Children's Medical Center, UT Southwestern Medical Center, Dallas, TX 75207, USA
* Corresponding author.
E-mail address: bowercharlesm@uams.edu

Otolaryngol Clin N Am 47 (2014) 631–649
http://dx.doi.org/10.1016/j.otc.2014.06.002
0030-6665/14/$ – see front matter © 2014 Elsevier Inc. All rights reserved.

Abbreviations	
AABR	Automated auditory brainstem response
ABR	Auditory brainstem response
EHDI	Early hearing detection and intervention
OAE	Otoacoustic emission
OME	Otitis media with effusion

of permanent hearing loss in infants and children on speech, language, and literacy have been well established, and are related to the severity of the hearing level.[2,3] Infants discovered and provided appropriate intervention before 6 months of age have significantly better language skills than those identified later.[4–7] Although randomized trials of hearing loss outcomes are not available,[8] the apparent benefits of early screening and intervention have resulted in dramatic growth in programs that address all aspects of hearing status and rehabilitation. All states have now established an early hearing detection and intervention (EHDI) program, with more than 98% of US infants now completing testing shortly after birth.[9,10] Early diagnosis and intervention is available for the majority of identified infants, and outcomes remain positive. However, many challenges remain in hearing screening programs. Some children are never screened, and of those screened, loss to follow-up rates can be unacceptably high (>50%).[11,12] The availability of pediatric audiology services for diagnostic testing and intervention remain limited in many locations.

Otolaryngologists play an important role in hearing screening and intervention, and can be critical to the success of local and regional programs. This role includes surveillance for and identification of infants who are deaf or hard of hearing, diagnosis and management of ear disease, assistance with referrals to appropriate services, and ongoing assessment of the success of intervention. Otolaryngologists are also important in hearing screening program development, quality improvement, and education for practitioners. They promote and participate in the advocacy for initiation, maintenance, and funding of hearing programs. Because of their key role in infant hearing, this article is a guide for pediatricians and otolaryngologists on infant hearing screening and early intervention.

Incidence and Program Development

Significant hearing loss occurs in approximately 1 to 3 per 1000 newborns with higher rates occurring in neonatal intensive care unit patients. The incidence quadruples by 16 years of age owing to late-onset and progressive conditions.[13] Thus, hearing loss is among the most common birth conditions, but is difficult to recognize without objective testing. Parents and professionals are poor judges of the degree of hearing loss in infants while waiting for signs of speech and language deficits may delay identification for several years. Although some patients have recognizable syndromes or malformations, many children with hearing loss have no distinguishing features.[14] Before the advent of routine hearing screening, a high-risk registry was used to select patients for further testing (**Box 1**). Unfortunately, the use of the high-risk registry still missed about one half of the patients with congenital hearing loss.[15,16] With the implementation of universal hearing screening the age of identification of hearing loss improved from 30 to 6 months.[17,18] In terms of childhood development and plasticity of the developing auditory cortex, the importance of screening and early intervention to improve long-term outcomes is clear.[19]

Objective hearing screening tools have made routine infant screening a realistic possibility. Infant hearing screening is now recommended by the American Academy

---

Box 1
Risk factors for hearing loss

1. Caregiver concern regarding hearing or speech

2. Family history of childhood hearing loss

3. Neonatal intensive care stay longer than 5 days, including extracorporeal membrane oxygenation

4. In utero infections, such as cytomegalovirus or toxoplasmosis

5. Craniofacial anomalies

6. Anomalies associated with syndromic hearing loss

7. Syndromes associated with hearing loss

8. Neurodegenerative disorders

9. Bacterial or viral meningitis

10. Head trauma, especially basal skull/temporal bone fracture

11. Chemotherapy

12. Recurrent or persistent otitis media for at least 3 months

13. Other considerations: Duration of stay in the intensive care unit, respiratory distress syndrome, retrolental fibroplasia, asphyxia, meconium aspiration, neurodegenerative disorders, chromosomal abnormalities, drug and alcohol abuse by the mother, maternal diabetes, multiple births, and lack of prenatal care

Adapted from American Academy of Pediatrics, Joint Committee on Infant Hearing. Year 2007 position statement: principles and guidelines for early hearing detection and intervention programs. Pediatrics 2007;120(4):898–921; and Kountakis SE, Skoulas I, Phillips D, et al. Risk factors for hearing loss in neonates: a prospective study. Am J Otolaryngol 2002;23(3):133–7.

---

of Pediatrics, the American Academy of Otolaryngology Head and Neck Surgery, and the American Speech-Hearing-Language Association. *Healthy People 2010* and the Joint Commission on Infant Hearing recommend that all babies be screened by 1 month of age. Secondary diagnostic testing for infants who do not pass their hearing screen must be complete by 3 months of age. For infants identified as deaf or hard of hearing, early intervention should be implemented by 6 months of age.[20] This timeline of identification to management is commonly referred to as the "1-3-6" guideline, and is an important initiative in infant hearing screening and intervention programs.[12]

Screening Tools

The 2 commonly used methods for infant hearing screenings are automated otoacoustic emissions (OAE) or automated acoustic brainstem response (AABR) systems (**Table 1**). Both tools allow for quick, cost-effective screening in the newborn nursery by easily trained technicians.[21] One or both systems may be used to assess a newborn. OAE takes less time to complete than AABR, but may not pass as many babies on the first attempt. OAEs are more sensitive to external ear canal obstruction and middle ear effusions, and may not pass in infants with what could be temporary conductive hearing loss.[22] OAEs do not measure the integrity of the VIIIth nerve or auditory brainstem pathways, and therefore may miss auditory neuropathy. AABR measures the integrity of the cochlea, auditory nerve, and brainstem, and is highly correlated with hearing sensitivity in the 1000 to 8000 Hz range.[23,24] AABR may take slightly longer and have a higher cost than OAE, but this is matched with a slightly higher pass rate.[25,26]

Table 1
Hearing screening tools: A variety of hearing screening tools are available depending on patient age and ability to cooperate with testing

Test	Protocol	Appropriate for
Otoacoustic Emissions (OAE)	10-min screening test of cochlear function	Any age
Automated Auditory Brainstem Response (ABR)	15-min screening test of cochlea and auditory pathways	Any age
Visual Reinforces Audiometry	Sound booth based conditioned hearing test	8 mo to 2.5 y
Play Audiometry	Ear specific hearing levels reinforced by gaming	>2.5 y
Audiometry	Ear specific hearing levels	>4 y

Many hospitals employ a 2-tiered hearing screening system, using both OAE and AABR as needed. However, infants in the neonatal intensive care unit should always be tested with AABR because of their increased risk of sensorineural hearing loss and auditory neuropathy.[27] Rescreening is commonly recommended within 1 month, especially if the infant initially underwent OAE and did not pass.[28,29] In comparison with 1-step OAE to 2-step OAE and AABR programs, the latter has been shown to decrease the audiology referral rate from 5.8% to 1.8%.[30] No significant difference was noted between the 2 methods in terms of the accuracy and identification rates of congenital hearing loss. The total costs (including expenditures and intangible costs) were also lower in the protocol with OAE plus AABR. Infants should be referred for diagnostic testing after no more than 2 to 3 screening tests are not passed. Repeated hearing screens delays definitive diagnostic testing, and can add to cost, inconvenience, and anxiety for families.[31] Benchmarks for hearing screening programs in birthing hospitals include screening a minimum of 95% of infants before 1 month of age, and maintaining a referral rate for diagnostic testing of less than 4%.[32]

Diagnostic Testing

Diagnostic hearing testing is conducted by audiologists with experience in infant hearing loss and should be completed by 3 months of age. A comprehensive test battery includes evaluating the child and taking a complete family history, as well as an electrophysiologic measure of hearing threshold OAEs (such as ABR using frequency-specific stimuli), and a measure of middle ear function, including frequency appropriate tympanograms, bone conduction ABR, and/or pneumatic otoscopy.[32,33] The cross-check principle applies to older infants and children, using visual reinforcement audiometry, otoacoustic emissions, and tympanometry to most effectively determine the degree, type, and configuration of hearing loss.[34] Diagnostic ABR is often performed under natural sleep in infants under 6 months of age, but sometimes requires sedation. ABR testing allows for testing across many hearing frequencies and levels, and differentiation of conductive from sensorineural hearing loss. This test may take up to an hour or more to complete, but provides the audiologist enough information to fit most infants with appropriate hearing aids. In a recent study, 68% of infants referred for diagnostic testing were confirmed to have permanent hearing loss.[16] Bilateral hearing loss was found in 58.6% of patients and unilateral in 41.4% with severe median thresholds in both unilateral and bilateral cases.

Owing to the duration of infant hearing tests, some infants require sedation. Thus, the ability to offer sedation for infants for hearing testing is an important component of hearing screening systems. If required, sedation should be performed by qualified practitioners who are not conducting the diagnostic test(s). Sedation in infants may require the use of an anesthesiologist with close monitoring and the ability to manage and rescue patients from deep sedation. Audiology practices differ in their ability to perform diagnostic tests for infants, and prolonged waits for an appointment or testing are challenges in some regions.[35–37] To optimize the referral process for primary care providers, a national database called EHDI Pediatric Audiology Links to Services is being implemented. This database allows practitioners to search for pediatric audiology services, and includes a description of the types of testing and interventions available at each clinic.[38] The referring physician can thereby match each patient with the appropriate audiologic service.

Follow-up Challenges

More than 98% of infants born in the United States are now screened for hearing loss.[39] All states now offer routine screening and many require it by law. A variety of different protocols have been mandated or implemented, but in general families are informed of their infant's screening results, and provided information necessary for appropriate follow-up. The state health department is typically notified of screening results to track and help manage patients until diagnosis and intervention are complete. However, many challenges exist in the process (**Box 2**). One of the most common problems is that many patients do not return for diagnostic testing and intervention. Loss to follow-up rates exceed 70% in some regions despite multiple attempts to address the problem.[11] Maternal sociodemographic features (poor, non-white, young) and access issues have been considered primary factors for lack of follow-up. However, 1 recent review found 2 program characteristics to be most important for poor follow-up: The lack of prenatal education about newborn hearing screening and the lack of hospital hearing information functionally integrated with Public Health.[40]

Primary care providers may not have readily available hearing screening results, and may not be aware of the need to refer to specialty services.[41] There remains a need to improve infrastructure for pediatric primary care providers to receive and request

---

Box 2
Hearing screening system challenges

Nonhospitalized births

Small hospitals without a screening program

Lack of or unavailable screening resources

Lack of screening failure follow-up

Overuse of repeat screens

Loss to follow-up

Lack of physician recognition of loss to follow-up

Lack of referral for definitive testing

Insufficient clinical resources for diagnostic testing

Insufficient resources for amplification

Lack of early intervention

Lack of long-term follow-up

Lack of rescreening for high-risk infants

infant hearing screening results, facilitate reporting, and coordinate follow-up services for infants identified with hearing loss. Lack of available audiology resources has also been shown to delay testing and early intervention.[42] Lack of early intervention has been documented in up to 30% of patients known to be deaf or hard of hearing.[43] Strategies implemented to decrease the lost to follow-up rate include providing families with good documentation, educating families and caregivers regarding the importance of diagnostic testing and intervention, working with primary care providers to identify and refer appropriate patients, and improving state-based tracking and referral services. Despite these efforts, many patients are still not diagnosed on a timely basis.

OTOLARYNGOLOGIST ROLE IN INFANT HEARING

Owing to their common involvement in infant care, otolaryngologists play an important role in infant hearing screening follow-up (**Box 3**). As a component of routine otolaryngologic care, hearing should always be addressed, including ascertaining the results of infant screening tests. The otolaryngologist is often in a good position to assist the family with definitive diagnostic testing and referrals, as well as providing medical diagnostics and intervention should hearing loss be identified. Otolaryngologists may see patients at various time points of the infant hearing screening process. If seen for any other purpose in the newborn nursery, otolaryngologists can help with early ear examination and cleaning if necessary. In some institutions, otolaryngologists are only consulted after completion of diagnostic testing. In this situation, otolaryngologists should be available to see patients with hearing loss expediently for assessment and facilitation of rehabilitation, in compliance with the developmental urgency of intervention as outlined in the 1-3-6 guideline. Our preference is to see patients immediately before sedated ABR when diagnostic testing is necessary, especially if

---

Box 3
Role of the otolaryngologist in hearing screening

Routine surveillance for hearing loss for all patients

  Confirmation of hearing screen results at the patient's first visit

  Referral for rescreening or definitive testing if required

  Review of the most recent diagnostic hearing tests

  Surveillance for ear canal and middle ear pathology

  Surveillance for possible hearing loss, including identification of risk factors

  Assessment of speech and language development

Ongoing screening for patient with known hearing loss

  Confirmation of any recent hearing screens or tests

  Reassessment of hearing as appropriate

  Confirmation of use of appropriate amplification

  Surveillance for ear canal and middle ear pathology

  Reassessment for any new confounding medical problems

  Reassessment of speech language delay

  Assessment for balance disturbance

  Confirmation of appropriate early intervention

there is any evidence of ear canal or middle ear abnormalities. This assessment allows for evaluation of the integrity of the ear canal and middle ear, and to defer testing if infection or middle ear effusion needs medical treatment. Risk of sedation (if required for hearing testing) can also be assessed while preparing parents regarding the need for sedation and the important nature of the hearing tests. A relationship with the family before testing can make later counseling easier should hearing loss be identified.

Whether or not hearing loss is the chief complaint for a physician visit, hearing status should always be assessed. A complete history and physical examination relating to possible hearing loss should be completed at each visit. It is important to remember that parents and physicians are typically not very good at judging the degree of hearing loss in infants. If any concerns regarding hearing exist, definitive objective diagnostic hearing testing is required. Ongoing monitoring for hearing loss using risk factors seems to have value in identifying postnatal hearing loss.[44] Caregiver concern is an extremely sensitive indicator of hearing loss, and should always prompt hearing testing. There are many other potential observations that can lead to concern for hearing loss and the need for objective hearing testing (**Box 4**).

A loss in hearing level can be associated with involvement of many organ systems. Nearly one third of infants with hearing loss may have a coexisting birth condition.[45] The pinna shape, position, and anomalies should be assessed. The ear canal may be small or filled with cerumen or debris. The tympanic membrane should be fully assessed for any anomalies, middle ear fluid or infection, perforations, cholesteatoma, or other problems. Pneumatic otoscopy is important to determine tympanic membrane mobility. Otomicroscopic examination of the tympanic membranes is a recommended practice in infants and older children with small ear canals, as a component of diagnostic assessment. Middle ear fluid may be subtle, and can easily be missed.[46] Otitis media with effusion (OME) has been shown to account for a large percent of failed hearing screens, and should be addressed as a component of definitive hearing testing.[47] Craniofacial malformations should be documented. The eyes should be assessed for coloboma, heterotopia, or other defects. Assessment for nasal patency

---

Box 4
Indications for objective hearing screening

Any parent or caregiver concern regarding hearing or speech

No or limited response to sound

Poor speech or language development, or both

Decline in previous language skills

Ear infections, pain, or pulling at ears

Turning up TV or radio volume

Difficulty understanding conversation

Inappropriate responses to questions or commands

Not replying when called

Poor school performance

Behavior problems

Family history of hearing loss

Presence of any high-risk registry risk factors

Medical problems associated with hearing loss

may require nasal endoscopy to rule out choanal atresia. Cervical pits or cysts may suggest branchial cleft anomalies. A complete cranial nerve evaluation is required. Assessment for cardiac anomalies (murmur), airway problems (stridor), and abdominal and genital defects, as well as spine and limb problems may also be helpful. The differential diagnosis of infants with congenitally hearing loss is extensive, and many patients with hearing loss are nonsyndromic (**Box 5**). However, physical examination stigmata of a syndrome associated with hearing loss may help to guide further diagnostic workup.

Middle Ear Effusion

A common cause of infant hearing screening referral is middle ear effusion. Effusions may be noted by high-frequency tympanograms performed as a component of audiologic testing, or by the primary care physician on physical examination. If present, referral to an otolaryngologist is recommended for management. Often, middle ear fluid is first suspected by the otolaryngologist using a microscope to assess the middle ear. Occasionally, infants will have an acute ear infection that needs treatment with antibiotics. More commonly, the middle ear effusion is not infected, and antibiotics do not play a role in management. Observation is recommended for infant (Arkansas Children's Hospital), OME because the middle ear fluid resolves in the majority of

---

Box 5
Differential diagnosis of hearing loss

Unknown causes (45%)

Defined causes (55%)

  Acquired (40%)

    Infectious: Toxoplasmosis, cytomegalovirus, herpes viruses, mumps, measles, meningitis, sepsis

    Metabolic: Asphyxia, Hyperbilirubinemia

    Toxic: Alcohol, thalidomide, quinine

    Birth trauma: Intracranial hemorrhage, skull trauma, noise

  Genetic causes (60%)

    Nonsyndromic (70%)

      Autosomal recessive (80%): GJB2 (connexin26) genes

      Autosomal dominant (17%)

      X-chromosomal (3%)

    Syndromic (30%)

      Alport syndrome (with progressive renal failure)

      Pendred syndrome (with goiter owing to faulty iodine metabolism)

      Cogan syndrome (with interstitial keratitis)

      Waardenburg syndrome (with partial albinism and lateral displacement of the lacrimal puncta)

      Usher syndrome (with retinitis pigmentosa)

From Declau F, Boudewyns A, Van den Ende J, et al. Etiologic and audiologic evaluations after universal neonatal hearing screening: analysis of 170 referred neonates. Pediatrics 2008;121(6):1119–26.

infants. Our institution does not recommend sedated ABR if OME is present early in life, but delays the test for no more than 3 months to allow OME to resolve. If the OME resolves by 3 months of age, then an ABR can be completed. If the OME is present for longer than 3 months, ear tubes may be recommended. We routinely coordinate examination of the ears under anesthesia with bilateral ear tube placement along with diagnostic ABR. This minimizes the number of sedations needed and completes diagnostic testing according to the 1-3-6 timeline. However, a mild conductive hearing loss is commonly present even after suctioning out the middle ear fluid during the procedure, especially if the OME is mucoid. Follow-up hearing tests after intraoperative ABR have demonstrated discrepancies in both positive and negative directions.[48] Although the mild conductive hearing loss frequently resolves over time, the variance in measured intraoperative thresholds should be taken into consideration when discussing the implications of the ABR.

Counseling and Follow-up

Once diagnosed with hearing loss, parents should be counseled regarding their child's hearing status and intervention opportunities. Significant reduction in parental quality of life and psychosocial stress are common after a child is identified as deaf or hard of hearing, which may be improved by social support.[49] Although the majority of parents were satisfied with the range and quality of audiology and therapy services available, parents identified gaps in the areas of service coordination, availability of information, and integration of social service and parent support into the system.[50] Counseling is best done with otolaryngology and audiology present, and optimized by the inclusion of a deaf parent support professional who can provide a much-needed perspective on being a healthy and socially integrated individual with hearing loss. Counseling is supplemented by the remainder of the team involved in children with hearing loss, including other medical specialists, speech pathologists, and educators. The quality of professional communication has been shown to be an important factor in the family's early experience after diagnosis.[51] Initial information that should be conveyed to the family is fairly comprehensive. Although the side and degree of hearing level are baseline data that need to be relayed, it is important to emphasize that hearing assessment is an ongoing process, and some variation may occur over time and with behavioral testing (audiometry). Just as important to the family are the implications of the child's level of hearing as it relates to language development and human interaction. The availability of rehabilitation options, costs associated with rehabilitation (including insurance coverage issues), and potential outcomes are important to families.

The ability to interact with another family should be encouraged. Several organizations are available to assist with family support. For example, Hands and Voices, a national parent-driven organization, has many articles available at the state level and provides meaningful connections between families of children who are deaf or hard of hearing. Diagnostic testing can also be discussed, but may be deferred to a follow-up visit. Follow-up ENT and pediatric audiology visits should be scheduled quickly to allow for hearing aid fitting, repeat hearing testing, speech evaluation and counseling, further diagnostic testing, and help with setting up early intervention. It is important to remember that families of patients with a false-positive hearing screen also have anxiety, and may have ongoing concern regarding their child's hearing.[52]

Ongoing consultation with a pediatric audiologist is critical to the success of newborn screening and intervention programs. Protocols for providing amplification to infants with hearing loss have been described.[53,54] Ongoing hearing assessment, selection of appropriate amplification, adjustment of hearing aid fittings, and monitoring for amplification effectiveness are components of this ongoing relationship.[55]

Infants identified as deaf or hard of hearing can be fit with amplification (ie, hearing aids) by an audiologist at virtually any age. However, challenges with amplification fitting and use are also common.[56] In a recent article, the top 3 challenges parents reported in obtaining hearing aids were (1) paying for hearing aids, (2) accepting the need for hearing aids, and (3) wait time for an appointment. Almost one half of the parents (48%) reported that they did not receive adequate support from their audiologist in how to check the function of their child's hearing aids.[57] Auditory neuropathy may account for 10% of infants with hearing loss, and remains challenging to rehabilitate, with variable language acquisition relative to their audiograms.[55] With appropriate early intervention, children who are deaf or hard of hearing and use spoken communication can attend mainstream elementary and secondary education classes.[58,59] For hard of hearing children who are not identified and provided services early services, special education may cost an additional $420,000. It has been estimated that being deaf has an estimated lifetime cost of approximately $1 million per individual in the United States. Similar findings have been reported in England.[60]

Diagnostic Testing and Referrals

Otolaryngologists should complete an appropriate diagnostic testing algorithm in patients with hearing loss. Diagnostic testing can be helpful to establish a cause of the hearing loss, which may help with prognosis, and identification of related medical issues. An etiologic factor is identifiable in about 60% of patients who are deaf or hard of hearing.[16] Of causes identified, about 60% are genetic, 20% peripartum events, and 18% congenital cytomegalovirus (CMV). Testing includes an electrocardiography if there is a family history of early cardiac dysrhythmias or death. Computed tomography or magnetic resonance imaging or both of the temporal bones, urinalysis, and genetic testing are commonly recommended.[61-63] CMV testing is best performed in the newborn nursery for hearing loss possibly associated with CMV infection.[64] Screening for CMV has been recommended but not fully implemented for all newborns.[65,66] Nonetheless, infants should be tested for CMV as soon as hearing loss is suspected.[67] Genetic testing is very useful because more than 60% of patients with nonsyndromic hearing loss have identifiable sequence variants in the GJB2 (connexin26) genes or other genes know to cause hearing loss. Even unilateral hearing loss may have a genetic basis, as well as an identifiable structural abnormality on imaging.[68] Stepwise testing is commonly recommended as being more efficient and cost effective.[69] One proposed algorithm for testing is shown in **Fig. 1.**

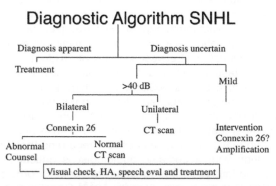

Diagnostic Algorithm SNHL

Diagnosis apparent · Diagnosis uncertain

Treatment

>40 dB · Mild

Bilateral · Unilateral

Connexin 26 · CT scan · Intervention Connexin 26? Amplification

Abnormal Counsel · Normal CT scan

Visual check, HA, speech eval and treatment

Fig. 1. A potential diagnostic testing algorithm for children with hearing loss. (*From* Greinwald JH Jr, Hartnick CJ. The evaluation of children with sensorineural hearing loss. Arch Otolaryngol Head Neck Surg 2002;128(1):86.)

Otolaryngologists should recommend referral to pediatric audiologists, speech/language pathologists, ophthalmologists, geneticists, and other indicated specialists for infants and children with hearing loss. Referral to a geneticist with interest in pediatric hearing loss can be very helpful if desired by the family, considering the broad range of genetic tests available and rapid advancements in this field. A good ophthalmologic examination with attention to the retina is important both for diagnostic reasons as well as to confirm function of the visual system.[70] Referral to other specialists (cardiology, nephrology, developmental pediatricians) may be indicated based on testing or diagnosis. The need for multidisciplinary evaluation is emphasized by a high rate of ophthalmologic findings (53%) among children with hearing loss.[71] Neurodevelopmental evaluations may reveal clinically significant findings in almost 70% of patients. Nearly 80% of patients may require speech/language intervention.

Management

Otolaryngologists should monitor hearing, external and middle ear status, and speech and language development in children with hearing loss. Otolaryngologists should establish a long and stable clinical relationship with patients who are deaf or hard of hearing. Although much of the process of rehabilitation with hearing aids is accomplished by audiology, otolaryngologists still play in important role. Cerumen impactions and otitis externa are common in hearing aid users, and frequently need to be treated by an otolaryngologist. Ear canal cleaning may be necessary for medical purposes, or to assist with ear mold impressions. Middle ear infections or OME are common in infants and often require management. Speech and language development should be monitored and, if inadequate, appropriate intervention implemented. This may include hearing aid adjustments, enhanced therapy, or consideration of alternative language strategies.

Otolaryngologists play an important role in ongoing surveillance of hearing status. Children may present at any age with a chief complaint of hearing difficulty or speech and language delays, which requires assessment with objective hearing testing. Parent concern, school and primary care screens that are not passed, and speech and language delay are the most common reasons for referral for further testing.[72] Hearing screening should be performed routinely throughout childhood, and patients may present to the otolaryngologist after a hearing screening that was not passed. Hearing should be tested for many medical problems, including potentially toxic therapy (chemotherapy), head or ear trauma, and ear surgery. Children who have already been identified as deaf or hard of hearing should be reassessed at least annually, because some forms of hearing loss are progressive.

Otolaryngologists should recommend appropriate surgical procedures for children with hearing loss. Surgical options may frequently be considered in infants with hearing loss. Recurrent ear infections or persistent middle ear effusions occur in patients with hearing loss. The consequences of middle ear effusion may be greater owing to decrease in hearing beyond the baseline loss. Although ear tube insertion should be considered for 3 months of persistent effusion with worsening hearing level, patients and families should be counseled on the added challenge of otorrhea, which seems to be more frequent and more challenging to address with early hearing aid molds occluding the ear canal. Surveillance for more critical problems such as cholesteatoma should also be performed. For patients with hearing loss at a profound level that is not adequately rehabilitated with hearing aids that meet appropriate criteria, cochlear implants may be discussed with the family and recommended.[73,74] Bone-anchored hearing aids have been shown to be helpful for conductive hearing loss, and benefit children with profound unilateral hearing loss.[75]

Early intervention

The Individuals with Disabilities Education Act governs states and public agencies regarding how to provide services and education to children with disabilities. Part C of the act specifically addresses how early intervention services are funded and provided to children with delays in development.[76] States individually define the criteria for determining the degree of developmental delay that qualifies a child to receive Part C services, but it is often based on a permanent condition that has the potential to impact the development of a child long-term. Children who are deaf or hard of hearing usually qualify under these guidelines to receive Part C early intervention services.

The involvement of early intervention is critical when providing deaf and hard of hearing children the best opportunity for optimal development. The importance of timely early intervention referral cannot be emphasized enough. The provision of early intervention services before 6 months of age to infants who are deaf or hard of hearing has a statistically significant positive impact on language and social-emotional development.[77,78] Unfortunately, sometimes children "slip through the cracks" and receive late referrals to early intervention services, or in the worst-case scenario, no referral at all. Children who are identified as deaf or hard of hearing see a number of providers including audiologists, otolaryngologists, and primary care providers, and therefore would presumably have multiple opportunities to be referred into the early intervention system. Yet there remain children who turn 3 years old, the age at which a child is no longer eligible for early intervention services, who were never referred and have missed out on developmental support services during critical early years of cognitive development. It is an easy trap to fall into to presume that the recommendation has already been made: When all the caregivers involved have assumed that someone else has made the referral, the child ends up with none.

Otolaryngologists, along with other health care providers, should feel empowered to make a referral to early intervention when necessary. Although an early intervention referral is not required to come specifically from a health care provider (eg, a parent can self-refer their child), physicians are often the ones who make the official referral. Each state has its own referral system for early intervention services, but it is usually a straightforward process that involves providing basic family demographic information to the early intervention office. The National Dissemination Center for Children with Disabilities has a directory of early intervention contact information by state available at http://nichcy.org/state-organization-search-by-state.

THE IMPORTANCE OF EARLY LANGUAGE ACCESS

Infants and young children learn language much more readily than adults. Synaptic connection development in the brain begins during prenatal development, and peaks by age 15 months. After this begins, a significant period of synaptic pruning occurs during which unused brain pathways are systematically eliminated. This period of pruning for sensory areas of the brain such as the visual and auditory cortex is usually complete between 4 and 6 years of age.[79] Language deprivation studies involving infants and young children in Romanian orphanages have shown that children who were deprived of linguistic and social communication had the potential to "catch up" if developmental enrichment such as foster care placement was instituted before the age of 2 years. However, those infants who remained deprived of language access for 2 years and longer demonstrated brain activity, language development, and measured IQ that did not return to a typical baseline function, even after enrichment was instituted.[80–82] Young infants and children who do not have quality language access during these critical first few years of life are at significant risk for serious developmental language delay, which in turn determines the quality of their future academic success, ability to form relationships, integration into the work force, and ability to become a successful member of society.

There is an unfortunate school of thought that still exists today: That exposing children who are deaf and hard of hearing to visual language will somehow delay their spoken language development. Parents anecdotally have reported being told by professionals not to sign with their deaf child because he/she would become "lazy" and not put energy into speaking. The current literature does not support this theory. Christine Yoshinaga-Itano has shown that children receiving early language services do not demonstrate language development differences, regardless of the mode of communication.[78] Rachel Mayberry demonstrated that either signed or spoken language, as long as it was accessible in early life, was linked with high levels of spoken language performance later in life.[83] Several small studies recently have looked at spoken language development specifically in children with cochlear implants, and examined those that had deaf signing parents providing their native language exposure in comparison with those who had hearing speaking parents. The children with natively signing deaf parents did not have reduced spoken language outcomes,[84] and 1 study demonstrated that spoken language outcomes in children with deaf signing parents exceeded that of their matched peers with hearing speaking parents.[85]

Health care providers can benefit a family with a child who is deaf or hard of hearing by focusing on overall early language access opportunities, as opposed to encouraging them to subscribe to 1 particular mode of communication. Amplification technologies such as hearing aids and cochlear implants are more advanced than ever. However, we do not possess the technology to predict which individual children will do best with any given resource or language mode. By supporting a family in providing a child with multiple language opportunities (both spoken and signed), we capitalize on a child's innate strengths, and allow him or her to "autoselect" what works best over time. Some children end up naturally gravitating toward spoken language, some toward sign language, and some retain both for the course of their lives. In this era when we routinely encourage our young children to learn multiple languages, and hearing children are more and more frequently being provided "baby sign language" to communicate their needs, it only makes sense that we would provide children who are deaf and hard of hearing those same opportunities.

ENT Community Education

Otolaryngologists have a critical role in advancing ear and hearing health in our communities. This includes working for individual patients, families, institutions, and regional and national groups. All patients and families should be counseled regarding the benefits of hearing screening and testing, and the importance of intervention should hearing loss be identified. Patients should be counseled on the importance of noise exposure prevention, including appropriate use of technology (earphones). Otolaryngologists should support the need for and be involved with quality improvement for the EHDI programs in their local institutions. Physicians may need to help with program setup, policy and procedure implementation, and ongoing management. Extending expertise to the development of hearing assessment and hearing health initiatives for community physician practices, schools, and other health care groups can help these programs to develop and thrive.

Otolaryngologists also can play a critical role in advocacy for hearing screening, diagnosis, and intervention. Otolaryngologists should be directly engaged in their local hospitals' screening program(s), with advocacy for the program, development of institutional policy and quality improvement, and availability for clinical care if needed. Otolaryngologists may be a good liaison between hospital screening programs and local diagnostic services. As mentioned, ENT can play an important role in the early diagnosis of external and middle ear problems in infants with possible hearing loss. ENT may also help with appropriate referrals for diagnostic services in collaboration with the medical home provider. Effective communication strategies are needed among the public health, primary care practice, referral/specialty service, and consumer advocacy communities to provide continuity of information required for medical decision making throughout prenatal, newborn, and early childhood periods of patient care.[86]

State health departments are usually in the position of development and management of hospital-based screening programs, and are often instrumental in follow-up and referrals. Infant hearing screening boards often require the services of otolaryngologists, as well as audiologists, speech pathologists, medical home providers, patients, and families. ENT can provide important guidance for state health departments in policy development and quality improvement programs.

Advocacy may to extend to state and national levels for maintenance and funding of hearing screening programs and early intervention services. In 2003, 76% of states with implemented Universal Newborn Hearing Screening legislation reported screening at least 95% of infants, compared with 26% in states without legislation.[87] These results demonstrate the potential gains that can be achieved with advocacy for legislation for hearing screening programs. Assurance of insurance reimbursement for appropriate diagnostic services, medical care, rehabilitation, and education is critical to the success of infant screening programs. Advocacy may occur in the context of national societies such as the American Academy of Pediatrics with its EHDI program and through the American Academy of Otolaryngology–Head and Neck Surgery or the American Society of Pediatric Otolaryngology with their dedication to otolaryngologic care of patients with hearing loss. Engagement with patient and family support programs, such as Hands and Voices, also strongly benefits patients and families.

SUMMARY

Infant hearing loss is common and infant hearing screening is now performed in more than 98% of infants in the United States. Screening is recommended for all infants by 1 month of age, with diagnostic testing completed by 3 months of age, and enrollment in early intervention services by 6 months of age (1-3-6 guideline). Otolaryngologists should routinely assess for hearing loss while ascertaining the results of infant hearing screening and diagnostics. Referral for hearing testing is required for any concern regarding hearing loss or speech and language development. Otolaryngologists should recognize the developmental urgency of hearing loss in infants and children and provide expedient clinical access for care. A complete history and physical examination, including otomicroscopy for assessment of the ear canal and middle ear, should be completed on all infants and children with known or suspected hearing loss. Diagnostic testing for the etiology of hearing loss may include electrocardiography, urinalysis, temporal bone imaging, genetic testing, and other indicated tests. When a child has been identified as deaf or hard of hearing, otolaryngologists should recommend referral to pediatric audiologists, speech/language pathologists, ophthalmologists, geneticists, and other indicated specialists. Surgical intervention may include tube insertion, ear canal or middle ear surgery, cochlear implantation, bone-anchored hearing aids, or other procedures. Otolaryngologists should routinely monitor for the success of intervention in children with hearing loss, and assess for newly developed or progressively declining hearing levels in all patients.

Otolaryngologists should be involved in the development and maintenance of hearing screening and intervention programs in their community and state.

REFERENCES

1. Haggard M. Screening children's hearing. Br J Audiol 1992;26(4):209–15.
2. Eisenberg LS. Current state of knowledge: speech recognition and production in children with hearing impairment. Ear Hear 2007;28(6):766–72.
3. Pimperton H, Kennedy CR. The impact of early identification of permanent childhood hearing impairment on speech and language outcomes. Arch Dis Child 2012;97(7):648–53.
4. Yoshinaga-Itano C, Apuzzo ML. Identification of hearing loss after age 18 months is not early enough. Am Ann Deaf 1998;143(5):380–7.
5. Yoshinaga-Itano C, Sedey AL, Coulter DK, et al. Language of early- and later-identified children with hearing loss. Pediatrics 1998;102(5):1161–71.
6. Kennedy CR, McCann DC, Campbell MJ, et al. Language ability after early detection of permanent childhood hearing impairment. N Engl J Med 2006; 354(20):2131–41.
7. Nelson HD, Bougatsos C, Nygren P, 2001 US Preventive Services Task Force. Universal newborn hearing screening: systematic review to update the 2001 US Preventive Services Task Force Recommendation. Pediatrics 2008;122(1): e266–76.
8. Puig T, Municio A, Meda C. Universal neonatal hearing screening versus selective screening as part of the management of childhood deafness. Cochrane Database Syst Rev 2005;(2):CD003731.
9. Centers for Disease Control and Prevention (CDC). Identifying infants with hearing loss - United States, 1999-2007. MMWR Morb Mortal Wkly Rep 2010; 59(8):220–3.
10. Centers for Disease Control and Prevention (CDC). CDC grand rounds: Newborn screening and improved outcomes. MMWR Morb Mortal Wkly Rep 2012;61(21):390–3.
11. Vohr B, Simon P, McDermott C, et al. Early hearing detection and intervention (EHDI) Rhode Island. Med Health R I 2002;85:369–72.
12. American Academy of Pediatrics, Joint Committee on Infant Hearing. Year 2007 position statement: principles and guidelines for early hearing detection and intervention programs. Pediatrics 2007;120(4):898–921.
13. Melvin LS, Folsom RC, Mancl LR. Prevalence of hearing impairment in school-aged children: an analysis of data from three Seattle-area school districts (Slides 7, 14 and 15). 2010; Available at: http://depts.washington.edu/lend/trainees/project/2010/melvin.pdf.
14. Bielecki I, Horbulewicz A, Wolan T. Risk factors associated with hearing loss in infants: an analysis of 5282 referred neonates. Int J Pediatr Otorhinolaryngol 2011;75(7):925–30.
15. Mauk GW, White KR, Mortensen LB, et al. The effectiveness of screening programs based on high-risk characteristics in early identification of hearing impairment. Ear Hear 1991;12(5):312–9.
16. Declau F, Boudewyns A, Van den Ende J, et al. Etiologic and audiologic evaluations after universal neonatal hearing screening: analysis of 170 referred neonates. Pediatrics 2008;121(6):1119–26.
17. Harrison M, Roush J. Age of suspicion, identification, and intervention for infants and young children with hearing loss: a national study. Ear Hear 1996;17(1):55–62.

18. Canale A, Favero E, Lacilla M, et al. Age at diagnosis of deaf babies: a retrospective analysis highlighting the advantage of newborn hearing screening. Int J Pediatr Otorhinolaryngol 2006;70(7):1283–9.

19. Cardon G, Campbell J, Sharma A. Plasticity in the developing auditory cortex: evidence from children with sensorineural hearing loss and auditory neuropathy spectrum disorder. J Am Acad Audiol 2012;23(6):396–411 [quiz: 495].

20. Healthy People 2010: Volume II (second edition). Available at: http://healthy people.gov/2020/topicsobjectives2020/objectiveslist.aspx?topicId=20.

21. Newborn hearing screening devices: sound advice on choosing the right technology. Health Devices 2005;34(10):350–6.

22. Doyle KJ, Burggraaff B, Fujikawa S, et al. Neonatal hearing screening with otoscopy, auditory brain stem response, and otoacoustic emissions. Otolaryngol Head Neck Surg 1997;116(6 Pt 1):597–603.

23. Gorga MP, Neely ST, Bergman B, et al. Otoacoustic emissions from normal-hearing and hearing-impaired subjects: distortion product responses. J Acoust Soc Am 1993;93(4 Pt 1):2050–60.

24. Hyde ML, Riko K, Malizia K. Audiometric accuracy of the click ABR in infants at risk for hearing loss. J Am Acad Audiol 1990;1(2):59–66.

25. Benito-Orejas JI, Ramirez B, Morais D, et al. Comparison of two-step transient evoked otoacoustic emissions (TEOAE) and automated auditory brainstem response (AABR) for universal newborn hearing screening programs. Int J Pediatr Otorhinolaryngol 2008;72(8):1193–201.

26. Korres SG, Balatsouras DG, Lyra C, et al. A comparison of automated auditory brainstem responses and transiently evoked otoacoustic emissions for universal newborn hearing screening. Med Sci Monit 2006;12(6):CR260–3.

27. Abdul Wahid SN, Md Daud MK, Sidek D, et al. The performance of distortion product otoacoustic emissions and automated auditory brainstem response in the same ear of the babies in neonatal unit. Int J Pediatr Otorhinolaryngol 2012;76(9):1366–9.

28. Korres S, Nikolopoulos TP, Peraki EE, et al. Outcomes and efficacy of newborn hearing screening: strengths and weaknesses (success or failure?). Laryngoscope 2008;118(7):1253–6.

29. Shoup AG, Owen KE, Jackson G, et al. The Parkland Memorial Hospital experience in ensuring compliance with Universal Newborn Hearing Screening follow-up. J Pediatr 2005;146(1):66–72.

30. Lin HC, Shu MT, Lee KS, et al. Comparison of hearing screening programs between one step with transient evoked otoacoustic emissions (TEOAE) and two steps with TEOAE and automated auditory brainstem response. Laryngoscope 2005;115(11):1957–62.

31. Mohd Khairi MD, Rafidah KN, Affizal A, et al. Anxiety of the mothers with referred baby during Universal Newborn Hearing Screening. Int J Pediatr Otorhinolaryngol 2011;75(4):513–7.

32. Year 2000 position statement: principles and guidelines for early hearing detection and intervention programs. Joint Committee on Infant Hearing. Am J Audiol 2000;9(1):9–29.

33. Prieve BA, Vander Werff KR, Preston JL, et al. Identification of conductive hearing loss in young infants using tympanometry and wideband reflectance. Ear Hear 2013;34(2):168–78.

34. Baldwin SM, Gajewski BJ, Widen JE. An evaluation of the cross-check principle using visual reinforcement audiometry, otoacoustic emissions, and tympanometry. J Am Acad Audiol 2010;21(3):187–96.

35. Munoz K, Nelson L, Goldgewicht N, et al. Early hearing detection and intervention: diagnostic hearing assessment practices. Am J Audiol 2011;20(2):123–31.
36. Park AH, Warner J, Sturgill N, et al. A survey of parental views regarding their child's hearing loss: a pilot study. Otolaryngol Head Neck Surg 2006;134(5): 794–800.
37. Windmill S, Windmill IM. The status of diagnostic testing following referral from universal newborn hearing screening. J Am Acad Audiol 2006;17(5):367–78 [quiz: 379–80].
38. Early Hearing Detection & Intervention - Pediatric Audiology Links to Services (EHDI PALS). Available at: http://www.ehdipals.org.
39. Centers for Disease Control and Prevention. Summary of 2009 National CDC EHDI Data. 2009 CDC EHDI hearing screening & follow-up survey. 2012; Available at: http://www.cdc.gov/ncbddd/hearingloss/2009-data/2009_ehdi_hsfs_summary_508_ok.pdf.
40. Todd NW. Universal newborn hearing screening follow-up in two Georgia populations: newborn, mother and system correlates. Int J Pediatr Otorhinolaryngol 2006;70(5):807–15.
41. Ross DS, Visser SN. Pediatric primary care physicians' practices regarding newborn hearing screening. J Prim Care Community Health 2012;3(4):256–63.
42. Larsen R, Munoz K, DesGeorges J, et al. Early hearing detection and intervention: parent experiences with the diagnostic hearing assessment. Am J Audiol 2012;21(1):91–9.
43. Gaffney M, Green DR, Gaffney C. Newborn hearing screening and follow-up: are children receiving recommended services? Public Health Rep 2010; 125(2):199–207.
44. Beswick R, Driscoll C, Kei J. Monitoring for postnatal hearing loss using risk factors: a systematic literature review. Ear Hear 2012;33(6):745–56.
45. Chapman DA, Stampfel CC, Bodurtha JN, et al. Impact of co-occurring birth defects on the timing of newborn hearing screening and diagnosis. Am J Audiol 2011;20(2):132–9.
46. Boone RT, Bower CM, Martin PF. Failed newborn hearing screens as presentation for otitis media with effusion in the newborn population. Int J Pediatr Otorhinolaryngol 2005;69(3):393–7.
47. Boudewyns A, Declau F, Van den Ende J, et al. Otitis media with effusion: an underestimated cause of hearing loss in infants. Otol Neurotol 2011;32(5): 799–804.
48. Yorgason JG, Park AH, Sturgill N, et al. The role of intraoperative auditory brainstem response testing for infants and difficult-to-test children. Otolaryngol Head Neck Surg 2010;142(1):36–40.
49. Burger T, Lohle E, Richter B, et al. "Your child is hard of hearing" - a longitudinal study of parental distress. Laryngorhinootologie 2008;87(8):552–9 [in German].
50. Fitzpatrick E, Angus D, Durieux-Smith A, et al. Parents' needs following identification of childhood hearing loss. Am J Audiol 2008;17(1):38–49.
51. Tattersall H, Young A. Deaf children identified through newborn hearing screening: parents' experiences of the diagnostic process. Child Care Health Dev 2006;32(1):33–45.
52. van der Ploeg CP, Lanting CI, Kauffman-de Boer MA, et al. Examination of long-lasting parental concern after false-positive results of neonatal hearing screening. Arch Dis Child 2008;93(6):508–11.
53. Bagatto M, Scollie SD, Hyde M, et al. Protocol for the provision of amplification within the Ontario infant hearing program. Int J Audiol 2010;49(Suppl 1):S70–9.

54. King AM. The national protocol for paediatric amplification in Australia. Int J Audiol 2010;49(Suppl 1):S64–9.
55. Berlin CI, Hood LJ, Morlet T, et al. Multi-site diagnosis and management of 260 patients with auditory neuropathy/dys-synchrony (auditory neuropathy spectrum disorder). Int J Audiol 2010;49(1):30–43.
56. Spivak L, Sokol H, Auerbach C, et al. Newborn hearing screening follow-up: factors affecting hearing aid fitting by 6 months of age. Am J Audiol 2009;18(1): 24–33.
57. Munoz K, Blaiser K, Barwick K. Parent hearing aid experiences in the United States. J Am Acad Audiol 2013;24(1):5–16.
58. Joint Committee on Infant Hearing, American Academy of Academy, American Academy of Pediatrics, et al. Year 2000 position statement: principles and guidelines for early hearing detection and intervention programs. Joint Committee on Infant Hearing, American Academy of Audiology, American Academy of Pediatrics, American Speech-Language-Hearing Association, and Directors of Speech and Hearing Programs in State Health and Welfare Agencies. Pediatrics 2000;106(4):798–817.
59. Verhaert N, Willems M, Van Kerschaver E, et al. Impact of early hearing screening and treatment on language development and education level: evaluation of 6 years of universal newborn hearing screening (ALGO) in Flanders, Belgium. Int J Pediatr Otorhinolaryngol 2008;72(5):599–608.
60. Schroeder L, Petrou S, Kennedy C, et al. The economic costs of congenital bilateral permanent childhood hearing impairment. Pediatrics 2006;117(4): 1101–12.
61. Cama E, Inches I, Muzzi E, et al. Temporal bone high-resolution computed tomography in non-syndromic unilateral hearing loss in children. ORL J Otorhinolaryngol Relat Spec 2012;74(2):70–7.
62. Joshi VM, Navlekar SK, Kishore GR, et al. CT and MR imaging of the inner ear and brain in children with congenital sensorineural hearing loss. Radiographics 2012;32(3):683–98.
63. Simons JP, Mandell DL, Arjmand EM. Computed tomography and magnetic resonance imaging in pediatric unilateral and asymmetric sensorineural hearing loss. Arch Otolaryngol Head Neck Surg 2006;132(2):186–92.
64. Avettand-Fenoel V, Marlin S, Vauloup-Fellous C, et al. Congenital cytomegalovirus is the second most frequent cause of bilateral hearing loss in young French children. J Pediatr 2013;162(3):593–9.
65. Barbi M, Binda S, Caroppo S, et al. Neonatal screening for congenital cytomegalovirus infection and hearing loss. J Clin Virol 2006;35(2):206–9.
66. Barkai G, Barzilai A, Mendelson E, et al. Newborn screening for congenital cytomegalovirus using real-time polymerase chain reaction in umbilical cord blood. Isr Med Assoc J 2013;15(6):279–83.
67. Bale JF Jr. Screening newborns for congenital cytomegalovirus infection. JAMA 2010;303(14):1425–6.
68. Dodson KM, Georgolios A, Barr N, et al. Etiology of unilateral hearing loss in a national hereditary deafness repository. Am J Otol 2012;33(5):590–4.
69. Preciado DA, Lawson L, Madden C, et al. Improved diagnostic effectiveness with a sequential diagnostic paradigm in idiopathic pediatric sensorineural hearing loss. Otol Neurotol 2005;26(4):610–5.
70. Nikolopoulos TP, Lioumi D, Stamataki S, et al. Evidence-based overview of ophthalmic disorders in deaf children: a literature update. Otol Neurotol 2006; 27(2 Suppl 1):S1–24 [discussion: S20].

71. Wiley S, Arjmand E, Jareenmeinzen D, et al. Findings from multidisciplinary evaluation of children with permanent hearing loss. Int J Pediatr Otorhinolaryngol 2011;75(8):1040–4.
72. Dedhia K, Kitsko D, Sabo D, et al. Children with sensorineural hearing loss after passing the newborn hearing screen. JAMA Otolaryngol Head Neck Surg 2013; 139(2):119–23.
73. Heman-Ackah SE, Roland JT Jr, Haynes DS, et al. Pediatric cochlear implantation: candidacy evaluation, medical and surgical considerations, and expanding criteria. Otolaryngol Clin North Am 2012;45(1):41–67.
74. Leigh J, Dettman S, Dowell R, et al. Evidence-based approach for making cochlear implant recommendations for infants with residual hearing. Ear Hear 2011;32(3):313–22.
75. Christensen L, Richter GT, Dornhoffer JL. Update on bone-anchored hearing aids in pediatric patients with profound unilateral sensorineural hearing loss. Arch Otolaryngol Head Neck Surg 2010;136(2):175–7.
76. National Dissemination Center for Children with Disabilities. 2012. Available at: http://nichcy.org/laws.
77. Yoshinaga-Itano C. Benefits of early intervention for children with hearing loss. Otolaryngol Clin North Am 1999;32(6):1089–102.
78. Yoshinaga-Itano C. From screening to early identification and intervention: discovering predictors to successful outcomes for children with significant hearing loss. J Deaf Stud Deaf Educ 2003;8(1):11–30.
79. Tierney AL, Nelson CA 3rd. Brain development and the role of experience in the early years. Zero Three 2009;30(2):9–13.
80. Marshall PJ, Reeb BC, Fox NA, et al. Effects of early intervention on EEG power and coherence in previously institutionalized children in Romania. Dev Psychopathol 2008;20(3):861–80.
81. Nelson CA 3rd, Zeanah CH, Fox NA, et al. Cognitive recovery in socially deprived young children: the Bucharest Early Intervention Project. Science 2007;318(5858):1937–40.
82. Windsor J, Glaze LE, Koga SF, Bucharest Early Intervention Project Core Group. Language acquisition with limited input: Romanian institution and foster care. J Speech Lang Hear Res 2007;50(5):1365–81.
83. Mayberry RI, Lock E, Kazmi H. Linguistic ability and early language exposure. Nature 2002;417(6884):38.
84. Park GY, Moon IJ, Kim EY, et al. Auditory and speech performance in deaf children with deaf parents after cochlear implant. Otol Neurotol 2013;34(2):233–8.
85. Hassanzadeh S. Outcomes of cochlear implantation in deaf children of deaf parents: comparative study. J Laryngol Otol 2012;126(10):989–94.
86. Downing GJ, Zuckerman AE, Coon C, et al. Enhancing the quality and efficiency of newborn screening programs through the use of health information technology. Semin Perinatol 2010;34(2):156–62.
87. Green DR, Gaffney M, Devine O, et al. Determining the effect of newborn hearing screening legislation: an analysis of state hearing screening rates. Public Health Rep 2007;122(2):198–205.

Contemporary Concepts in Management of Acute Otitis Media in Children

Eleni Rettig, MD[a], David E. Tunkel, MD[b],*

KEYWORDS

- Acute otitis media • Middle ear effusion • Tympanostomy tubes
- Clinical practice guidelines • Ear infections

KEY POINTS

- Acute otitis media (AOM) should be distinguished from chronic otitis media with effusion.
- Clinical practice guidelines have been updated to refine the "observation" option for treatment of AOM, with an emphasis on precise diagnosis.
- The bacteriology of AOM has been changed by the use of pneumococcal vaccines, but high dose amoxicillin or amoxicillin–clavulanate are good choices when initial antibiotic therapy is prescribed for AOM.
- Tympanostomy tubes are an option for children with recurrent AOM, particularly when there is evidence of ongoing Eustachian tube dysfunction.
- Complications of AOM are rare, but must be detected early to avoid serious morbidity.

INTRODUCTION AND DEFINITIONS

Acute otitis media (AOM) is a common disorder of early childhood, and among the most common reasons for referral of a young child to the otolaryngologist. Although the majority of children with AOM are managed by primary care providers without the need for specialty consultation, children with recurrent episodes, severe symptoms, or complications of AOM can require prompt otolaryngologic evaluation and surgical treatment. Although AOM affects many children, and tympanostomy tube placement is the most commonly performed operative procedure in young children, consensus is still being reached about the most appropriate use of surgery for children with AOM.

Disclosure: The authors have nothing to disclose.
[a] Department of Otolaryngology-Head and Neck Surgery, Johns Hopkins University School of Medicine, 601 North Caroline Street, Baltimore, MD 21287, USA; [b] Division of Pediatric Otolaryngology, Department of Otolaryngology-Head and Neck Surgery, Johns Hopkins University School of Medicine, 601 North Caroline Street, Room 6161B, Baltimore, MD 21287-0910, USA
* Corresponding author.
E-mail address: dtunkel@jhmi.edu

Otolaryngol Clin N Am 47 (2014) 651–672
http://dx.doi.org/10.1016/j.otc.2014.06.006
0030-6665/14/$ – see front matter © 2014 Elsevier Inc. All rights reserved.

We review the relevant concepts in the management of AOM in children, with an emphasis on changes in microbiology over the last 2 decades. We also discuss management paradigms for AOM advanced by evidence-based clinical practice guidelines published in 2013. Surprisingly, these guidelines are the first to recommend tympanostomy tube placement as an option for children with recurrent AOM, despite decades of tympanostomy tube placement for this indication. New emphasis is placed on accurate diagnosis based on strict criteria, with additional refinement of the selection of children most appropriate for observation without antibiotics at initial diagnosis of AOM. This review focuses on AOM and recurrent AOM, and we do not directly discuss management of middle ear effusion (MEE) that is asymptomatic other than hearing loss (otitis media with effusion [OME]). It is important to distinguish AOM from OME, which are separate entities with unique management considerations (**Table 1**).

EPIDEMIOLOGY

AOM is a common disease in children. In the United States, 8.8 million children (11.8%) under the age of 18 were reported to have ear infections in 2006, with an estimated total treatment cost of $2.8 billion.[5] Antibiotics are prescribed for AOM more frequently than for any other illness of childhood.[6] The epidemiology of AOM has evolved over the past decade, with a decrease in clinician visits for suspected AOM by 33% from 1995–1996 to 2005–2006.[6] The reasons for the decrease in clinician visits is unclear, with possible explanations including financial considerations, health care access issues, public educational campaigns about the viral etiology of most upper respiratory tract infections, the introduction of the 7-valent pneumococcal vaccine (PCV7) and influenza vaccines, and publication and implementation of clinical practice guidelines.[7]

Interestingly, clinician prescribing patterns have not changed significantly for children with AOM, with the rate of antibiotic prescription per visit remaining approximately stable (80% in 1995–1996 to 76% in 2005–2006).[6,8] More recent study of prescribing patterns for AOM shows treatment strategy may vary among medical disciplines, with 1 report showing a drop in early antibiotic use for AOM by pediatricians and otolaryngologists between 2002 and 2009, but an increase in antibiotic use by

Table 1 Classification of otitis media	
Term	**Definition**
Acute otitis media (AOM)	The rapid onset of signs and symptoms of inflammation of the middle ear Symptoms include otalgia, irritability, insomnia, anorexia Signs include fever, otorrhea, full or bulging opaque TM, impaired TM mobility, TM erythema
Recurrent acute otitis media (RAOM)	Three or more well-documented and separate AOM episodes in the past 6 mo, or ≥4 well-documented and separate AOM episodes in the past 12 mo with ≥1 in the past 6 mo
Otitis media with effusion (OME)	The presence of fluid in the middle ear without signs or symptoms of acute ear infection (AOM)
Chronic otitis media with effusion (COME)	OME persisting for ≥3 mo from the date of onset (if known) or from the date of diagnosis (if onset unknown)

Abbreviation: TM, tympanic membrane.
Adapted from Refs.[1–4]

family practitioners over the same period.[9] However, with now almost 10 years since the advancement of the concept that prompt antibiotic treatment is not needed for many children with AOM, observation of selected children with a diagnosis of AOM without initial antibiotics has become more accepted by both caregivers and providers. Additionally, physician adherence to the treatment recommendations from clinical practice guidelines may be improved with performance feedback and decision support systems using electronic health records.[10]

PATHOPHYSIOLOGY AND MICROBIOLOGY

AOM is often, although not always, preceded by a viral upper respiratory tract infection.[11] Inflammation leads to edema in the nasal cavities and nasopharynx, causing functional obstruction of the Eustachian tube and the development of negative pressure in the middle ear from a lack of equilibration. Microbe-containing secretions from the upper airway mucosa move into the middle ear owing to the pressure differential, where they become trapped. Bacterial replication and infection may ensue.[12–14] Young children are at particularly increased risk for AOM because of increased viral exposure, immunologic naiveté, and impaired Eustachian tube function even at baseline.[15]

With sensitive assays including culture, polymerase chain reaction and antigen detection, bacteria, viruses, or both, are detected in middle ear fluid in up to 96% of AOM cases. A study of middle ear fluid in 79 children with AOM and indwelling tympanostomy tubes found that 66% had bacteria and viruses, 27% had bacteria alone, and 4% had only viruses.[16]

The microbiology of AOM has changed over the last 2 decades with increasing penetration of pneumococcal vaccination programs. The most common bacterial species that cause AOM continue to be *Streptococcus pneumoniae*, nontypeable *Haemophilus influenza*, and *Moraxella catarrhalis*.[17] The heptavalent *S pneumoniae* vaccine (PCV7) was introduced in 2000, shortly after which the frequency of *S pneumoniae* recovery in tympanocentesis studies of AOM decreased relative to that of the other microbes.[18] The *S pneumoniae* serotypes contained in PCV7 continued to decline in AOM patients, and were in fact nearly absent by 2007 through 2009.[17] However, they have been replaced by nonvaccine pneumococcal serotypes in both tympanocentesis and nasopharyngeal colonization studies, so that the incidence of *S pneumoniae* was approximately equal to that of *H influenza*, with *M catarrhalis* less frequent.[17,19] The new 13-valent *S pneumoniae* vaccine, PCV13, was licensed in 2010[20] and will undoubtedly additionally shift the microbiological landscape of AOM.

DIAGNOSIS

Because there is no gold standard for the diagnosis of AOM, short of tympanocentesis and culture of middle ear fluid, there is controversy about the best clinical means to accurately diagnose acute middle ear infection. Diagnostic accuracy is challenging because of the wide spectrum of signs and symptoms that develop throughout the course of the disease, the difficulties in examining the ears of young children who may be uncooperative or have occluding cerumen, and the overlap of symptoms (fever, otalgia, irritability, insomnia) with other entities such as viral illness. In one study of 469 patients ages 6 to 35 months who were suspected by their caregivers to have AOM, only 237 (50%) actually met strict defined criteria for this diagnosis.[21] Additionally, the distinction between AOM and chronic OME is unclear to many caregivers and even to many medical professionals.

The diagnostic accuracy for children with AOM is important when we strategize for treatment of children with AOM. Children with upper respiratory infections and chronic OME generally should not be treated with antibiotics.[22–24] Many children with AOM do not require antibiotics for cure because the natural history of AOM is in general favorable.[25] When we interpret studies of treatment of AOM with antibiotics compared with placebo, those studies that include children with AOM diagnosed less stringently are more likely to include children with respiratory tract infections and OME rather than AOM. Treatment differences may be affected (made smaller) by use of less stringent diagnostic criteria. However, the "real-world" diagnosis of AOM in young children is unfortunately often far from precise, and the conclusions of those studies may be quite applicable to a cohort of children with presumed AOM.

The 2013 American Academy of Pediatrics (AAP) guideline on the management of AOM emphasized diagnostic criteria that focused on otoscopic examination (Table 2). This guideline proposed that AOM should be diagnosed in children with moderate to severe bulging of the tympanic membrane (TM) or new onset of otorrhea, or in children with mild bulging of the TM with recent onset of ear pain or intense TM erythema. In addition, AOM should not be diagnosed in children without a MEE.[7] This represents a new emphasis on precise diagnosis compared with the 2004 guidelines, which did not require a bulging TM and made management suggestions when there was an "uncertain diagnosis."[26]

Such strict diagnostic criteria were used in 2 randomized, controlled trials of antibiotics for AOM, both of which found benefit of antibiotic compared with placebo. In prior studies, antibiotic therapy resulted in clinical improvement in approximately 6% to 12% of children with AOM. In these 2 recent trials the rate of clinical improvement was 26% to 35%, likely owing to accurate diagnosis of AOM on entry as well as the nature of the measures of clinical improvement.[7,27,28]

Hoberman and colleagues[28] randomized 291 patients 6 to 23 months old with AOM to receive either amoxicillin–clavulanate or placebo for 10 days and recorded symptomatic response with the Acute Otitis Media Severity of Symptoms scale, as well as treatment failure. Diagnostic criteria included (1) onset of symptoms within 48 hours with score of 3+ on the Acute Otitis Media Severity of Symptoms scale, (2) MEE, and (3) moderate or marked bulging of TM, or slight bulging with either otalgia or marked erythema of TM. The treatment group had a lower Acute Otitis Media Severity of Symptoms scale score at 7 days ($P = .04$), with a lower treatment failure rate at days 4 or 5 and 10 through 12 (4% vs 24% [$P<.001$] and 16% vs 51% [$P<.001$], respectively). Tahtinen and colleagues[27] randomized 319 patients 6 to 35 months old with AOM to receive either amoxicillin–clavulanate or placebo for 7 days and measured time to treatment failure. Diagnostic criteria were (1) MEE, (2) signs of acute inflammation in TM, and (3) acute symptoms such as fever, ear pain, or respiratory symptoms. Treatment failure occurred in 18.6% of the treatment group, which was significantly lower than the 44.0% treatment failure rate for the placebo group ($P<.001$).

We should consider that these studies used amoxicillin–clavulanate rather than amoxicillin in the treatment arms. We should also consider that the treatment benefits of antibiotics over placebo were small, with debate about the clinical significance of some outcome measures in these studies.[29,30] Of course, small benefits of antibiotics must be assessed in light of side effects, most commonly diarrhea or yeast infections, as well as concerns about antibiotic overuse and bacterial resistance.[7,27,28,31,32]

Otoscopy

Note that the "red eardrum," or the ear "with fluid," is not diagnostic for AOM in the absence of bulging or otorrhea, according to the 2013 AAP guideline. MEE is necessary but alone not sufficient for the diagnosis of AOM, because OME is distinct from AOM (see **Table 1**). Although OME may precede or follow an episode of AOM, it is not an acute infectious process and in general should not be treated with antibiotics.[7,33] The appearance of the TM evolves over the course of the disease, and a change in clinical status warrants repeat examination.

In addition to examination of the color, position, and contour of the TM, pneumatic otoscopy to assess TM mobility is an important component of otoscopy. Absent or reduced TM mobility are diagnostic features of a MEE, as is an air–fluid level behind the TM. Tympanometry, when available, can also provide more quantitative information about TM mobility and middle ear compliance.[34]

Otoscopy can be challenging in children. Uncooperative patients, cerumen impaction, inadequate instrumentation, and even lack of expertise are common difficulties. Despite these challenges, the 2013 guideline underscores the importance of a thorough physical examination in the management of AOM, and reinforces the need for training pediatric clinicians in otoscopic and pneumatic otoscopic skills.[7] Suggestions for cerumen removal can be found in the American Academy of Otolaryngology–Head and Neck Surgery (AAO-HNS) Clinical Practice guidelines on cerumen impaction.[35] Diagnostic difficulties may lead to referral to an otolaryngologist for cerumen removal and examination of the ears with the otomicroscope (**Box 1**).

MANAGEMENT

Management goals for AOM are to decrease severity and duration of symptoms, principally by controlling pain and fever, to improve hearing outcomes, and to prevent complications.[7,36]

Analgesia

The assessment and treatment of pain is an important but possibly overlooked component of pediatric care. Poorly controlled pain is associated with suffering and can be emotionally traumatic, causing anxiety for patients and their caregivers.[37] Pain control should be actively addressed whether initial treatment included immediate antibiotics or not, because the antibiotics may not begin to provide pain relief for more than 24 hours.[7,31,38] Although there are many options for treatment of otalgia, including oral, topical, and homeopathic agents, few have been well studied.[7,39]

Oral acetaminophen and ibuprofen are commonly used to treat pain in children with AOM. A randomized, blinded, placebo-controlled trial found that both ibuprofen and acetaminophen improved pain control over placebo, but only ibuprofen resulted in a significant increase over placebo, with continued pain in 7%, 10%, and 24% of patients receiving ibuprofen, acetaminophen, and placebo, respectively ($P<.01$ for ibuprofen).[40] Topical drops, both anesthetic and naturopathic, have been found in small trials to improve pain symptoms, but a Cochrane review concluded that there is insufficient evidence to make any statement about their efficacy.[39,41,42] The selection of pain medication, as well as the dosing and schedule for administration, should be discussed with the caregivers, who may have valuable experience and preferences.[37]

Antibiotic Therapy

Antibiotic therapy is intended to target the bacteria present in the MEE of children with AOM.[16] Two key decisions regarding antibiotic use occur with every diagnosis of AOM: (1) Should antibiotics be used immediately, and (2) if antibiotics are used, which antibiotic is the best choice for treatment?

Table 2
Key differences in the 2004 and 2013 American Academy of Pediatrics guidelines for the diagnosis and management of acute otitis media (AOM)

Subject	2004	2013	Rationale for 2013 Changes
Children <6 mo	Treat with antibiotic therapy	No recommendations	
Diagnosis of AOM	Acute onset of signs and symptoms Presence of MEE Signs and symptoms of middle ear inflammation[a]	Moderate to severe bulging of TM, or new-onset otorrhea not owing to acute otitis externa Mild bulging of TM and recent[b] onset ear pain[c] or intense TM erythema Must have MEE	2004 criteria allowed less precise diagnosis, provided treatment recommendation when diagnosis was uncertain.
Uncertain diagnosis	Expected and included in treatment guidelines	Excluded	Emphasized need for diagnosis of AOM for best management.
Initial observation option instead of initial antibiotic therapy	Option for observation: 6 mo–2 y: Option if uncertain diagnosis and nonsevere illness[d] ≥2 y: Option if nonsevere[d] and certain diagnosis Observation recommended: ≥2 y and uncertain diagnosis	Option for observation: 6 mo–2 y: Unilateral OM without otorrhea ≥2 y: Unilateral or bilateral AOM without otorrhea Observation recommended: None	Favorable natural history overall. Evidence of small benefit of antibiotics in recent trials that used stringent diagnostic criteria.

Initial antibiotic therapy recommended	Antibiotics recommended: <6 mo: All cases 6 mo–2 y: Certain diagnosis, or uncertain diagnosis if severe[e] illness ≥2 y: Certain diagnosis and severe[e] illness Antibiotics an option: 6 mo–2 y: Uncertain diagnosis and nonsevere[d] illness ≥2 y: Certain diagnosis and nonsevere[d] illness	Antibiotics recommended: 6 mo–2 y: Otorrhea or severe[e] illness or bilateral without otorrhea ≥2 y: Otorrhea or severe[e] illness Antibiotics an option: 6 mo–2 y: Unilateral without otorrhea ≥2 y: Bilateral without otorrhea or unilateral without otorrhea	More stringent diagnostic guidelines in 2013 should lead to greater antibiotic benefit. Greater antibiotic benefit for bilateral disease, AOM with otorrhea. Two recent studies show small benefit of antibiotics for age 6–24 mo.
Recurrent AOM	No recommendations	Do not prescribe prophylactic antibiotics May offer tympanostomy tubes	Minimal benefit for prophylaxis and antibiotics come with risks (antibiotic resistance and adverse effects). Modest reduction in AOM with tubes.

Abbreviations: MEE, middle ear effusion; TM, tympanic membrane.

[a] Signs and symptoms of middle ear inflammation include distinct erythema of TM or distinct otalgia ('discomfort clearly referable to the ear[s] that results in interference with or precludes normal activity or sleep').

[b] Recent: <48 hours.

[c] Ear pain may be indicated by holding, tugging, or rubbing of the ear in a nonverbal child.

[d] Nonsevere illness defined as mild otalgia and fever <39°C in the past 24 hours in the 2004 guideline; the 2013 guideline modifies this to "mild otalgia for less than 48 hours and temperature less than 39°C."

[e] Severe signs or symptoms include moderate or severe otalgia or temperature ≥39°C in 2004 guideline; the 2013 guideline also includes otalgia for ≥48 hours.

Adapted from Lieberthal AS, Carroll AE, Chonmaitree T, et al. The diagnosis and management of acute otitis media. Pediatrics 2013;131(3):e964–99; and American Academy of Pediatrics Subcommittee on Management of Acute Otitis Media. Diagnosis and management of acute otitis media. Pediatrics 2004;113(5):1451–65.

Box 1
Acute otitis media (AOM): when to refer to the otolaryngologist

Referral to an otolaryngologist should be considered for the following reasons:

Inability to examine the ear

Unexplained, progressive, or irreversible tympanic membrane abnormality

Poor response to therapy

Recurrent AOM

Associated hearing difficulties that persist or progress

Recurrent AOM in the "at-risk child"

Suspected complication of AOM

The decision of whether or not to treat with initial antibiotics is based on age, severity of symptoms, the presence of otorrhea, and laterality (**Box 2**, see **Table 2**).[7] In the 2013 AAP guideline, antibiotics are recommended for any child with otorrhea, or severe symptoms, or both, and for children younger than 2 years with bilateral AOM. There is an option for initial observation instead of initial antibiotics if children are younger than 2 years old with unilateral disease and no otorrhea, or 2 years or older with either bilateral or unilateral disease and no otorrhea (see **Table 2**).

The concept of initial observation, without immediate antibiotic treatment, of children diagnosed with AOM was advanced in Europe before the 2004 recommendations of the AAP did so here in the United States. The favorable natural history of AOM, the potential overdiagnosis of AOM, and the potential consequences of antibiotics, including frequent side effects and the emergence of drug resistant microbes, are all considerations here.[7,27,28,31,32]

A recent Cochrane review found that up to 82% of children with AOM improve spontaneously. Although there is a slight improvement in symptoms associated with antibiotics (relative risk [RR], 0.70; 95% CI, 0.57–0.86 and RR, 0.79; 95% CI 0.66–0.95 for 2–3 days and 4–7 days, respectively), 20 children would need to receive antibiotics to prevent 1 child from experiencing ear pain at 2 to 7 days.[31] Antibiotics did significantly reduce TM perforations and contralateral AOM episodes; however, there was no effect on tympanometry findings at 4 weeks to 3 months, or on the number of AOM

Box 2
Initial antibiotic therapy or observation for acute otitis media (AOM)

The decision to treat AOM with antibiotics at time of diagnosis or to observe with close follow-up should include:

Parental/caregiver input and informed shared decision making

Ability to follow patients for improvement or deterioration

Understanding that young children (<6 months of age), children with bilateral AOM, and children with otorrhea should be treated with antibiotics

Understanding that children with severe symptoms (moderate or severe otalgia or otalgia for at least 48 hours, or temperature 39°C [102.2°F] or higher) should be treated with antibiotics

Understanding the controversies about the need to use antibiotics in children between 6 and 24 months who have AOM with mild or moderate symptoms.

recurrences. Antibiotics also increased the relative risk of adverse events by 34% (95% CI, 16%–55%), most commonly vomiting, diarrhea, and rash.[31]

The decision to observe without immediate antibiotics should be made in conjunction with caregivers, with a plan for pain management at the outset and a mechanism for follow-up within 48 to 72 hours so antibiotics can be started for persistent or worsening symptoms.[7] There is evidence that in the proper setting this strategy does not increase complication rates.[43] Clinicians may also give caregivers an antibiotic prescription with instructions to have it filled only under certain circumstances, the so-called wait-and-see prescription (WASP).[44] This approach seems to avoid antibiotic use in up to two thirds of children selected for observation.[44,45]

Antibiotic Choice

If antibiotic treatment is used for a child with AOM, the choice of antibiotic is based on the most common pathogens and their susceptibility patterns as well as the side effect profile of the drug. High-dose amoxicillin (90 mg/kg per day) is the recommended first-line agent in the 2013 guidelines, with the addition of beta-lactamase coverage for cases in which the patient has recently received amoxicillin, has concurrent purulent conjunctivitis, or has recurrent AOM unresponsive to amoxicillin.[7] S pneumoniae is 83 to 87% susceptible to high-dose amoxicillin, and H influenza is 58% to 82% susceptible.[7] Interestingly, more than 90% of M catarrhalis is beta-lactamase positive,[46] but a high rate of spontaneous clinical improvement and low rate of suppurative complications with AOM from this organism makes amoxicillin treatment an appropriate first choice.[7,47,48]

For penicillin-sensitive patients, second- or third-generation cephalosporins, including intramuscular ceftriaxone, may be used. Other useful agents, particularly for penicillin-sensitive patients or amoxicillin failures, include second- and third-generation cephalosporins and clindamycin. Patients who do not improve in 48 to 72 hours on their first-line regimen should be reassessed, and alternative therapy considered.[7] In this instance, amoxicillin–clavulanate and intramuscular or intravenous ceftriaxone are considered first line, with alternatives including clindamycin or combination treatment with both clindamycin and a third-generation cephalosporin. In difficult cases, tympanocentesis may be considered for drainage and culture-directed therapy.[7]

COMPLICATIONS

AOM can progress to severe complications, including acute mastoiditis, meningitis, and intracranial abscess. Complications can be thought of as (a) intracranial, extratemporal, (b) intratemporal, extracranial, and (c) extratemporal, extracranial (Table 3). The most common complication seen by the clinician is TM perforation with suppuration and otorrhea, but a busy clinician can expect to see facial nerve paralysis or acute mastoiditis (Fig. 1) in a young child with AOM as well. Such suppurative complications require prompt referral to the appropriate surgical specialists (ie, an otolaryngologist or neurosurgeon) for aggressive antibiotic therapy and for surgical drainage when indicated. Although a full discussion of such complications is beyond the scope of this review, the presentations and diagnostic schemes for such conditions are detailed in Table 3. Importantly, the recommendation of initial observation of AOM without antibiotics in selected children has not caused a substantial increase in suppurative complications such as mastoiditis.[43,51]

RECURRENT AOM AND TYMPANOSTOMY TUBES

Recurrent AOM is defined as at least 3 episodes of AOM in 6 month or 4 episodes in 1 year, with one of these episodes in the preceding 6 months.[7] Risk factors that have

Table 3
Complications of acute otitis media (AOM)

Complication	Presentation	Diagnostic Tests	Treatment Options
Intracranial, extratemporal			
Meningitis	Headache, altered mental status, nausea, vomiting, lethargy, poor oral intake, seizures, meningismus, focal neurologic deficits	LP after CT or MRI to exclude other intracranial complications	Antibiotics Myringotomy ± tympanostomy tube
Intracranial abscess		CT first-line and for follow-up MRI more sensitive	Antibiotics Myringotomy ± tympanostomy tube
Subdural or epidural abscess		CT first-line and for follow-up MRI more sensitive	Neurosurgical consultation
Otitic hydrocephalus (nonobstructing mural thrombus of transverse sinus)	Headache, vomiting, blurred vision, seizures, abducens palsy	LP to measure ICP, after CT to exclude mass effect: high ICP and normal cytology	Antibiotics Measures to decrease ICP
Thrombosis of dural venous sinuses (lateral or sigmoid sinus thrombophlebitis)	Headache, neck stiffness, fever, otalgia, postauricular pain & erythema	CT-contrast enhanced, MRI/MRA/MRV	Antibiotics ± anticoagulation Myringotomy ± tympanostomy tube ± Mastoidectomy Consider clot removal
Extracranial, intratemporal			
Acute mastoiditis (see **Fig. 1**)	Postauricular erythema, tenderness, edema, protrusion of pinna	CT: bony erosion, destruction of mastoid air cells	Antibiotics Myringotomy ± tympanostomy tube Mastoidectomy or aspiration of subperiosteal abscess

Subperiosteal abscess	Postauricular erythema, tenderness, fluctuance	CT: fluid collection adjacent to eroded mastoid cortex	Antibiotics Myringotomy ± tympanostomy tube Mastoidectomy or needle aspiration of abscess
Petrositis (Gradenigo's syndrome)	Abducens palsy and retrobulbar pain	CT first-line MRI for nerve involvement, apical petrositis	Antibiotics Myringotomy ± tympanostomy tube Mastoidectomy
Facial nerve palsy	Often incomplete acute onset facial weakness on affected side	CT to assess extent of disease and rule out cholesteatoma or other lesion	Antibiotics Myringotomy ± tympanostomy tube
Labyrinthitis	Acute onset SNHL and vertigo	Physical examination	Antibiotics Myringotomy ± tympanostomy tube Consider steroids if SNHL persists
TM perforation	Otorrhea	Physical examination	Antibiotics Close follow-up to determine for surgical repair
Extracranial, extratemporal			
Sepsis	Fever, lethargy, tachycardia, hypotension	Physical examination	Antibiotics Myringotomy ± tympanostomy tube

Abbreviations: CT, computed tomography scan; ICP, intracranial pressure; LP, lumbar puncture; MRA, magnetic resonance angiography; MRI, magnetic resonance imaging; MRV, magnetic resonance venography; SNHL, sensorineural hearing loss; TM, tympanic membrane.
Adapted from Refs. [3,49,50]

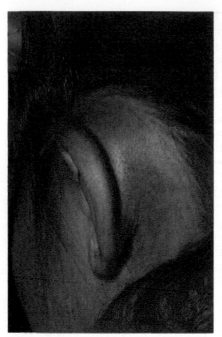

Fig. 1. Acute mastoiditis, characterized by postauricular erythema and swelling.

been identified for recurrent AOM include group child care attendance, male gender, winter season, passive smoking, pacifier uses, presence of siblings, lack of breast-feeding, and symptoms for longer than 10 days at presentation.[52] The 2013 AAP guideline examines the role of both prophylactic antibiotic therapy and tympanostomy tube placement for prevention of recurrent AOM. Prophylactic antibiotics do reduce the incidence of AOM by approximately 0.5 to 1.5 episodes per 12 months of treatment per child, and the treatment of 5 children for 1 year would prevent 1 child from developing AOM during therapy.[53] However, given the cost, side effects, potential for antibiotic resistance, and scant clinical benefit with a large number needed to treat to avoid a single episode of AOM, a recommendation against the routine administration of antibiotic prophylaxis for children with recurrent AOM was made in the 2013 AAP AOM guideline.[7]

Tympanostomy Tubes

Tympanostomy tubes are placed in 667,000 children under the age of 15 every year in the United States.[54] One out of 15 children, or 6.8% of the population, had tympanostomy tubes placed before the age of 3 years.[55] The health care costs of tympanostomy tubes are enormous, at an estimated cost of $2200 per patient[56] for a total of nearly $1.5 billion annually in the United States.

Tympanostomy tubes are most commonly placed for persistent MEE with associated hearing difficulties (OME) or for recurrent AOM. This surgery is less commonly performed for AOM treatment failure, impending complications of AOM, or structural TM changes associated with long-term Eustachian tube dysfunction.[57] Indications for tympanostomy tube placement have been subject to recent scrutiny. Possible overuse of tympanostomy tubes has been identified, particularly for children with MEEs of short duration and for children with infrequent or poorly documented episodes of

AOM.[58] These issues have been addressed by a national "overuse" summit that included tympanostomy tube placement as 1 of the 5 potentially overused treatments,[59] as well as by the recent publication of a multidisciplinary clinical practice guideline on the use of tympanostomy tubes in children.[1]

Most studies of the benefits of tympanostomy tubes focus on utility for MEEs and conductive hearing loss.[60,61] The literature studying the use of tympanostomy tubes for recurrent AOM is scant; few studies exclude children with long-term MEE. The reduction of AOM by tube placement is likely modest.

One trial of recurrent AOM treatment that excluded children with MEE randomized children to tympanostomy tube placement, amoxicillin prophylaxis, or placebo and followed them for 2 years. The tympanostomy tube group did not show a decrease in episodes of AOM.[2] However, several randomized trials of tympanostomy tubes for recurrent AOM that included children with MEE at entry did show a modest reduction in AOM episodes from 0.55 to 2.5 episodes per child-year.[62–64] A recent Cochrane review included 2 of these studies of tympanostomy tubes for recurrent AOM, and concluded that tympanostomy tubes reduced AOM episodes by 1.5 in the 6 months after surgery.[65] A systematic review that included 5 studies of recurrent AOM and tympanostomy tubes concluded that 2 to 5 children needed to be treated with tubes to prevent 1 episode of AOM over a 6-month period.[66]

A recent study of tympanostomy tube insertion with or without adenoidectomy in children 10 months to 2 years with recurrent AOM, and no evidence of chronic OME, showed a modest benefit in preventing recurrent AOM in the 12 months after tube surgery, with a decrease in treatment failure of 13% in the tympanostomy tubes group (95% CI, −25% to −1%) and 18% in the tympanostomy tubes and adenoidectomy group (95% CI, −30% to −6%) compared with controls.[62]

Children (and caregivers) with AOM may experience improved quality of life after tympanostomy tube insertion. Children with middle ear disease, including OME, recurrent AOM, or both, had improved disease-specific quality of life measures in several studies of tympanostomy tube placement, including improvement in physical suffering, hearing, speech, caregiver concerns, and emotional distress domains.[56,67–69]

The 2013 AAP AOM guideline states that "clinicians may offer tympanostomy tubes for recurrent AOM."[7] Few if any prior guidelines have included tympanostomy tube placement for this indication, despite widespread accepted use of tubes for recurrent AOM. The use of tympanostomy tubes for recurrent AOM is additionally refined in the recently published AAO-HNS Clinical Practice guideline for Tympanostomy Tubes in Children.[1]

This AAO-HNS tympanostomy tube guideline contains a key action statement that "clinicians should NOT perform tympanostomy tube insertion in children with recurrent AOM who do not have a MEE in either ear at the time of assessment." This recommendation is based on evidence from the trials that studied antibiotic prophylaxis for recurrent AOM that excluded children with MEE, where children in the placebo groups improved with fewer subsequent ear infections.[25] This may reflect a favorable natural history of recurrent AOM, and also may reflect uncertainties in the diagnosis of AOM in referred children.[70] Importantly, this guideline recommendation did not apply to "at-risk" children, or those children who are immunocompromised, had severe or persistent AOM, a prior complication of AOM, or antibiotic allergies/intolerances. Such children may need tympanostomy tubes inserted for prevention of AOM more urgently, even in the absence of obvious ear disease.[57]

This same guideline contains a key action statement that "clinicians should offer bilateral tympanostomy tube insertion in children with RAOM who have unilateral or bilateral middle ear effusion at the time of assessment." In these children, the presence of the effusion provides some confidence in the history of AOM, and it suggests ongoing Eustachian tube dysfunction that could lead to more AOM. The tubes provide a small benefit in the reduction of the number of AOM episodes, and perhaps additional benefits with quality of life measures, as well reduction of pain and fever with subsequent infection. Note that this statement is an "offer" of tympanostomy tubes, with the decision to place the tubes based on shared decision making with caregivers.[1]

Tympanostomy tube insertion is a safe procedure performed on an outpatient basis with risks related mostly to short- and long-term effects on the TM and potential complications of general anesthesia. One quarter of patients experience transient otorrhea while the tympanostomy tube is in place. At least 2% of children may develop persistent TM perforations, and up to one third will develop tympanosclerosis. Other short-term and long-term complications include granulation tissue, premature extrusion or displacement of tympanostomy tubes, focal atrophy, and increased risk of cholesteatoma (RR, 2.6; 95% CI, 1.5–4.4).[71]

To better understand the potential risks of anesthesia, 1 study of 3198 children undergoing tympanostomy tube placement with general anesthesia at a tertiary care children's hospital found that 9% had minor complications (upper airway obstruction, agitation, prolonged recovery, and emesis) and 1.9% had major complications (laryngospasm, desaturation, bradycardia, dysrhythmia, and stridor). Rates were significantly increased in patients with acute or chronic illnesses (odds ratio, 2.78; $P<.001$).[72] However another study of 4979 outpatient otolaryngologic procedures at an ambulatory surgical center, including 2045 (41.1%) tympanostomy tube placements, found a complication rate of just 0.2% overall, the majority of which occurred in those who had adenoidectomy and/or tonsillectomy.[73] Complications of tympanostomy tube insertion are infrequent but are not negligible, and should be taken into consideration in clinical decision making.

Tympanostomy Tube Otorrhea

An advantage of tympanostomy tube insertion is the ability to deliver topical antibiotic therapy in the place of systemic medication should AOM occur after tube placement. In children with tympanostomy tubes, AOM is often manifested by acute tympanostomy tube otorrhea (TTO), discharge from the middle ear through the tympanostomy tube into the external auditory canal. TTO is also a common postoperative complication of tympanostomy tube insertion,[71] defined as such if it occurs within 4 weeks postoperatively. Beyond 4 weeks after surgery, TTO is referred to as delayed otorrhea. It may also be chronic ($\geq$3 months) or recurrent ($\geq$3 episodes).[57]

Acute TTO is generally caused by the same pathogens as AOM in children without tympanostomy tubes, such as, S pneumonia, H influenza, or M catarrhalis.[16] In older children and those with a history of water exposure, pathogens may include Pseudomonas aeruginosa and Staphylococcus aureus.[1,74] The AAO-HNS tympanostomy tube guideline contains a strong recommendation that clinicians "should prescribe topical antibiotic eardrops only, without oral antibiotics, for children with uncomplicated acute tympanostomy tube otorrhea."[1] This is based on randomized, controlled trials comparing topical with systemic oral antibiotics that demonstrated superiority for topical therapy in treatment, eradication of bacterial pathogens, and patient satisfaction.[75–77] Approved topical drops include ofloxacin or ciprofloxacin–dexamethasone. In general, aminoglycoside-containing drops should be avoided owing to the potential for ototoxicity. Systemic antibiotics should be considered if TTO persists despite adequate ototopical therapy, if delivery of the ear drops is impeded by an obstructed external auditory canal or uncooperative child, or if there is concern for more severe disease (ie, cellulitis, fever, severe otalgia, concurrent sinusitis or pharyngitis, immune compromise). Oral antibiotics may be given concurrently with topical antibiotics.[1]

PREVENTION

Several anticipatory health interventions and environmental factors can reduce the incidence of AOM and are endorsed in the 2013 AAP guideline. Vaccination with the conjugate pneumococcal vaccine (PCV7) decreased physician visits for AOM, although there was a subsequent trend toward serotype replacement where AOM (and complications) were caused by nonvaccine serotypes.[17,19] Vaccination with the more recent PCV13, which covers 6 additional S pneumoniae serotypes, should be encouraged.[17,19,20,78] The influenza vaccine is recommended for all children over 6 months of age.[79] AOM frequently complicates influenza owing to predisposing inflammation of the upper respiratory mucosa, and this vaccination can reduce the frequency of AOM with up to 55% efficacy.[7,80–83]

Exclusive breastfeeding for 4 to 6 months after birth reduces frequency of AOM and recurrent AOM.[84,85] Passive tobacco smoke exposure significantly increases the risk of middle ear disease,[86,87] and parental smoking cessation is a preventative measure that should be addressed by clinicians. Group childcare attendance and pacifier use are other modifiable risk factors that have also been associated with OM.[87,88]

The literature does contain low-level evidence that nutritional supplementation may have a role in preventing OM.[89,90] A large, randomized, placebo-controlled trial in Bangladesh of weekly zinc supplementation found a significant reduction in suppurative otitis media in the group receiving zinc (RR, 0.58; 95% CI, 0.41–0.82; $P = .002$), although the significance of these results in developed countries is unclear. A recent randomized, placebo-controlled trial of vitamin D supplementation taking place in Italy enrolled 116 children with a history of recurrent AOM and randomized to 4 months of either vitamin D or placebo. Fewer children in the treatment group experienced 1 or more episode of AOM ($P = .03$). It was also noted that the likelihood of AOM was significantly lower among patients with higher serum concentrations of vitamin D ($\geq$30 ng/mL).[89] Additional well-designed, randomized trials are necessary to further define the role of nutritional supplementation in the prevention of AOM.

COMPLEMENTARY AND ALTERNATIVE MEDICINE

Although many dietary modifications and complementary and alternative medicine options have been proposed and are available for prevention and treatment of AOM, high-quality evidence does not exist to support their use. Naturopathic herbal extracts have been used as topical analgesics and have been found to provide similar rates of pain relief to conventional anesthetic ear drops,[41] although good evidence of benefit is lacking.[39]

A randomized, double-blind, placebo-controlled study involving 328 Israeli children examined the impact on upper respiratory infections of a mixture of Echinacea with several other substances including propolis and vitamin C in an elixir called "Chizukit" administered twice daily during the winter months. This study found a 68% reduction in AOM in the treatment group (19.4% vs 43.5% incidence AOM; $P<.001$).[91] Additional studies of individual components of such mixtures using more rigorous study design are necessary before routine recommendation of such for prevention of AOM.

The general health benefits of probiotics have been widely endorsed but sparsely studied. Studies of probiotics given to children in milk, capsule form, nasal sprays, and formula have conflicting results, but some have found a modest benefit in the prevention of AOM.[92] One placebo-controlled study of probiotic formula supplementation for infants from younger than 2 months through 12 months of age found a significantly decreased frequency of AOM, with fewer antibiotic prescriptions, in the first 7 months of life in the treatment group.[93] Other randomized, controlled trials, however, have found no difference in the frequency of AOM.[94,95]

Xylitol is a natural sugar found in fruit and administered as a gum, syrup, or lozenge that has been extensively studied as a preventative compound for AOM. It decreases microbial adherence to nasopharyngeal cells, and alters Streptococcus pneumoniae gene expression.[92] A recent Cochrane review found a 25% reduced risk of AOM (RR, 0.75; 95% CI, 0.65–0.88) in otherwise healthy children receiving xylitol compared with controls.[96] Despite these findings, the clinical relevance of xylitol is limited by the need for frequent dosing (5 times daily in most studies), frequent gastrointestinal side effects, and poor compliance.

The 2013 AAP guideline calls for additional research to compare complementary and alternative medicine therapies with the observation option for AOM. Clinicians should take appropriate caution when discussing complementary and alternative medicine therapies, given the lack of supporting evidence for many approaches, potential side effects, and costs.[92] Of course, any study of such interventions should be interpreted in light of our knowledge of the inconsistencies in diagnosis of AOM as well as the general favorable natural history of children identified as having recurrent AOM.

"AT-RISK" CHILDREN AND OTITIS MEDIA

Children with medical comorbidities, neurocognitive and/or communication impairment, and craniofacial anomalies that affect Eustachian tube function may be at increased risk for frequent AOM or consequences of middle ear disease and associated conductive hearing loss. These children are usually excluded from clinical trials that evaluate the management and outcomes of otitis media, and in fact are excluded from the 2013 AAP AOM guideline recommendations. The AAO-HNS Clinical Practice guideline on Tympanostomy Tubes in Children specifically recommended identification of such "at-risk" children, with acknowledgment that these children may need more urgent and chronic management of otitis media, often with tympanostomy tubes.

At-risk children include those with underlying hearing loss, autism spectrum and other developmental disorders, Down syndrome, craniofacial disorders with cognitive delays, vision impairment, cleft palate with or without an associated syndrome, and developmental delay.[22] Children with craniofacial disorders, Down syndrome, cleft palate, and many other syndromes often have anatomic and functional impairment of the Eustachian tubes that increase the risk of AOM.[97,98] Underlying immune dysfunction and unique group care settings may further exacerbate middle ear disease in these patients. Physical examination and hearing assessment may be difficult in these children because of behavioral and communication issues. Some have stenotic external auditory canals, particularly children with Down syndrome, prone to cerumen impaction and difficult otoscopy.[99]

The AAO-HNS 2004 guideline for Otitis Media with Effusion and the 2013 guideline for Tympanostomy Tubes in Children acknowledge the special needs of this population and encourage the optimization of conditions for hearing, speech and language.[1,22] Some of these "at-risk" children have medical issues that increase the risk of general anesthesia, a consideration when tympanostomy tubes are recommended. General anesthesia for tympanostomy tube placement carries an higher rate of complications in children with chronic illnesses.[72] Children with developmental abnormalities have high rates of sleep apnea, which increases the risks of general anesthesia, and skeletal deformities may present airway management challenges during anesthesia.[98,100] These risks should be taken into account when planning for tympanostomy tube insertion.

SUMMARY

Management of AOM requires keen diagnostic skills to recognize the signs, symptoms, and severity of the illness and to determine the otoscopic hallmarks of acute middle ear infection. Recent clinical practice guidelines emphasize the need for precise diagnosis, whereas understanding the generally favorable natural history of AOM may allow many children to be observed without initial antibiotic treatment. Prevention of AOM can include vaccinations, environmental modifications, maintenance of breastfeeding, as well as other interventions. Tympanostomy tubes may modestly lower the number of infections in children with recurrent AOM, and improve disease-related quality of life for children as well.

REFERENCES

1. Rosenfeld RM, Schwartz SR, Pynnonen MA, et al. Clinical practice guideline: tympanostomy tubes in children. Otolaryngol Head Neck Surg 2013;149(Suppl 1): S1–35.
2. Casselbrant ML, Kaleida PH, Rockette HE, et al. Efficacy of antimicrobial prophylaxis and of tympanostomy tube insertion for prevention of recurrent acute otitis media: results of a randomized clinical trial. Pediatr Infect Dis J 1992;11(4): 278–86.
3. Bluestone CD, Klein JO. Otitis media in infants and children. 4th edition. Hamilton (Ontario): BC Decker; 2007.
4. Rosenfeld RM, Bluestone CD. Evidence-based otitis media. 2nd edition. Hamilton (Ontario); Lewiston (NY): B.C. Decker; 2003.
5. Soni A. Ear infections (otitis media) in children (0-17): use and expenditures, 2006. Rockville (MD): Agency for Healthcare Research and Quality; 2008. Statistical Brief No. 228.
6. Grijalva CG, Nuorti JP, Griffin MR. Antibiotic prescription rates for acute respiratory tract infections in US ambulatory settings. JAMA 2009;302(7):758–66.
7. Lieberthal AS, Carroll AE, Chonmaitree T, et al. The diagnosis and management of acute otitis media. Pediatrics 2013;131(3):e964–99.
8. Coco A, Vernacchio L, Horst M, et al. Management of acute otitis media after publication of the 2004 AAP and AAFP clinical practice guideline. Pediatrics 2010;125(2):214–20.
9. Grossman Z, Silverman BG, Miron D. Physician specialty is associated with adherence to treatment guidelines for acute otitis media in children. Acta Paediatr 2013;102(1):e29–33.
10. Forrest CB, Fiks AG, Bailey LC, et al. Improving adherence to otitis media guidelines with clinical decision support and physician feedback. Pediatrics 2013; 131(4):e1071–81.
11. Winther B, Alper CM, Mandel EM, et al. Temporal relationships between colds, upper respiratory viruses detected by polymerase chain reaction, and otitis media in young children followed through a typical cold season. Pediatrics 2007; 119(6):1069–75.
12. Rovers MM, Schilder AG, Zielhuis GA, et al. Otitis media. Lancet 2004;363(9407): 465–73.

13. Chonmaitree T, Heikkinen T. Role of viruses in middle-ear disease. Ann N Y Acad Sci 1997;830:143–57.
14. Heikkinen T, Chonmaitree T. Importance of respiratory viruses in acute otitis media. Clin Microbiol Rev 2003;16(2):230–41.
15. Bluestone CD, Swarts JD. Human evolutionary history: consequences for the pathogenesis of otitis media. Otolaryngol Head Neck Surg 2010;143(6):739–44.
16. Ruohola A, Meurman O, Nikkari S, et al. Microbiology of acute otitis media in children with tympanostomy tubes: prevalences of bacteria and viruses. Clin Infect Dis 2006;43(11):1417–22.
17. Casey JR, Adlowitz DG, Pichichero ME. New patterns in the otopathogens causing acute otitis media six to eight years after introduction of pneumococcal conjugate vaccine. Pediatr Infect Dis J 2010;29(4):304–9.
18. Grubb MS, Spaugh DC. Microbiology of acute otitis media, Puget sound region, 2005-2009. Clin Pediatr 2010;49(8):727–30.
19. O'Brien KL, Millar EV, Zell ER, et al. Effect of pneumococcal conjugate vaccine on nasopharyngeal colonization among immunized and unimmunized children in a community-randomized trial. J Infect Dis 2007;196(8):1211–20.
20. Centers for Disease Control and Prevention. Licensure of a 13-valent pneumococcal conjugate vaccine (PCV13) and recommendations for use among children - Advisory Committee on Immunization Practices (ACIP), 2010. MMWR Morbid Mortal Wkly Rep 2010;59(9):258–61.
21. Laine MK, Tahtinen PA, Ruuskanen O, et al. Symptoms or symptom-based scores cannot predict acute otitis media at otitis-prone age. Pediatrics 2010;125(5): e1154–61.
22. Rosenfeld RM, Culpepper L, Doyle KJ, et al. Clinical practice guideline: otitis media with effusion. Otolaryngol Head Neck Surg 2004;130(Suppl 5):S95–118.
23. Centers for Disease Control and Prevention. Get smart: know when antibiotics work. Available at: http://www.cdc.gov/getsmart/campaign-materials/about-campaign.html. Accessed September 26, 2013.
24. Weissman J, Besser RE. Promoting appropriate antibiotic use for pediatric patients: a social ecological framework. Semin Pediatr Infect Dis 2004;15(1):41–51.
25. Rosenfeld RM, Kay D. Natural history of untreated otitis media. Laryngoscope 2003;113(10):1645–57.
26. American Academy of Pediatrics Subcommittee on Management of Acute Otitis Media. Diagnosis and management of acute otitis media. Pediatrics 2004; 113(5):1451–65.
27. Tahtinen PA, Laine MK, Huovinen P, et al. A placebo-controlled trial of antimicrobial treatment for acute otitis media. N Engl J Med 2011;364(2):116–26.
28. Hoberman A, Paradise JL, Rockette HE, et al. Treatment of acute otitis media in children under 2 years of age. N Engl J Med 2011;364(2):105–15.
29. Newman DH, Shreves AE. Treatment of acute otitis media in children. N Engl J Med 2011;364(18):1775 [author reply: 1777–8].
30. Darby-Stewart A, Graber MA, Dachs R. Antibiotics for acute otitis media in young children. Am Fam Physician 2011;84(10):1095–7.
31. Venekamp RP, Sanders S, Glasziou PP, et al. Antibiotics for acute otitis media in children. Cochrane Database Syst Rev 2013;(1):CD000219.
32. Pichichero ME, Casey JR. Evolving microbiology and molecular epidemiology of acute otitis media in the pneumococcal conjugate vaccine era. Pediatr Infect Dis J 2007;26(Suppl 10):S12–6.
33. Rosenfeld RM, Culpepper L, Yawn B, et al. Otitis media with effusion clinical practice guideline. Am Fam Physician 2004;69(12):2776, 2778–9.

34. Onusko E. Tympanometry. Am Fam Physician 2004;70(9):1713–20.
35. Roland PS, Smith TL, Schwartz SR, et al. Clinical practice guideline: cerumen impaction. Otolaryngol Head Neck Surg 2008;139(3 Suppl 2):S1–21.
36. Shaikh N, Hoberman A, Paradise JL, et al. Development and preliminary evaluation of a parent-reported outcome instrument for clinical trials in acute otitis media. Pediatr Infect Dis J 2009;28(1):5–8.
37. American Academy of Pediatrics, Committee on Psychosocial Aspects of Child and Family Health, Task Force on Pain in Infants, Children, and Adolescents. The assessment and management of acute pain in infants, children, and adolescents. Pediatrics 2001;108(3):793–7.
38. Burke P, Bain J, Robinson D, et al. Acute red ear in children: controlled trial of non-antibiotic treatment in general practice. BMJ 1991;303(6802):558–62.
39. Foxlee R, Johansson A, Wejfalk J, et al. Topical analgesia for acute otitis media. Cochrane Database Syst Rev 2006;(3):CD005657.
40. Bertin L, Pons G, d'Athis P, et al. A randomized, double-blind, multicentre controlled trial of ibuprofen versus acetaminophen and placebo for symptoms of acute otitis media in children. Fundam Clin Pharmacol 1996;10(4):387–92.
41. Sarrell EM, Mandelberg A, Cohen HA. Efficacy of naturopathic extracts in the management of ear pain associated with acute otitis media. Arch Pediatr Adolesc Med 2001;155(7):796–9.
42. Bolt P, Barnett P, Babl FE, et al. Topical lignocaine for pain relief in acute otitis media: results of a double-blind placebo-controlled randomised trial. Arch Dis Child 2008;93(1):40–4.
43. Marcy M, Takata G, Chan LS, et al. Management of acute otitis media. Evid Rep Technol Assess (Summ) 2000;(15):1–4.
44. Spiro DM, Tay KY, Arnold DH, et al. Wait-and-see prescription for the treatment of acute otitis media: a randomized controlled trial. JAMA 2006;296(10):1235–41.
45. McCormick DP, Chonmaitree T, Pittman C, et al. Nonsevere acute otitis media: a clinical trial comparing outcomes of watchful waiting versus immediate antibiotic treatment. Pediatrics 2005;115(6):1455–65.
46. Doern GV, Jones RN, Pfaller MA, et al. Haemophilus influenzae and Moraxella catarrhalis from patients with community-acquired respiratory tract infections: antimicrobial susceptibility patterns from the SENTRY antimicrobial Surveillance Program (United States and Canada, 1997). Antimicrobial Agents Chemother 1999;43(2):385–9.
47. Palmu AA, Herva E, Savolainen H, et al. Association of clinical signs and symptoms with bacterial findings in acute otitis media. Clin Infect Dis 2004;38(2):234–42.
48. Petersen CG, Ovesen T, Pedersen CB. Acute mastoidectomy in a Danish county from 1977 to 1996 with focus on the bacteriology. Int J Pediatr Otorhinolaryngol 1998;45(1):21–9.
49. Naseri I, Sobol SE. Regional and intracranial complications of acute otitis media. In: Bell LM, editor. Pediatric otolaryngology: the requisites in pediatrics. 1st edition. Philadelphia: Mosby, Inc; 2007. p. 105–17.
50. Ropposch T, Nemetz U, Braun EM, et al. Management of otogenic sigmoid sinus thrombosis. Otol Neurotol 2011;32(7):1120–3.
51. Thompson PL, Gilbert RE, Long PF, et al. Effect of antibiotics for otitis media on mastoiditis in children: a retrospective cohort study using the United kingdom general practice research database. Pediatrics 2009;123(2):424–30.
52. Damoiseaux RA, Rovers MM, Van Balen FA, et al. Long-term prognosis of acute otitis media in infancy: determinants of recurrent acute otitis media and persistent middle ear effusion. Fam Pract 2006;23(1):40–5.

53. Leach AJ, Morris PS. Antibiotics for the prevention of acute and chronic suppurative otitis media in children. Cochrane Database Syst Rev 2006;(4):CD004401.
54. Cullen KA, Hall MJ, Golosinskiy A. Ambulatory surgery in the United States, 2006. Natl Health Stat Report 2009;(11):1–25.
55. Kogan MD, Overpeck MD, Hoffman HJ, et al. Factors associated with tympanostomy tube insertion among preschool-aged children in the United States. Am J Public Health 2000;90(2):245–50.
56. Mui S, Rasgon BM, Hilsinger RL Jr, et al. Tympanostomy tubes for otitis media: quality-of-life improvement for children and parents. Ear Nose Throat J 2005; 84(7):418, 420–2, 424.
57. Rosenfeld RM, Schwartz SR, Pynnonen MA, et al. Clinical practice guideline: tympanostomy tubes in children–executive summary. Otolaryngol Head Neck Surg 2013;149(1):8–16.
58. Keyhani S, Kleinman LC, Rothschild M, et al. Overuse of tympanostomy tubes in New York metropolitan area: evidence from five hospital cohort. BMJ 2008;337: a1607.
59. Advisory Panel Work Group for Tympanostomy Tubes. Tympanostomy tubes for middle ear effusion of brief duration. Paper presented at: The National Summit on Overuse. Oakbrook Terrace, September 24, 2012.
60. Browning GG, Rovers MM, Williamson I, et al. Grommets (ventilation tubes) for hearing loss associated with otitis media with effusion in children. Cochrane Database Syst Rev 2010;(10):CD001801.
61. Agency for Healthcare Research and Quality (AHRQ). Number 101, otitis media with effusion: comparative effectiveness of treatments, executive summary. Rockville (MD): Agency for Healthcare Research and Quality; 2013.
62. Kujala T, Alho OP, Luotonen J, et al. Tympanostomy with and without adenoidectomy for the prevention of recurrences of acute otitis media: a randomized controlled trial. Pediatr Infect Dis J 2012;31(6):565–9.
63. Gebhart DE. Tympanostomy tubes in the otitis media prone child. Laryngoscope 1981;91(6):849–66.
64. Gonzalez C, Arnold JE, Woody EA, et al. Prevention of recurrent acute otitis media: chemoprophylaxis versus tympanostomy tubes. Laryngoscope 1986;96(12): 1330–4.
65. McDonald S, Langton Hewer CD, Nunez DA. Grommets (ventilation tubes) for recurrent acute otitis media in children. Cochrane Database Syst Rev 2008;(4):CD004741.
66. Lous J, Ryborg CT, Thomsen JL. A systematic review of the effect of tympanostomy tubes in children with recurrent acute otitis media. Int J Pediatr Otorhinolaryngol 2011;75(9):1058–61.
67. Rosenfeld RM, Bhaya MH, Bower CM, et al. Impact of tympanostomy tubes on child quality of life. Arch Otolaryngol Head Neck Surg 2000;126(5):585–92.
68. Witsell DL, Stewart MG, Monsell EM, et al. The Cooperative Outcomes Group for ENT: a multicenter prospective cohort study on the effectiveness of medical and surgical treatment for patients with chronic rhinosinusitis. Otolaryngol Head Neck Surg 2005;132(2):171–9.
69. Witsell DL, Stewart MG, Monsell EM, et al. The Cooperative Outcomes Group for ENT: a multicenter prospective cohort study on the outcomes of tympanostomy tubes for children with otitis media. Otolaryngol Head Neck Surg 2005;132(2): 180–8.
70. Pichichero ME. Acute otitis media: part I. Improving diagnostic accuracy. Am Fam Physician 2000;61(7):2051–6.

71. Kay DJ, Nelson M, Rosenfeld RM. Meta-analysis of tympanostomy tube sequelae. Otolaryngol Head Neck Surg 2001;124(4):374–80.
72. Hoffmann KK, Thompson GK, Burke BL, et al. Anesthetic complications of tympanostomy tube placement in children. Arch Otolaryngol Head Neck Surg 2002; 128(9):1040–3.
73. Shah RK, Welborn L, Ashktorab S, et al. Safety and outcomes of outpatient pediatric otolaryngology procedures at an ambulatory surgery center. Laryngoscope 2008;118(11):1937–40.
74. Dohar J. Microbiology of otorrhea in children with tympanostomy tubes: implications for therapy. Int J Pediatr Otorhinolaryngol 2003;67(12):1317–23.
75. Dohar J, Giles W, Roland P, et al. Topical ciprofloxacin/dexamethasone superior to oral amoxicillin/clavulanic acid in acute otitis media with otorrhea through tympanostomy tubes. Pediatrics 2006;118(3):e561–9.
76. Goldblatt EL, Dohar J, Nozza RJ, et al. Topical ofloxacin versus systemic amoxicillin/clavulanate in purulent otorrhea in children with tympanostomy tubes. Int J Pediatr Otorhinolaryngol 1998;46(1–2):91–101.
77. Heslop A, Lildholdt T, Gammelgaard N, et al. Topical ciprofloxacin is superior to topical saline and systemic antibiotics in the treatment of tympanostomy tube otorrhea in children: the results of a randomized clinical trial. Laryngoscope 2010; 120(12):2516–20.
78. Centers for Disease Control and Prevention. Invasive pneumococcal disease in young children before licensure of 13-valent pneumococcal conjugate vaccine - United States, 2007. MMWR Morb Mortal Wkly Rep 2010;59(9):253–7.
79. Committee on Infectious Diseases. Recommendations for prevention and control of influenza in children, 2013-2014. Pediatrics 2013;132:e1089–104.
80. Block SL, Heikkinen T, Toback SL, et al. The efficacy of live attenuated influenza vaccine against influenza-associated acute otitis media in children. Pediatr Infect Dis J 2011;30(3):203–7.
81. Heikkinen T, Ruuskanen O, Waris M, et al. Influenza vaccination in the prevention of acute otitis media in children. Am J Dis Child 1991;145(4):445–8.
82. Clements DA, Langdon L, Bland C, et al. Influenza A vaccine decreases the incidence of otitis media in 6- to 30-month-old children in day care. Arch Pediatr Adolesc Med 1995;149(10):1113–7.
83. Marchisio P, Cavagna R, Maspes B, et al. Efficacy of intranasal virosomal influenza vaccine in the prevention of recurrent acute otitis media in children. Clin Infect Dis 2002;35(2):168–74.
84. Duncan B, Ey J, Holberg CJ, et al. Exclusive breast-feeding for at least 4 months protects against otitis media. Pediatrics 1993;91(5):867–72.
85. Scariati PD, Grummer-Strawn LM, Fein SB. A longitudinal analysis of infant morbidity and the extent of breastfeeding in the United States. Pediatrics 1997;99(6):E5.
86. Jones LL, Hassanien A, Cook DG, et al. Parental smoking and the risk of middle ear disease in children: a systematic review and meta-analysis. Arch Pediatr Adolesc Med 2012;166(1):18–27.
87. Lubianca Neto JF, Hemb L, Silva DB. Systematic literature review of modifiable risk factors for recurrent acute otitis media in childhood. J Pediatr (Rio J) 2006; 82(2):87–96.
88. Jackson JM, Mourino AP. Pacifier use and otitis media in infants twelve months of age or younger. Pediatr Dent 1999;21(4):255–60.
89. Marchisio P, Consonni D, Baggi E, et al. Vitamin D supplementation reduces the risk of acute otitis media in otitis-prone children. Pediatr Infect Dis J 2013;32: 1055–60.

90. Elemraid MA, Mackenzie IJ, Fraser WD, et al. Nutritional factors in the pathogenesis of ear disease in children: a systematic review. Ann Trop Paediatr 2009; 29(2):85–99.
91. Cohen HA, Varsano I, Kahan E, et al. Effectiveness of an herbal preparation containing Echinacea, propolis, and vitamin C in preventing respiratory tract infections in children: a randomized, double-blind, placebo-controlled, multicenter study. Arch Pediatr Adolesc Med 2004;158(3):217–21.
92. Levi JR, Brody RM, McKee-Cole K, et al. Complementary and alternative medicine for pediatric otitis media. Int J Pediatr Otorhinolaryngol 2013;77(6):926–31.
93. Rautava S, Salminen S, Isolauri E. Specific probiotics in reducing the risk of acute infections in infancy–a randomised, double-blind, placebo-controlled study. Br J Nutr 2009;101(11):1722–6.
94. Hatakka K, Savilahti E, Ponka A, et al. Effect of long term consumption of probiotic milk on infections in children attending day care centres: double blind, randomised trial. BMJ 2001;322(7298):1327.
95. Hatakka K, Blomgren K, Pohjavuori S, et al. Treatment of acute otitis media with probiotics in otitis-prone children-a double-blind, placebo-controlled randomised study. Clin Nutr 2007;26(3):314–21.
96. Azarpazhooh A, Limeback H, Lawrence HP, et al. Xylitol for preventing acute otitis media in children up to 12 years of age. Cochrane Database Syst Rev 2011;(11):CD007095.
97. Sando I, Takahashi H. Otitis media in association with various congenital diseases. Preliminary study. Ann Otol Rhinol Laryngol Suppl 1990;148:13–6.
98. Lyford-Pike S, Hoover-Fong J, Tunkel DE. Otolaryngologic manifestations of skeletal dysplasias in children. Otolaryngol Clin North Am 2012;45(3):579–98, vii.
99. Shott SR, Joseph A, Heithaus D. Hearing loss in children with Down syndrome. Int J Pediatr Otorhinolaryngol 2001;61(3):199–205.
100. Rosen D. Management of obstructive sleep apnea associated with Down syndrome and other craniofacial dysmorphologies. Curr Opin Pulm Med 2011;17(6): 431–6.

Pediatric Tonsillectomy
An Evidence-Based Approach

Glenn Isaacson, MD[a],*

KEYWORDS

- Adenotonsillectomy • Complications • Pain management • Tonsillectomy
- Wound healing

KEY POINTS

- Tonsillectomy decreases the frequency of severe recurrent sore throats in children who meet the "Paradise criteria."
- Adenotonsillectomy improves symptoms of sleep disordered breathing in children with adenotonsillar hypertrophy.
- Polysomnography is a useful adjunct in selecting children for surgery, especially when the diagnosis is in doubt or risks of surgery are increased because of young age or comorbid conditions.
- Obese children with sleep disordered breathing may not be cured by surgery.
- Ibuprofen is safe after tonsillectomy and provides good pain relief with fewer side effects than narcotics.

INTRODUCTION

The tonsillectomy operation has changed in recent years. More children are operated on for sleep disordered breathing and fewer for recurrent pharyngitis. New instruments now permit less invasive surgery. Systematic reviews by the Cochrane Collaboration and others have helped to define best practices for preoperative assessment and postoperative care.

Approximate 100 million tonsillectomies have been performed worldwide in the century since the procedure was popularized. Pediatric tonsillectomy with or without adenoidectomy is an effective operation for obstructive sleep apnea and sleep

Funding: None.
Financial Disclosures: None.
Conflicts of Interest: None.
[a] Departments of Otolaryngology – Head & Neck Surgery and Pediatric, Temple University School of Medicine, 3400 North Broad Street, Philadelphia, PA 19140, USA
* Department of Otolaryngology – Head & Neck Surgery, Temple University School of Medicine, 1077 Rydal Road, Suite 201, Rydal, PA 19046.
E-mail address: glenn.isaacson@temple.edu

Abbreviations	
AAO-HSN	American Academy of Otolaryngology – Head and Neck Surgery Foundation
IL	Interleukin
PANDAS	Pediatric autoimmune neuropsychiatric disorders associated with streptococcal infections

disorder breathing. It can decrease the incidence of sore throat in children who have frequent throat infections and may be effective for children who suffer from peritonsillar cellulitis or abscess, pediatric autoimmune neuropsychiatric disorders associated with streptococcal infections (PANDAS), "chronic" tonsillitis, febrile seizures, halitosis, dental malocclusion, cryptic tonsils, or hemorrhagic tonsillitis. It has a role in the prevention of recurrences of rheumatic fever, and in controlling chronic pharyngeal carriage of group A beta-hemolytic streptococci. Yet despite a century of experience with this operation, tonsillectomy remains a traumatic experience for children and their families. In the best of hands, tonsillectomy has a 1% to 5% risk of immediate or delayed hemorrhage[1] and a 1:35,000 death rate.[2] The surgery produces separation anxiety, postoperative edema, dysphagia, weight loss, and night terrors. Nausea and vomiting remain common despite pharmacologic advances and everyone suffers from pain. Even when well-treated with opioid and nonopioid analgesics, most children still rate their pain as moderate to severe.

This article reviews current knowledge of the science of pediatric tonsillectomy—developmental anatomy of the tonsil, physiology of the operation, and wound healing after surgery. It outlines indications for surgery and best practices for intraoperative and postoperative care as described in the American Academy of Otolaryngology–Head and Neck Surgery Foundation (AAO-HSN) clinical practice guideline: Tonsillectomy in Children. Finally, it discusses areas of uncertainty in the field and opportunity for future improvement.

DEVELOPMENTAL ANATOMY

Developmental anatomy describes when the tonsil becomes immunologically active, how its structure changes, when it enlarges, and when it involutes. An appreciation of the fetal development of the tonsil and the changes it undergoes in the first decade of life can aid in surgical decision making (**Table 1**).

Intrauterine Development

The epithelium that covers the tonsil's medial surface and lines the tonsillar crypts arises from the second branchial (pharyngeal) pouch. The outer edges of this outpouching go on to form the faucial arches and mucosa plicae. In the embryo, solid epithelial cores form in the lateral walls of each pouch and grow outward into the surrounding mesenchymal tissue. These epithelial cores branch and subsequently canalize. The branches ultimately become the primary and secondary tonsillar crypts (**Fig. 1**A).[3] Transmission electron microscopy has demonstrated that the mature crypt epithelium is porous and allows the protrusion of lymphocytes that mediate the immune response.[4]

The mucosa of the tonsillar fossa is similar in microscopic structure to the lining of the oropharynx. Its surface is nonkeratinizing squamous epithelium with an underlying lamina propria. The pharyngeal tonsils are a part of the mucosa-associated lymphatic tissue system and develop their monocellular populations in a fashion much like the

Table 1
Fetal development of the tonsil and the changes it undergoes

Observation	Implications for Intracapsular Tonsillectomy
The tonsil epithelium arises before the lymphoid component. Lymphoid cells infiltrate the lamina propria then proliferate.	The crypt epithelium runs full thickness through the tonsil; thus, superficial treatment of the crypts is unlikely to be effective.
The tonsil is arranged in lymphoepithelial fronds. Lymphoid elements are arranged around a fibrovascular core in each frond. The fronds are surrounded by crypt epithelium.	Crypt epithelium and lymphoid elements are intimately associated and cannot be treated independently.
Germinal center activation occurs after birth when the immune system is exposed to stimulating antigens.	The tonsil is an immunologically active structure. It is insignificant in mass in most infants.
Rapid germinal center proliferation is the most conspicuous event of the first decade of tonsil development and accounts for most of tonsillar enlargement.	Surgery that leaves significant amounts of residual lymphoid tissue may lead to recurrent hyperplasia.
The tonsil has no core.	It is not possible to perform a tonsil "core" biopsy without contamination by epithelial elements. The concept of bacterial sequestration in the tonsil "core" is not valid.
The tonsil capsule is contiguous with the trabeculae and frond fibrovascular cores.	There is no natural surgical plane between the tonsil parenchyma and the capsule.
The tonsil capsule surrounds the tonsil except on the medial crypt surface.	Powered intracapsular tonsillectomy, proceeding outward from the crypt area, can remove all of the lymphoid and epithelial elements. The appearance of thick trabeculae signals the approach of the capsule. Marginal incisions around the crypt area are made in intracapsular tonsillectomy with bipolar electrosurgical scissors or plasma excision. Such incisions will encompass all tonsil epithelial elements.
The tonsil expands, rather than invades, surrounding structures as it grows.	Removal of the parenchyma of the tonsil allows collapse of expanded normal tissues, minimize wound surface area.
The tonsillar pillars and plicae do not contain bulky lymphoid elements or crypt epithelium.	The tonsil pillars and all plica mucosa can be preserved for healing without compromising surgical goals.
Involution of lymphoid elements is characteristic of the second decade of life.	More conservative tonsil resection (or avoidance of surgery) may be preferable in older children.
Prominent fibrosis of the capsule and trabeculae is typical of the third decade and beyond.	Techniques applicable to young children may work less well in the fibrotic tonsils of adults.

From Isaacson G, Parikh T. Developmental anatomy of the tonsil and its implications for intracapsular tonsillectomy. Int J Pediatr Otorhinolaryngol 2008;72(1):89–96; with permission.

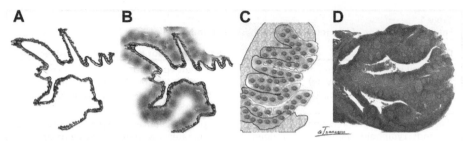

Fig. 1. Development of the tonsil (*A*) epithelial evagination, (*B*) lymphoid infiltration of the lamina propria, (*C*) primary germinal centers develop before birth, and (*D*) hyperplastic tonsil of childhood. (*From* Isaacson G, Parikh T. Developmental anatomy of the tonsil and its implications for intracapsular tonsillectomy. Int J Pediatr Otorhinolaryngol 2008;72(1):89–96; with permission.)

Peyer's patches in the gut.[5] Around the 16th week postconception, the lamina propria is invaded by wandering lymphocytes and lymphoid stem cells of bone marrow origin (see **Fig. 1**B).[6] The lymphatic tissue surrounding the crypts becomes organized into a cellular architecture resembling that of lymph nodes and includes B-cell follicles, primary germinal centers, and extrafollicular T-cell areas (see **Fig. 1**C).[7] Unlike lymph nodes, tonsils lack afferent lymphatics. Instead, the epithelium that lines the crypts contains dendritic cells that can transport exogenous antigens to extrafollicular T-cell areas and to B-cell follicles. The intimate relationship between the crypt epithelium and lymphoid component continues through life.

Immune stimulation begins shortly after birth in response to exogenous antigens. Terminal differentiation of effector B-cells to extrafollicular plasma cells can be seen first at approximately 2 weeks postnatally.[8] This results in the development of secondary follicles with active germinal centers. The proliferation of these germinal centers is the outstanding event of the first decade of life and accounts for the rapid growth of the tonsil in the young child (see **Fig. 1**D). This hyperplasia expands the tonsil at the expense of the surrounding soft tissues and the oropharyngeal space. The tonsils behave like other benign mass lesions, expanding rather than invading the surrounding tissues.

The tonsillar capsule arises from deep layers of the lamina propria. The deepest layers are pushed aside by the enlarging lymphoid component of the tonsil and condense to form a thin, compact membrane or capsule. The capsule surrounds the tonsil mass on all sides, except on its medal, cryptic surface. The more superficial fibers coalesce into trabeculae between the branching crypts. The tonsillar capsule is continuous with these trabeculae. Thus, there is no natural surgical plane between the tonsil's parenchyma and its capsule.

Unlike a lymph node, the tonsil is not a mass of lymphoid tissue with a central core and surrounding capsule. Rather, the tonsil parenchyma is a series of densely packed fingerlike fronds. Each frond is based on a fibrovascular core, surrounded by a layer of lymphoid tissue and covered by crypt epithelium. These fronds extend from the capsule to the medial cryptic surface (**Fig. 2**A). The crypt epithelium runs full thickness through the tonsil and lymphoid tissue and is present throughout the tonsil parenchyma.

In the second decade of life, the B-cell component of the tonsil begins to involute.[9] Germinal centers become smaller and there is a proliferation of fibrous tissue in the trabeculae and capsule. The tonsil decreases in mass and regresses, disappearing behind the anterior tonsillar pillar, much as it appeared at birth. By the seventh decade,

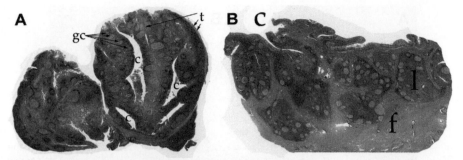

Fig. 2. (*A*) Hyperplastic tonsil of a 3 year old. C, tonsillar crypt; gc, germinal centers; t, trabeculae (stain: hematoxylin and eosin; original magnification: ×3). (*B*) Tonsil of a 67 year old at autopsy. C, crypt; f, fibrosis of capsule and trabeculae; l, lymphoid element (stain: hematoxylin and eosin; original magnification: ×1). (*From* Isaacson G, Parikh T. Developmental anatomy of the tonsil and its implications for intracapsular tonsillectomy. Int J Pediatr Otorhinolaryngol 2008;72(1):89–96; with permission.)

fibrous connective tissue surrounds the lymphoid fronds making the outline of the tonsil less distinct (see **Fig. 2**B). Fatty degeneration begins at about 25 years of age and progresses with age.[10]

TONSILLECTOMY HEALING

Most of the complications and all of the misery associated with pediatric tonsillectomy come from the injury of surgery and the inflammatory process of second intention healing resulting from an open pharyngeal wound. Although there is progressive improvement from the first day after surgery, pain does not resolve and the risk of bleeding remains until the tonsillar fossae are fully healed at about 2 weeks after surgery. There has been much research into the mechanism of cutaneous wound healing. Healing in the oral cavity is less well studied. Oral mucosal wounds proceed through the same healing stages as seen in the skin, including hemostasis, inflammation, proliferation, and remodeling of the collagen matrix. Oral mucosal healing is more rapid than skin repair and less likely to produce scar.

Several animal studies have focused on the effects of different cutting instruments (lasers,[11] ultrasound, electrosurgical devices, etc) on oral wound healing. Most show that cold steel incision produces the lowest level of collateral tissue damage and leads to the most rapid healing and ultimate tensile strength.[12] Ultrasound, bipolar and monopolar electrosurgery, and carbon dioxide laser (in that order) cause greater injury to surrounding tissues. Such injury results in delayed epithelialization.[13] In a dog tonsil model, microdebrider tonsillectomy resulted in less inflammation and more rapid healing than monopolar electrosurgery.[14]

Serial photography of the healing human tonsillar fossa suggests that mucosal injury and healing follows the pattern described in animal experiments (**Fig. 3**).[15] In human oral wounds, as in the porcine model, polymorphonuclear infiltrates appear quickly. Inflammation is greatest on days 3 through 7, resolving by day 14. Granulation tissue (stroma) forms in the pig cheek defect and is gradually covered by advancing epithelium, as demonstrated in serial human photographs.

Studies of pharyngeal wounding and healing help to explain posttonsillectomy complications, including edema, pain, and hemorrhage. Thermal spread to the tonsillar fossa prevents bleeding by thrombosing blood vessels, but also damages

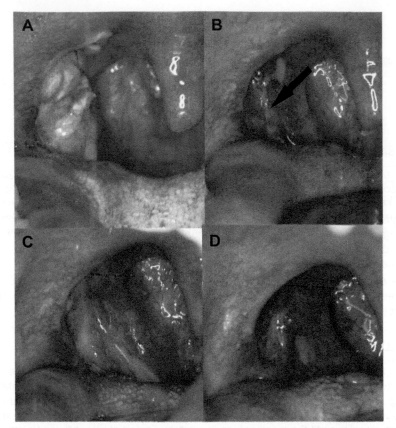

Fig. 3. Serial photographs of 1 patient after tonsillectomy. (*A*) Postoperative day (POD) 5. Exuberant fibrin clot fills the tonsillar fossa protruding beyond the tonsillar pillars. (*B*) POD 7. The fibrin clot has separated from the tonsillar fossa. New stroma lines the tonsillar fossa. Initial ingrowth of posterior pillar epithelium is discernible (*arrow*). (*C*) POD 9. The bridge of epithelium has widened, advancing laterally across the stomal bed. (*D*) POD 17. The tonsillar fossa is covered by a layer of epithelium. The initial epithelial bridge has thickened and resembles normal mucosa. (*From* Isaacson G. Tonsillectomy healing. Ann Otol Rhinol Laryngol 2012;121(10):645–9; with permission.)

lymphatics at the base of the uvula,[16] producing annoying edema and occasional airway obstruction.[17]

The same inflammatory mediators responsible for stimulating the monocellular influx that clears necrotic wound debris cause injury-associated pain. In a mouse incisional model, increasing postoperative pain was strongly correlated with neutrophil infiltration. Skin samples harvested from these mice show enhanced levels of 5 cytokines: interleukin (IL)-1β, IL-6, tumor necrosis factor alpha, granulocyte colony stimulating factor, and keratinocyte-derived cytokine.[18] After tonsillectomy, analog pain scores decrease linearly from postoperative days 1 through 10. This progression is often interrupted by a 'bump' in pain[19] on days 3 through 5, coincident with maximum inflammation and fibrin clot accumulation.[20]

Capillary development in the stoma is greatest at the end of the first postoperative week. This stomal development precedes epithelial ingrowth. With separation of the fibrin clot, capillaries in the vascular stoma are exposed and vulnerable to minor trauma and bleeding. Involution of the vascular stoma (presumably from decreasing levels of vascular endothelial growth factor and cellular apoptosis) coincides with the decreasing risk of secondary hemorrhage in the second week after surgery.[1]

CLINICAL DECISION MAKING
Indications

Tonsillectomy, when performed for the right reasons, can:

- Decrease upper airway resistance;
- Ameliorate or cure obstructive sleep apnea and sleep disordered breathing;
- Decrease the incidence of recurrent pharyngitis; and
- Improve child health status and quality of life.

Debate rages about what constitutes the "right reasons." For each child, the potential benefits of tonsillectomy (usually in combination with adenoidectomy) must be weighed against its substantial discomforts and occasional, but real risks.

Adenotonsillar hypertrophy is most pronounced between ages of 3 and 6 years. Tonsils involute in most children after age 8. This sequence accounts for the appearance and natural resolution of snoring and sleep disordered breathing in many children.[3]

Obstructive sleep apnea
There is little doubt that, for children with true obstructive sleep apnea secondary to adenotonsillar enlargement, the negative aspects of surgery are far outweighed by its benefits to health and function. As the severity of the sleep disorder breathing spectrum decreases, the risk–benefit balance shifts. Most pediatric otolaryngologists would not recommend an adenotonsillectomy for a well child troubled only by snoring. By the same token, the child with suspected sleep disordered breathing who also suffers from growth retardation, poor school performance, enuresis, or certain behavioral problems may derive greater benefit from surgery. When uncertainty exists, formal polysomnography can help to quantitate the severity of disease and correlate sleep disruption with symptoms.[21,22]

Recurrent severe sore throat
Similarly, one must weigh the pros and cons of tonsillectomy versus continued medical management for recurrent sore throats. It is clear that a child undergoing tonsillectomy for frequent severe sore throats will experience fewer sore throats in years to come. It is less clear that the tonsillectomy is the reason for the improvement. For most children, recurrent severe sore throats (characterized by temperature >38.3°C, cervical adenopathy, tonsillar exudate, or positive test for group A beta-hemolytic streptococci) resolve spontaneously within a few years. In a prospective, randomized trial of adenotonsillectomy for severe recurrent sore throats (7 episodes in a year, or 5 in 2 consecutive years, or 3 in 3 consecutive years—also known as "the Paradise criteria") children derived benefit from surgery for at least 2 years compared with nonoperative controls.[23] In a second, similar trial of moderately affected children (number of episodes, severity or documentation relaxed), surgery slightly decreased the frequency of sore throats compared with controls. The subsequent number of sore throats was so low in both arms as to mute the clinical impact of tonsillectomy.[24] There is likely a subgroup of children with recurrent sore throats who do not improve over time and who might receive greater benefit from surgery.[25] Unfortunately, there is no way to distinguish such patients in advance.

Other relative indications for tonsillectomy include:

- Peritonsillar cellulitis or abscess;
- PANDAS;
- "Chronic" tonsillitis;
- Febrile seizures;
- Halitosis;
- Dental malocclusion;
- Cryptic tonsils;
- Hemorrhagic tonsillitis;
- Prevention of recurrences of rheumatic fever; and
- Chronic pharyngeal carriage of group A beta-hemolytic streptococci.

The role of tonsillectomy in the management of these disorders has not undergone rigorous scientific study.[21]

PROCEDURE

It is likely many more tonsillectomies would be performed were it not such a morbid procedure. To reach the oropharynx and overcome strong protective reflexes requires deep general anesthesia in nearly all children. Such anesthetics often lead to transient postoperative disorientation, nausea, and vomiting.[26] Even in the best of hands, classic tonsillectomy is complicated by immediate (0.2%–2%) and delayed (1%–5%) hemorrhage. Incomplete ligation or coagulation of peritonsillar arteries or veins can lead to bleeding immediately after surgery. Delayed bleeding occurs during the inflammatory phase of healing, usually 7 to 10 days after surgery.[1,27] Bleeding can be controlled safely in most cases but usually requires a second, potentially more dangerous general anesthetic.[28] If bleeding is severe or the child is far from a medical facility, exsanguination may occur requiring transfusion or leading to death.[2] Other less common tonsillectomy sequelae include facial burns, airway fires, airway edema, postobstructive pulmonary edema, sepsis, disorders of taste, velopharyngeal insufficiency, and nasopharyngeal stenosis.[29]

Which Tonsillectomy to Do

Extracapsular tonsillectomy

Standard extracapsular tonsillectomy consists of the en bloc excision of the palatine tonsil and its enveloping capsule, usually including a portion of the anterior tonsillar pillar for exposure.[30,31] It removes the tonsil quickly and completely, leaving little chance of tonsillar regrowth or future peritonsillar abscess. Extracapsular tonsillectomy produces a relatively large oropharyngeal wound that exposes the superior and middle constrictor muscles, bridging tonsillar arteries, and the tonsillar venous plexus.[32] The glossopharyngeal nerve, peritonsillar fat, and tongue base muscles are nearby structures that are occasionally exposed during excision (**Fig. 4**A).[33] This complete extracapsular procedure has been the gold standard operation since the early 20th century, employed in all major studies of the effectiveness of tonsillectomy.

Surgeons and engineers have devised dozens of instruments to facilitate tonsil removal and subsequent hemostasis. Each has its champions and detractors. In general, surgical methods are divided into "cold" and "hot" techniques. In cold tonsillectomy, sharp instruments are used to incise the anterior tonsillar pillar and blunt ones separate the tonsillar capsule from the superior constrictor muscle. Bridging tonsillar vessels are interrupted and left to bleed. Thus, the extirpative phase must be done

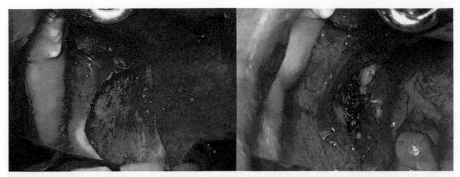

Fig. 4. Tonsillar fossa at completion of surgery. (*Left*) Extracapsular tonsillectomy. (*Right*) Intracapsular complete tonsillectomy. (*From* Isaacson G. Inside-out complete tonsillectomy: extended intracapsular tonsillectomy for severe sore throat. Ann Otol Rhinol Laryngol 2005;114(10):757–61; with permission.)

swiftly and hemostasis achieved separately. Bleeding is controlled with pressure from tonsil sponges, suture ligation of vessels, or chemical cautery.

Hot techniques use electrosurgical or thermal instruments for incision, excision, and control of bleeding. These include monopolar electrosurgical (Bovie, Clear Water, FL) tonsillectomy, bipolar electrosurgical scissors or forceps, and bipolar radiofrequency ionic dissociation (coblation). Various lasers, plasma knife, ultrasound, and molecular resonance technologies have all been tried. Each has advantages; none is consistently superior in terms of postoperative pain, wound healing, or post-tonsillectomy hemorrhage.[34,35] These instruments allow excision of the tonsils and simultaneous coagulation of bridging vessels, thus avoiding the intraoperative blood loss of cold techniques. These instruments seal blood vessel by heating and coagulating proteins in the vessel walls. They cause variable amounts of thermal damage to surrounding normal tissues in the process. The most effective coagulators tend to have the greatest thermal spread. Surgeons like these instruments despite their negative aspects because they permit rapid, controlled tonsil removal, usually without blood loss.

Intracapsular tonsillectomy and tonsillotomy

En bloc tonsillectomy is an oncologically sound way to remove tonsillar cancer. It may be a more radical operation than is required to relieve upper airway obstruction and prevent recurrent tonsillar infection. Tonsillectomy evolved in the 1910s when pediatric anesthesia was dangerous and hemostatic devices were limited. At that time, the masters of surgery denounced existing partial tonsillectomy techniques (tonsillotomy), claiming they led to unacceptable rates of immediate posttonsillectomy hemorrhage and persistent pharyngeal infection.[36] This dogma remains strongly ingrained in the collective memory of otolaryngologists despite advances in anesthesia and instrumentation that make controlled, graded tonsillar excision feasible.

Several investigators have explored less radical approaches to tonsil surgery.[37,38] In 2002, Peter Koltai and his colleagues[39] published a series of 150 "intracapsular" tonsillectomies in children with sleep disordered breathing. In this technique a microdebrider,[39] bipolar electrosurgical scissors,[40] or a coblation wand[41] are used to debulk most of the tonsil. The residual tonsil parenchyma is then electrodesiccated, preserving the surrounding normal tissue (see **Fig. 4**B). Prospective, randomized trials and case series with long-term follow-up now reinforce the notion that partial tonsillectomy techniques are less morbid than extracapsular tonsillectomy.[42] Moreover, there seems to be a correlation between the amount of tonsil left behind and the reduction of pain and posttonsillectomy hemorrhage. Surgeons who remove only the exophytic portion of the tonsil (tonsillotomy)[43] report slightly better results in terms of pain and bleeding than those who remove all (intracapsular complete tonsillectomy)[44] or most (intracapsular partial tonsillectomy)[39] of the tonsil. Multicenter series describe a low incidence of peritonsillar abscess or need for revision surgery with intracapsular techniques.[45,46] A few series have addressed the adequacy of intracapsular tonsillectomy for the control of recurrent sore throat. Although small in scale, these reports suggest that intracapsular surgery is not inferior.[47]

It is curious that the vast majority of tonsillectomies undertaken in the United States are still extracapsular given the growing body of evidence supporting less extensive surgery. A recent survey of pediatric otolaryngologists found that 73% always use extracapsular tonsillectomy for sleep disordered breathing and 97% choose it for control of recurrent sore throats.[48] Lingering concerns about the effectiveness of intracapsular tonsillectomy and fear of liability (for "inadequate" resection)[49] may drive this surgical inertia.

How to Prevent and Manage Posttonsillectomy Problems

Perioperative care

Perioperative tonsillectomy problems come from the disorders that necessitate surgery as well as the anesthetic and surgical procedures. Children with obstructive sleep apnea as an indication for surgery often exhibit continued upper airway obstruction and respiratory drive abnormalities for some time after surgery.[50] Although most tonsillectomy patients are treated in an ambulatory setting (same-day discharge or inpatient observation for <24 hours), some may require more protracted inpatient care and/or intensive care unit observation,[51] including:

- Children younger than age 3 years;
- Children with severe obstructive sleep apnea; and
- Children with comorbid conditions (obesity, sickle cell disease, coagulopathies, congenital heart disease, arrhythmias, craniofacial abnormalities).

Balanced anesthesia techniques that minimize postoperative respiratory suppression are favored in children with significant obstructive sleep apnea. Placement of a nasopharyngeal airway[17] and selective use of postoperative endotracheal intubation may decrease the risk of airway obstruction in the immediate postoperative period. The AAO-HNS guideline recommends a single dose of intraoperative dexamethasone to decrease postoperative nausea and vomiting. A systematic review from the Cochrane Collaboration showed that children receiving dexamethasone were less likely to vomit in the first 24 hours than children receiving placebo and more likely to advance to a soft or solid diet on postoperative day 1.[52] Selective serotonin 3 antagonists and other antiemetics are useful adjuvants.[53] Perioperative antibiotics are of little value in reducing pain or bleeding and have associated risks.[54] They are best reserved for treatment of infections rather than for prophylaxis.

For children over the age of 4 years without severe upper airway obstruction or comorbidities, observational studies suggest no increased risk of complications with outpatient tonsillectomy.[55] A minimum safe observational period after tonsillectomy has not been established,[56] nor are there generally accepted discharge criteria. Intravenous hydration with isotonic solutions[57] and administration of oral analgesics are recommended.[58] Need to tolerate oral intake before discharge is controversial. Cessation of operative bleeding, absence of upper airway obstruction, and control of pain and nausea should be documented.[59] In some series, stays as short as 1 to 2 hours were sufficient.[60]

Pain

Pain after tonsillectomy is universal, stereotypic in pattern, and variable from child to child. Most studies describe intense pain on the day of surgery, gradually decreasing over the first week but not disappearing until the end of the second week. Referred ear pain is common during this same period and is significantly greater after monopolar electrosurgical tonsillectomy.[61,62] Pain tends to be more intense in the morning. Anxiety, previous painful experience, and age affect the perception of pain.[63]

Remarkably little is known of the mechanism of posttonsillectomy pain. Stimulation of pain fibers by hypotonic solutions, stretch during chewing and swallowing, and release of inflammatory mediators are all potential culprits.[64] Several authors implicate spasm of pharyngeal muscles as a cause of pain, but this has never been proven.[65] Neural plasticity may play as important a role as gradual healing in the stepwise resolution of pain.[66]

Local anesthetics intraoperatively Intraoperative injection of local anesthetics has been advocated to decrease posttonsillectomy pain. A Cochrane review found no evidence that perioperative infiltration of local anesthetic in the tonsillar fossae improves postoperative pain control.[67]

Oral analgesics posttonsillectomy Oral analgesics form the cornerstone of posttonsillectomy pain control. Traditionally, acetaminophen with codeine has been the most widely used preparation. However, both its value and safety have been called into question in recent years. In a prospective, randomized trial, acetaminophen with codeine did not provide superior control of pain compared with acetaminophen alone.[19] This peculiar finding may be due in part to inconsistent metabolism of codeine to morphine—its activity metabolite, by the cytochrome P4502D6. Individuals may be slow, normal, rapid, or ultra-rapid metabolizers, depending on cytochrome P450 polymorphisms.[68] Slow metabolizers may derive little or no analgesic effect from codeine. Ultra-rapid metabolizers are at risk for toxicity with associated respiratory depression. Recently, the Food and Drug Administration issued a "boxed" warning against the used of codeine preparations after pediatric tonsillectomy.[69] Between 1% and 29% of all children may be ultra-rapid metabolizers, depending on ethnicity. Other oral narcotics may be susceptible to the same variable metabolism.[70] Further, postoperative nausea, vomiting, and constipation are increased with narcotic use. Unfortunately, acetaminophen alone may provide inadequate analgesia for many children.

Based on these observation and strong safety data, the AAO-HNS guideline now recommends the routine use of ibuprofen after tonsillectomy. A review from the Cochrane Collaboration with nearly 1000 children from 13 randomized, controlled trials found that nonsteroidal antiinflammatory drugs (other than ketorolac and aspirin) did not significantly alter postoperative bleeding compared with placebo or other analgesics.[71] Dosing schedules for oral analgesics remain controversial. In a recent study of acetaminophen with codeine, time-contingent (straight order) dosing resulted in administration of more medication and lower pain scores than as-needed dosing.[72]

Nonpharmacologic pain relief posttonsillectomy Good hydration and correction of dehydration are both associated with decreased pain.[73] Parents of younger children report holding the child on their lap as the most effective nonpharmacologic method of postoperative pain alleviation used at home.[74]

Bleeding

Posttonsillectomy hemorrhage is alarming to families, consumptive of health care resources, and occasionally lethal. Although most bleeding episodes can be handled with efficiency and safety, the sight of a child and parent arriving covered with blood is one that otolaryngologists struggle to avoid. Busy pediatric hospitals expend a significant part of their emergency resources caring for bleeding tonsillectomy patients.[75,76]

Coagulopathies Although children with significant coagulopathies are at increased risk for posttonsillectomy hemorrhage,[77] routine coagulation testing in children with no personal or family history of such a disorder is not cost effective.[78] Despite this recommendation, a recent survey found that 35% of general otolaryngologists and 10% of pediatric otolaryngologists still order a partial thromboplastin time and a prothrombin time before tonsillectomy.[79] Children with von Willebrand disease[80] and other treatable disorders of coagulation[81] benefit from perioperative hematologic consultation and intervention. Additional monitoring may be warranted in this population given the increased risk of early bleeding and of side effects from medication (eg, hyponatremia from desmopressin).[82]

Diet and activity Most otolaryngologists limit diet and activity after tonsillectomy, seeking to decrease the risk of posttonsillectomy hemorrhage. Prospective studies comparing restricted with unrestricted diet and activity fail to show a significant difference in bleeding incidence.[83] This does not mean these activities are risk free; most posttonsillectomy patients, freed from restriction, voluntarily avoid rough foods and vigorous activity.[84]

Emergency care Deaths associated with posttonsillectomy bleeding result from both exsanguination and anesthesia complications.[85] Surgery in older children and for acute peritonsillar abscess is more likely to lead to bleeding. Several studies identify electrosurgery as a risk factor for both bleeding and severe bleeding.[86] Thermal or mechanical injury to tongue base vessels can produce pseudoaneurysms that may bleed massively.[87]

There is considerable variation in the management of posttonsillectomy bleeding. Most major centers caring for small children advocate physical examination for any observed bleeding rather than reassurance over the telephone.[88] Minor bleeding rates may exceed 15%.[89] This imposes a burden on families, physicians, and hospitals. Still, parents may tend to overestimate or minimize bleeding severity, necessitating impartial evaluation.

On arrival in the emergency department, the child is assessed for hemodynamic stability and active bleeding. Most children are not actively bleeding on arrival.[90] Those with evidence of significant bleeding or a visible clot in the tonsillar fossa are usually treated surgically.[81] Those with no evidence of bleeding are observed. Patients with minor bleeding had a 41% rate of severe bleeding within 24 hours in 1 large, prospective series.[15]

Adults and some teenagers may tolerate cautery (chemical or electrosurgical) under local anesthesia.[91] Young children with significant bleeding require surgical management under general anesthesia.[92] Fluid resuscitation with isotonic solutions (or blood products in cases of severe anemia) should precede general anesthesia.[16] Rapid sequence induction with cricoid pressure is recommended given the risk of aspiration of swallowed blood.[93]

Once the airway is secured, the site of bleeding is identified and controlled, usually with monopolar electrocoagulation. Topical hemostatic agents can help with minor bleeding from granulation. Old blood should be evacuated from the stomach by warm saline lavage. Arterial bleeding from large vessels or ruptured pseudoaneurysms may require endovascular control[94] or, rarely, major vessel ligation.

SUMMARY

Things we know (or are pretty sure we know):
1. Tonsillectomy decreases the frequency of severe recurrent sore throats in children who meet the "Paradise criteria." It has little benefit in less severely affected children.
2. Tonsillectomy improves symptoms of sleep disordered breathing and adenotonsillar hypertrophy. It improves quality of life in appropriately selected children.
3. Polysomnography is a useful adjunct in selecting children for surgery, especially when the diagnosis is in doubt or risks of surgery are increased because of young age or comorbid conditions.
4. Obese children with sleep disordered breathing may not be cured by surgery. Repeat polysomnography and adjuvant measures (especially continuous positive airway pressure) may be needed.
5. Ibuprofen is safe after tonsillectomy and provides good pain relief with fewer side effects than narcotics.
6. Antibiotics are of little benefit in routine posttonsillectomy care and have associated risk.
7. A single dose of intraoperative dexamethasone decreases nausea and vomiting after tonsillectomy.

Things we believe (and may well be true):
1. Tonsillectomy is beneficial for children with severe recurrent sore throats who do not meet the "Paradise criteria" if they have certain other conditions (eg, multiple antibiotic allergy/intolerance, periodic fever, aphthous stomatitis, pharyngitis, and adenitis, or a history of peritonsillar abscess).
2. Adenotonsillar hypertrophy is most pronounced between ages of 3 and 6. Tonsils involute in most children after age 8, so snoring and sleep disordered breathing may resolve with time.
3. Children with suspected hematologic disorders should be assessed and, when appropriate, treated before surgery.
4. Compared with cold surgical techniques, hot techniques decrease operative time and immediate bleeding, but increase delayed hemorrhage rates and slow the healing process.
5. Intracapsular tonsillectomy is less painful and less frequently complicated by delayed hemorrhage than extracapsular tonsillectomy.
6. Children under the age of 3, those with severe obstructive sleep apnea, coagulopathy, or certain comorbid conditions (neuromuscular disorders, prematurity, obesity, failure to thrive, craniofacial anomalies) benefit from in-hospital observation.
7. Time-contingent (straight-order) pain medication has advantages in controlling posttonsillectomy pain during the first week after surgery.
8. Children should be cautioned to avoid sharp-edged foods, to avoid vigorous activity, and to remain near a hospital equipped to treat posttonsillectomy bleeding during the healing phase.
9. Good hydration and appropriate rehydration in volume-depleted children improves recovery.

10. Children who bleed after tonsillectomy should undergo physical examination and prompt surgical care if there has been significant bleeding or if they are at risk for further bleeding.

Things we do not know (and really should):
1. Whether some children with recurrent sore throats benefit more from tonsillectomy than the general population (ie, would continue to have severe symptoms for years without surgery).
2. Whether tonsillectomy is the best choice for poorly validated indications, for example, PANDAS, periodic fever, aphthous stomatitis, pharyngitis, and adenitis, halitosis, febrile seizures, and dental malocclusion.
3. Whether partial tonsillectomy is equivalent to total tonsillectomy for long-term control of sore throat and upper airway obstruction and if so, how much tonsil can be spared without compromising results.
4. What tonsillectomy instruments result in best healing, least pain, and fewest bleeding complications.
5. Whether some topical or injected agents can lessen pain after surgery.

REFERENCES

1. Sarny S, Ossimitz G, Habermann W, et al. Hemorrhage following tonsil surgery: a multicenter prospective study. Laryngoscope 2011;121(12):2553–60.
2. Stevenson AN, Myer CM 3rd, Shuler MD, et al. Complications and legal outcomes of tonsillectomy malpractice claims. Laryngoscope 2012;122(1): 71–4.
3. Isaacson G, Parikh T. Developmental anatomy of the tonsil and its implications for intracapsular tonsillectomy. Int J Pediatr Otorhinolaryngol 2008; 72(1):89–96.
4. Choi G, Suh YL, Lee HM, et al. Prenatal and postnatal changes of the human tonsillar crypt epithelium. Acta Otolaryngol Suppl 1996;523:28–33.
5. Boyaka PN, Wright PF, Marinaro M, et al. Human nasopharyngeal-associated lymphoreticular tissues. Functional analysis of subepithelial and intraepithelial B and Tcells from adenoids and tonsils. Am J Pathol 2000; 157:2023–35.
6. von Gaudecker B. Development and functional anatomy of the human tonsilla palatina. Acta Otolaryngol Suppl 1988;454:28–32.
7. Brandtzaeg P. Immunology of tonsils and adenoids: everything the ENT surgeon needs to know. Int J Pediatr Otorhinolaryngol 2003;67(Suppl 1):S69–76.
8. Wilson S, Norton P, Haverson K, et al. Development of the palatine tonsil in conventional and germ-free piglets. Dev Comp Immunol 2005;29:977–87.
9. Siegel G, Linse R, Macheleidt S. Factors of tonsillar involution: age-dependent changes in B-cell activation and Langerhans' cell density. Arch Otorhinolaryngol 1982;236(3):261–9.
10. Harada K. The histopathological study of human palatine tonsils——especially age changes. Nippon Jibiinkoka Gakkai Kaiho 1989;92(7):1049–64.
11. Carew JF, Ward RF, LaBruna A, et al. Effects of scalpel, electrocautery, and CO2 and KTP lasers on wound healing in rat tongues. Laryngoscope 1998;108(3): 373–80.
12. Sinha UK, Gallagher LA. Effects of steel scalpel, ultrasonic scalpel, CO2 laser, and monopolar and bipolar electrosurgery on wound healing in guinea pig oral mucosa. Laryngoscope 2003;113(2):228–36.

13. Liboon J, Funkhouser W, Terris DJ. A comparison of mucosal incisions made by scalpel, CO2 laser, electrocautery, and constant-voltage electrocautery. Otolaryngol Head Neck Surg 1997;116(3):379–85.
14. Johnson K, Vaughan A, Derkay C, et al. Microdebrider vs electrocautery: a comparison of tonsillar wound healing histopathology in a canine model. Otolaryngol Head Neck Surg 2008;138(4):486–91.
15. Isaacson G. Tonsillectomy healing. Ann Otol Rhinol Laryngol 2012;121(10):645–9.
16. Nasr VG, Bitar MA, Chehade JM, et al. Postoperative severe uvular edema following tonsillectomy in a child with a history of obstructive sleep apnea. Paediatr Anaesth 2008;18(7):673–5.
17. Isaacson G. Avoiding airway obstruction after pediatric adenotonsillectomy. Int J Pediatr Otorhinolaryngol 2009;73(6):803–6.
18. Clark JD, Shi X, Li X, et al. Morphine reduces local cytokine expression and neutrophil infiltration after incision. Mol Pain 2007;3:28.
19. Moir MS, Bair E, Shinnick P, et al. Acetaminophen versus acetaminophen with codeine after pediatric tonsillectomy. Laryngoscope 2000;110(11):1824–7.
20. Sutters KA, Isaacson G. Prevention and management of post-tonsillectomy pain in children. Am J Nurs 2014;114(2):36–42.
21. Roland PS, Rosenfeld RM, Brooks LJ, et al, American Academy of Otolaryngology—Head and Neck Surgery Foundation. Clinical practice guideline: polysomnography for sleep-disordered breathing prior to tonsillectomy in children. Otolaryngol Head Neck Surg 2011;145(Suppl 1):S1–15.
22. Aurora RN, Zak RS, Karippot A, et al, American Academy of Sleep Medicine. Practice parameters for the respiratory indications for polysomnography in children. Sleep 2011;34(3):379–88.
23. Paradise JL, Bluestone CD, Bachman RZ, et al. Efficacy of tonsillectomy for recurrent throat infection in severely affected children. Results of parallel randomized and nonrandomized clinical trials. N Engl J Med 1984;310(11):674–83.
24. Paradise JL, Bluestone CD, Colborn DK, et al. Tonsillectomy and adenotonsillectomy for recurrent throat infection in moderately affected children. Pediatrics 2002;110(1 Pt 1):7–15.
25. Burton MJ, Isaacson G, Rosenfeld RM. Extracts from The Cochrane Library: tonsillectomy for chronic/recurrent acute tonsillitis. Otolaryngol Head Neck Surg 2009;140(1):15–8.
26. Pieters BJ, Penn E, Nicklaus P, et al. Emergence delirium and postoperative pain in children undergoing adenotonsillectomy: a comparison of propofol vs sevoflurane anesthesia. Paediatr Anaesth 2010;20(10):944–50.
27. Blakley BW. Post-tonsillectomy bleeding: how much is too much? Otolaryngol Head Neck Surg 2009;140(3):288–90.
28. Fields RG, Gencorelli FJ, Litman RS. Anesthetic management of the pediatric bleeding tonsil. Paediatr Anaesth 2010;20(11):982–6.
29. Leong SC, Karkos PD, Papouliakos SM, et al. Unusual complications of tonsillectomy: a systematic review. Am J Otolaryngol 2007;28:419–22.
30. Thomson SC. Removal of the tonsils in disease of the nose and throat. London: Cassell & Co; 1912. p. 359–69.
31. Ballenger WL. Diseases of the nose, throat and ear. Philadelphia: Lea & Febiger, Co; 1911. p. 412–38.
32. Hollingshead WH. Anatomy for surgeons. 3rd edition. Philadelphia: Harper & Row; 1982. p. 397.
33. Gnepp DR, Souther J. Skeletal muscle in routine tonsillectomy specimens: a common finding. Hum Pathol 2000;31(7):813–6.

34. Pinder DK, Wilson H, Hilton MP. Dissection versus diathermy for tonsillectomy. Cochrane Database Syst Rev 2011;(3):CD002211.
35. Mink JW, Shaha SH, Brodsky L. Making sense out of the tonsillectomy literature. Int J Pediatr Otorhinolaryngol 2009;73(11):1499–506.
36. Sluder G. The method of tonsillectomy by means of the alveolar eminence of the mandible and guillotine. JAMA 1916;67:2005–7.
37. Krespi YP, Ling EH. Laser-assisted serial tonsillectomy. J Otolaryngol 1994;23: 325–7.
38. Linder A, Markstrom A, Hultcrantz E. Using the carbon dioxide laser for tonsillotomy in children. Int J Pediatr Otorhinolaryngol 1999;50:31–6.
39. Koltai PJ, Solares CA, Mascha EJ, et al. Intracapsular partial tonsillectomy for tonsillar hypertrophy in children. Laryngoscope 2002;112(8 Pt 2 Suppl 100):17–9.
40. Isaacson G. Pediatric intracapsular tonsillectomy with bipolar electrosurgical scissors. Ear Nose Throat J 2004;83(10):702, 704–6.
41. Friedman M, Wilson MN, Friedman J, et al. Intracapsular coblation tonsillectomy and adenoidectomy for the treatment of pediatric obstructive sleep apnea/hypopnea syndrome. Otolaryngol Head Neck Surg 2009;140(3):358–62.
42. Gallagher TQ, Wilcox L, McGuire E, et al. Analyzing factors associated with major complications after adenotonsillectomy in 4776 patients: comparing three tonsillectomy techniques. Otolaryngol Head Neck Surg 2010;142(6):886–92.
43. Ericsson E, Graf J, Hultcrantz E. Pediatric tonsillotomy with radiofrequency technique: long-term follow-up. Laryngoscope 2006;116(10):1851–7.
44. Isaacson G. Inside-out complete tonsillectomy: extended intracapsular tonsillectomy for severe sore throat. Ann Otol Rhinol Laryngol 2005;114(10):757–61.
45. Solares CA, Koempel JA, Hirose K, et al. Safety and efficacy of powered intracapsular tonsillectomy in children: a multi-center retrospective case series. Int J Pediatr Otorhinolaryngol 2005;69(1):21–6.
46. Doshi HK, Rosow DE, Ward RF, et al. Age-related tonsillar regrowth in children undergoing powered intracapsular tonsillectomy. Int J Pediatr Otorhinolaryngol 2011;75(11):1395–8.
47. Schmidt R, Herzog A, Cook S, et al. Powered intracapsular tonsillectomy in the management of recurrent tonsillitis. Otolaryngol Head Neck Surg 2007;137(2):338–40.
48. Walner DL, Parker NP, Miller RP. Past and present instrument use in pediatric adenotonsillectomy. Otolaryngol Head Neck Surg 2007;137(1):49–53.
49. Simonsen AR, Duncavage JA, Becker SS. A review of malpractice cases after tonsillectomy and adenoidectomy. Int J Pediatr Otorhinolaryngol 2010;74(9):977–9.
50. Fiorino EK, Brooks LJ. Obesity and respiratory diseases in childhood [review]. Clin Chest Med 2009;30(3):601–8, x.
51. Baugh RF, Archer SM, Mitchell RB, et al, American Academy of Otolaryngology-Head and Neck Surgery Foundation. Clinical practice guideline: tonsillectomy in children. Otolaryngol Head Neck Surg 2011;144(Suppl 1):S1–30.
52. Steward DL, Welge J, Myer C. Steroids for improving recovery following tonsillectomy in children. Cochrane Database Syst Rev 2003;(1):CD003997.
53. Islam MR, Haq MF, Islam MA, et al. Preoperative use of granisetron plus dexamethasone and granisetron alone in prevention of post operative nausea and vomiting in tonsillectomy. Mymensingh Med J 2011;20(3):386–90.
54. Dhiwakar M, Clement WA, Supriya M, et al. Antibiotics to reduce post-tonsillectomy morbidity. Cochrane Database Syst Rev 2010;(7):CD005607.
55. Bhattacharyya N. Ambulatory pediatric otolaryngologic procedures in the United States: characteristics and perioperative safety. Laryngoscope 2010; 120(4):821–5.

56. Brigger MT, Brietzke SE. Outpatient tonsillectomy in children: a systematic review. Otolaryngol Head Neck Surg 2006;135:1–7.
57. Choong K, Arora S, Cheng J, et al. Hypotonic versus isotonic maintenance fluids after surgery for children: a randomized controlled trial. Pediatrics 2011;128(5): 857–66.
58. Segerdahl M, Warrén-Stomberg M, Rawal N, et al. Children in day surgery: clinical practice and routines. The results from a nation-wide survey. Acta Anaesthesiol Scand 2008;52(6):821–8.
59. Kingdon B, Newman K. Determining patient discharge criteria in an outpatient surgery setting. AORN J 2006;83(4):898–904.
60. Jaryszak EM, Lander L, Patel AK, et al. Prolonged recovery after out-patient pediatric adenotonsillectomy. Int J Pediatr Otorhinolaryngol 2011;75(4):585–8.
61. Warnock FF, Lander J. Pain progression, intensity and outcomes following tonsillectomy. Pain 1998;75:37–45.
62. Lister MT, Cunningham MJ, Benjamin B, et al. Microdebrider tonsillotomy vs electrosurgical tonsillectomy: a randomized, double-blind, paired control study of postoperative pain. Arch Otolaryngol Head Neck Surg 2006;132(6):599–604.
63. Crandall M, Lammers C, Senders C, et al. Children's tonsillectomy experiences: influencing factors. J Child Health Care 2009;13(4):308–21.
64. Hanafiah Z, Potparic O, Fernandez T. Addressing pain in burn injury. Curr Anaesth Crit Care 2008;19(5–6):287–92.
65. Hanif J, Frosh A. Effect of chewing gum on recovery after tonsillectomy. Auris Nasus Larynx 1999;26(1):65–8.
66. Reichling DB, Levine JD. Critical role of nociceptor plasticity in chronic pain. Trends Neurosci 2009;32(12):611–8.
67. Hollis L, Burton MJ, Millar J. Perioperative local anaesthesia for reducing pain following tonsillectomy. Cochrane Database Syst Rev 1999;(4):CD001874.
68. Williams DG, Patel A, Howard RF. Pharmacogenetics of codeine metabolism in an urban population of children and its implications for analgesic reliability. Br J Anaesth 2002;89(6):839–45.
69. FDA Drug Safety Communication: codeine use in certain children after tonsillectomy and/or adenoidectomy may lead to rare, but life-threatening adverse events or death. Available at: http://www.fda.gov/Drugs/DrugSafety/ucm313631.htm. Accessed July 24, 2014.
70. Isaacson G. Further concerns regarding opioids after tonsillectomy in children. Otolaryngol Head Neck Surg 2013;148(5):892.
71. Cardwell ME, Siviter G, Smith AF. Non-steroidal anti-inflammatory drugs and perioperative bleeding in paediatric tonsillectomy. Cochrane Database Syst Rev 2005;(2):CD003591.
72. Sutters KA, Miaskowski C, Holdridge-Zeuner DW, et al. A randomized clinical trial of the efficacy of scheduled dosing of acetaminophen and hydrocodone for the management of postoperative pain in children after tonsillectomy. Clin J Pain 2010;26:95–103.
73. Klemetti S, Kinnunen I, Suominen T, et al. The effect of preoperative fasting on postoperative pain, nausea and vomiting in pediatric ambulatory tonsillectomy. Int J Pediatr Otorhinolaryngol 2009;73:263–73.
74. Kankkunen P, Vehvilainen-Julkunen K, Pietila AM, et al. Is the sufficiency of discharge instructions related to children's postoperative pain at home after day surgery? Scand J Caring Sci 2003;17:365–72.
75. Peterson J, Losek JD. Post-tonsillectomy hemorrhage and pediatric emergency care. Clin Pediatr (Phila) 2004;43(5):445–8.

76. Sun GH, Harmych BM, Dickson JM, et al. Characteristics of children diagnosed as having coagulopathies following posttonsillectomy bleeding. Arch Otolaryngol Head Neck Surg 2011;137(1):65–8.
77. Witmer CM, Elden L, Butler RB, et al. Incidence of bleeding complications in pediatric patients with type 1 von Willebrand disease undergoing adenotonsillar procedures. J Pediatr 2009;155(1):68–72.
78. Cooper JD, Smith KJ, Ritchey AK. A cost-effectiveness analysis of coagulation testing prior to tonsillectomy and adenoidectomy in children. Pediatr Blood Cancer 2010;55(6):1153–9.
79. Wieland A, Belden L, Cunningham M. Preoperative coagulation screening for adenotonsillectomy: a review and comparison of current physician practices. Otolaryngol Head Neck Surg 2009;140(4):542–7.
80. Rodriguez KD, Sun GH, Pike F, et al. Post-tonsillectomy bleeding in children with von Willebrand disease: a single-institution experience. Otolaryngol Head Neck Surg 2010;142(5):715–21.
81. Watts RG, Cook RP. Operative management and outcomes in children with congenital bleeding disorders: a retrospective review at a single haemophilia treatment centre. Haemophilia 2011. http://dx.doi.org/10.1111/j.1365-2516.2011.02667.x.
82. Dunn AL, Cox Gill J. Adenotonsillectomy in patients with desmopressin responsive mild bleeding disorders: a review of the literature. Haemophilia 2010;16(5):711–6.
83. Brodsky L, Radomski K, Gendler J. The effect of post-operative instructions on recovery after tonsillectomy and adenoidectomy. Int J Pediatr Otorhinolaryngol 1993;25(1–3):133–40.
84. Thomas PC, Moore P, Reilly JS. Child preferences for post-tonsillectomy diet. Int J Pediatr Otorhinolaryngol 1995;31(1):29–33.
85. Morris LG, Lieberman SM, Reitzen SD, et al. Characteristics and outcomes of malpractice claims after tonsillectomy. Otolaryngol Head Neck Surg 2008;138(3):315–20.
86. Tomkinson A, Harrison W, Owens D, et al. Risk factors for postoperative hemorrhage following tonsillectomy. Laryngoscope 2011;121(2):279–88.
87. Windfuhr JP, Sesterhenn AM, Schloendorff G, et al. Post-tonsillectomy pseudoaneurysm: an underestimated entity? J Laryngol Otol 2010;124(1):59–66.
88. Wintrak BJ, Woolley AL. Pharyngitis and adenotonsillar disease. In: Cummings CW, editor. Pediatric otolaryngology–head & neck surgery, vol. 5, 3rd edition. St Louis (MO): Mosby; 1998. p. 208–9.
89. Doshi J, Damadora M, Gregory S, et al. Post-tonsillectomy morbidity statistics: are they underestimated? J Laryngol Otol 2008;122(4):374–7.
90. Attner P, Haraldsson PO, Hemlin C, et al. A 4-year consecutive study of post-tonsillectomy haemorrhage. ORL J Otorhinolaryngol Relat Spec 2009;71(5):273–8.
91. Steketee KG, Reisdorff EJ. Emergency care for posttonsillectomy and postadenoidectomy hemorrhage. Am J Emerg Med 1995;13(5):518–23.
92. Liu JH, Anderson KE, Willging JP, et al. Posttonsillectomy hemorrhage: what is it and what should be recorded? Arch Otolaryngol Head Neck Surg 2001;127(10):1271–5.
93. Goldsmith AR, Rosenfeld RM. Tonsillectomy, adenoidectomy and UPPP. In: Bluestone CD, Rosenfeld RM, editors. Surgical atlas of pediatric otolaryngology. Hamilton (Ontario): BC Decker Inc; 2002. p. 395–6.
94. van Cruijsen N, Gravendeel J, Dikkers FG. Severe delayed posttonsillectomy haemorrhage due to a pseudoaneurysm of the lingual artery. Eur Arch Otorhinolaryngol 2008;265(1):115–7.

Oropharyngeal Dysphagia in Children

Mechanism, Source, and Management

Venkata S.P.B. Durvasula, MD, FRCS ENT[a], Ashley C. O'Neill, MS[b],
Gresham T. Richter, MD[a],*

KEYWORDS

- Oropharyngeal dysphagia • Dysphagia • Pediatric dysphagia
- Swallowing disorders • Microaspiration • Aspiration • Children • Pharyngeal

KEY POINTS

- Oropharyngeal dysphagia (OPD) is the presence of laryngeal penetration or aspiration of food contents, predominately liquid, during oral ingestion.
- The incidence of OPD in children is on the rise due to increasing life expectancy of premature infants and children with complex medical conditions.
- Identification and resolution of OPD in children is best determined by the presence or absence of symptoms, including wet respirations and coughing and choking during drinking.
- An initial clinical evaluation of feeding and swallowing is instrumental in assessment of OPD in children whereas video fluoroscopic swallow studies (VFSSs) and fibreoptic endoscopic evaluations of swallowing (FEES) remain the best tools for confirming aspiration in infants and children.
- Persistent OPD in neurologically normal children demands careful evaluation for potential etiologies and is best managed by a dedicated multidisciplinary team.

INTRODUCTION

Swallowing disorders can be identified at all ages. Coughing, choking, and wet respirations with feeding are all evidence of feeding problems in newborns and children. When left undiscovered or untreated, recurrent cough, bronchiectasis, reactive airway disease, and pneumonias may ensue. The cycle of symptoms and sickness is

Disclosures: Nil.
Funding Sources: Nil.
[a] Department of Pediatric Otolaryngology and Head and Neck surgery, Arkansas Children's Hospital, 1 Children's Way, Slot #836, Little Rock, AR 72202, USA; [b] Department of Audiology and Speech Pathology, Arkansas Children's Hospital, 1 Children's Way, Slot #113, Little Rock, AR 72202, USA
* Corresponding author.
E-mail address: GTRichter@uams.edu

frequently stressful to patients and their caretakers who simply want their child to eat normally. The duration of dysphagia and difficulty in identifying the source compounds this anxiety. Unfortunately, epidemiologic data and sound diagnostic and treatment protocols for dysphagia are not well established.

Swallowing disorders in infants and children are common, with 25% of the pediatric population reported to experience some type of nonspecific feeding difficulty.[1] OPD is the most commonly encountered feeding disorder and refers to the dysfunction of the oral and pharyngeal phase of swallowing that results in laryngeal penetration and aspiration of solid or liquid food. As expected, higher rates of OPD are discovered in children with prematurity, upper aerodigestive tract anomalies, central nervous system (CNS) malformations, neurodevelopmental delays, and craniofacial syndromes. OPD is rarely an isolated event, however, and occurs in both developmentally delayed and normal children.

Recent advances in neonatal medicine have improved the survival of premature infants (<37 weeks' gestation) and those with complex medical conditions, thereby increasing the number of children in the community with residual difficulties with feeding and OPD.[2,3] The correlation between prematurity, complex medical conditions and feeding disorders in children is well established.[4,5] Pediatricians and otolaryngologists now see a greater number of children with persistent OPD. This includes developmentally normal and neurologically intact children who, as demonstrated by Sheikh and colleagues,[6] can present with chronic aspiration. The impact of OPD on the health of developmentally normal children emphasizes the importance of an extensive work-up and effective algorithm for treatment. Subtle inflammatory and anatomic problems are frequently present in otherwise healthy children with OPD.

Delayed reflexes, hypotonia, and generalized discoordination complicate the control of normal swallowing function in neurologically or developmentally affected children. Alternative feeding options or modified diets help maintain nutrition in this population pending improvement in function and strength. Gastrostomy tubes are frequently necessary to achieve fluid and nutritional goals. Depending on the underlying neurologic condition, dysphagia may take many years to improve and may never reach a normal state. Nonetheless, inflammatory and anatomic conditions, such as reflux, generalized respiratory illness, and upper aerodigestive anatomic anomalies, need to be assessed for in neurologically affected children because they may exacerbate their OPD.

The psychological impact of OPD on the family complicates early intervention because significant dysfunctional interactions between mothers and their infants with feeding disorders have been found.[7,8] The chronic nature of OPD with associated complications and the strain on the child and the family requires a dedicated team that caters to the medical, social, and dietary needs of these patients. Such a multidisciplinary team should consist of, with varying degrees of involvement, a pediatric otolaryngologist, pulmonologist, gastroenterologist, pediatric surgeon, speech and language pathologist (SLP), radiologist, nutritionist, occupational therapist, psychologist, and social worker. The objective of this clinical review is to provide pediatricians and otolaryngologists a global understanding of the potential causes of dysphagia and to provide an algorithm for diagnosing and treating infants and children with complicated or persistent OPD.

MECHANISM OF NORMAL AND DYSFUNCTIONAL SWALLOWING

Normal swallowing is a complex process that involves both voluntary and involuntary mechanisms. It includes 4 phases: oral preparatory, oral transit, pharyngeal, and esophageal. The oral preparatory phase involves grinding or chewing the food and mixing with saliva, creating a food bolus of appropriate size and consistency. The food bolus is voluntarily pushed backwards into the oropharynx. The backward movement to the oropharynx triggers the reflex pharyngeal phase.

The pharyngeal phase of swallowing is reflex mediated by the stimulation of the afferent receptors along the anterior tonsillar pillars, base of tongue, and epiglottis. The resultant efferent motor muscular activity is mediated by the glossopharyngeal (cranial nerve [CN] IX) and vagus (CN X) nerves. This muscular activity is a complex and coordinated contraction involving a series of muscle groups to ensure quick bolus passage across the relaxed cricopharyngeal or upper esophageal sphincter (UES) while simultaneously protecting the airway. The bolus is directed posteriorly by the voluntary propulsion of the tongue and then by the sequential reflex contractions of pharyngeal constrictors. The soft palate moves against the posterior pharyngeal wall to close the nasopharyngeal port. At the same time, the hyoid is advanced anteriorly by contraction of the strap muscles while pulling the larynx anteriorly and superiorly. In the process, the epiglottis is retroflexed to cover the laryngeal introitus.

During the pharyngeal phase, various measures protect the airway to prevent aspiration. The pharyngoglottal closure reflex is initiated by the sensory and chemoreceptors in the pharynx and larynx and is mediated by the CN IX and CN X nerves. When stimulated, adduction of true vocal cords and approximation of arytenoid cartilages occurs by contraction of the thyroarytenoid and interarytenoid muscles, thereby closing the laryngeal inlet.[9,10]

The swallow center of the CNS is located in the medulla along the nucleus tractus solitarius and the nuclei of the reticular system of the fourth ventricle. The supranuclear connections are relayed from the swallow center via the hypothalamus to the cerebral cortex. The swallow center is the area for coordination of the afferent and efferent activity in swallowing and transmits inhibitory impulses to the adjacent respiratory center, located in the medulla, thus inhibiting respiration during swallowing. The afferent oropharyngeal, pharyngeal, and laryngeal receptors relay information via afferent nerves in CN IX and CN X and the efferent arm is relayed via the same nerves from nuclei located in the nucleus ambiguus (**Fig. 1**).

The laryngeal adductor reflex (LAR) is the second protective reflex that is more specific to the supraglottic portion of larynx. It is mediated by the internal sensory division of the superior laryngeal nerve (CN X) supplying the mucosal surface of the epiglottis, aryepiglottic folds, and posterior larynx above the vocal cords. The LAR coordinates the sensory input from these areas and relays them to the medulla. The efferent return through the recurrent laryngeal nerve (CN X) causes contraction of the thyroarytenoid and interarytenoid muscles, which results in reflex closure and protection of the airway.

The significance of normal laryngopharyngeal sensation is demonstrated by recent studies using FEES with sensory testing. Evidence suggests that laryngopharyngeal sensation is reduced or inhibiting in pediatric and adult patients with OPD.[11]

The stimulation of the swallow center in the medulla inhibits the adjacent respiratory center that results in a temporary cessation of respiration, which accompanies the laryngeal upward movement, the closure of epiglottis, and the reflex closure of the larynx during the process of deglutition. The temporal coordination of breathing and pharyngeal phase of swallow is critical. Unfortunately this process can be severely disrupted in children with neurologic conditions[12] and chronic lung disease associated with prematurity,[13] thus increasing the risk of aspiration in these groups.

The movement of the food bolus below the pharynx occurs with opening of the UES, primarily by reflex relaxation of the cricopharyngeus muscle, and aided by the upward

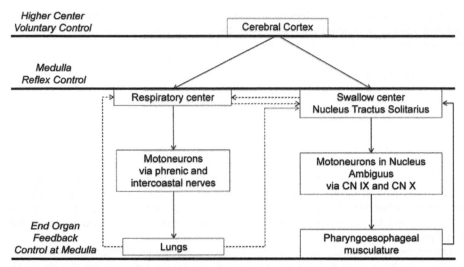

Fig. 1. The neural regulation of swallow. Cerebral cortex is involved in voluntary control of both respiratory and swallows centers located in the medulla. Dotted lines indicate inhibitory influence and continuous lines indicate stimulatory effect. Inflation of lungs inhibits both centers. Stimulation of pharyngoesophageal musculature stimulates deglutition. Both medullary centers have inhibitory influence on one another.

and anterior movement of larynx. This is followed by the esophageal phase of swallowing, which is reflex mediated under the influence of the autonomic nervous system of cervical and thoracic ganglia.

Age-Related Differences—Maturation of Swallow with Age

All the phases of swallowing are demonstrable in children, adolescents, and adults. There are some inherent differences, however, in swallowing between neonates, infants and adolescents. The oral phase in neonates and infants is a primitive sucking reflex. The buccal pads are prominent to aid sucking; the tongue protrudes whereas the perioral muscles, including the lips, cheeks, tongue, and palate act rhythmically and synergistically like a single organ to compress the nipple and express its contents. In the first 3 months, infants fail to differentiate consistency between solids and liquids and use the same suck reflex for both. Furthermore, the pharyngeal phase in infants lasts longer than in adults.[14] In spite of the longer duration of the pharyngeal phase in infants, no aspiration is noticed in a majority, possibly due to a more efficient laryngeal closure owing to the softer cartilaginous framework.[15,16]

The coordination between breathing and swallowing, as described previously in adults, translates into a coordinated suck-swallow-breathe sequence in infants, so that they can suck efficiently and swallow rapidly with minimal interruption in airflow. Poor coordination of this sequence is associated with prematurity[17] and patients with cerebral palsy (CP).[12] Upper airway obstruction in neonates and infants may interrupt this sequence mainly by breathlessness and prolonged sucking when infants are unable to generate a sufficient suction pressure in the presence of obstruction. This subtle discoordination between eating and breathing contributes to OPD in infants with upper airway obstruction.[18]

As an infant matures, the jaw grows and the buccal pads are absorbed to increase the intraoral space. The protrusion of tongue, which is an important component of suckling, is gradually lost by 6 months and replaced by raising and lowering of the tongue. This is coupled with increasing use of tongue intrinsic musculature, which is responsible for the development of propulsive action.[19] At this stage, the infants may be fed with solids as their voluntary swallow function starts to mature beyond the primitive suckling. The rhythmic biting in response to stimulation of the alveolar ridge gradually develops into mastication with the development of deciduous teeth. This stage represents a maturation of swallowing that may continue to 24 months of age.[20] These changes represent a continuum of development in response to stimulation in the form of changing oral feeding habits. Lack of development is often noticed in infants on gastrostomy feeds who develop oral aversion and OPD if oral stimulation is not attempted.[21]

ETIOLOGY OF OROPHARYNGEAL DYSPHAGIA

Efficient and effective swallowing relies on 2 important steps. The voluntary oral skills that involve preparation of the food bolus and the reflex patterned motor actions of swallowing. This combination results in the coordinated action and inhibition of the muscle groups located around the oropharynx and esophagus responsible for the passage of food into the stomach. As discussed previously, voluntary oral skills are not present until 6 months of age and may be a primary source of dysfunction in this age group. This is especially true if neonatal hospitalization and chronic illness prevents normal oral intake and stimulation at this key developmental age.

Frequently, OPD is multifactorial (**Box 1**). Developmental and neurologic delays can result in discoordination of swallow and contribute to OPD. Inflammatory, obstructive, and anatomic conditions may also be involved and are more frequently seen in developmentally normal individuals. Contributing factors may be grossly apparent at presentation or only through meticulous investigation. For example, prematurity and laryngomalacia can both independently contribute to OPD but premature patients have more prolonged symptoms than seen in those with laryngomalacia alone.[22] Contributing factors in children with OPD are outlined.

Prematurity

A functionally appropriate feeding pattern in neonates and young infants involves a coordinated suck-swallow-breathing rhythm so that an infant can suck efficiently and swallow rapidly with minimal airflow interruption. Due to neurologic immaturity, prematurity less than 34 weeks may be associated with poor coordination of this rhythm. Prematurity contributes to a delay in the pharyngeal phase of swallowing as demonstrated on high-resolution manometry studies of neurologically normal preterm infants at 31 to 32 weeks. Poor pharyngeal pressures coupled with poor coordination of pharyngeal propulsion and UES relaxation were found compared with term infants.[23] Weaker pharyngeal pressures were presumably related to neurologic immaturity in the premature infants.

Premature infants also have a weak suck reflex.[24] A sucking pattern consists of suckling bursts. An immature pattern may include a short burst of 4 to 6 sucks at 1 to 1.5 sucks/s and a mature pattern may consist of approximately 30 sucks at 2 sucks/s.[25] The number of sucking bursts gradually increases by term gestation.[26] These suckling bursts should be coordinated with breathing and swallowing. A poorly coordinated suck-swallow-breathe sequence is found in infants born before 34 weeks of gestation due to lack of myelination in the medulla.[27] A mature sucking pattern is characterized by prolonged suckling bursts of more than 10 sucks with suck-swallow-breathe in equal proportions with a ratio of 1:1:1. A delay in maturation of the swallow and sucking reflex is reported in patients born very early when sucking

Box 1
Common contributors to oropharyngeal dysphagia in infants and children

Neuromuscular
- Cerebral palsy (CP)
- Head trauma
- Mild developmental delays
- Hypoxic injury
- Arnold-Chiari malformations
- Muscular dystrophy
- Prematurity

Larynx and trachea-bronchial tree
- Vocal cord paralysis
- Glottic/subglottic stenosis
- Laryngeal cleft
- Tracheoesophageal fistula

Anatomic

Nasal and nasopharyngeal
- CHARGE[a] syndrome
- Narrow piriform aperture

Oral cavity and oropharynx
- Cleft lip and cleft palate
- Ranula, etc.
- Lymphatic malformations
- Down syndrome
- Beckwith-Wiedemann syndrome

Craniofacial syndromes
- Crouzon syndrome
- Treacher Collins syndrome
- Goldenhar syndrome
- Pierre Robin syndrome

Hypopharnyx/supraglottis
- Congenital cysts
- Laryngomalacia

Neoplastic
Benign
- Vascular malformations of aerodigestive tract
- Leiomyoma
Malignant
- Lymphoma
- Rhabdomyosarcoma

Esophagus
- Esophageal atresia
- Vascular rings/anomalies
- Achalasia

Physiologic
- Gastroesophageal reflux disease (GERD)/ Laryngopharyngeal reflux (LPR)
- Eosinophilic esophagitis (EoE)
- Sinonasal secretions

Postsurgical
- Strictures of esophagus
- Nerve injury
- Tracheostomy
- Laryngotracheal reconstruction

Acquired
- Foreign body
- Chemical injury—ingestion of alkali, acid, corrosive, etc
- Medication induced
- Adenotonsillar hypertrophy

Behavioral
- Poor conditioning
- Oral aversion
- Globus
- Solid food dysphagia

[a] CHARGE stands for coloboma of the eye, heart defects, atresia of the nasal choanae, retardation of growth and/or development, genital abnormalities, and ear abnormalities.

patterns were analyzed at a corrected age of 40 weeks. Extremely preterm infants born at 24 to 29 weeks' gestation generate significantly fewer bursts and sucks per burst than more mature preterm infants (30–32 weeks) and those born at term.[28] This causes preterm infants to have a tendency to aspirate easily and fatigue quickly. This can make breastfeeding difficult and accounts for more desaturations in preterm infants when feeding.[24]

Preterm infants are also more likely to suffer anoxia or hypoxia at birth. This can result in permanent, but sometimes subtle, neurologic damage, including dysfunctional feeding patterns. A higher incidence of CP is found in preterm infants with lower gestational age (24–26 weeks) compared with those born later.[29] These patients primarily suffer with poor and noncoordinated oral skills required for sucking. They also exhibit poor head control, uncoordinated tongue movements, impaired palatal function, poor gag reflex, and laryngopharyngeal hyposensitivity; all of which increase the risk of OPD and aspiration. Subtle and radiographically undetectable hypoxic injury to the swallowing and respiratory centers in premature infants may help explain the increased incidence of OPD in these children.

Intubation as a newborn can also contribute to OPD in this population. The presence of an endotracheal tube and the resultant remodeling of the soft palate can lead to palatopharyngeal incompetence, nasal reflux, or a defective integration of the suck-swallow mechanism.[30] On the other hand, the presence of a tracheostomy tube in a newborn can prevent the normal rise of subglottic pressure and laryngeal elevation necessary for an effective pharyngeal phase of swallowing.

Neurologic Disorders

The manifestation, course, and possible resolution of OPD in neurologically affected children are determined by the nature, site, and evolution of the CNS defect. The prognosis for recovery also is influenced strongly by whether the underlying neurologic condition is static or progressive. Static neurologic conditions include CP, cerebrovascular accident, Arnold-Chiari malformation, syringomyelia, congenital viral infections with varicella, cytomegalovirus, tumors, and injuries to the brainstem. Progressive neurologic disorders are not limited to but include myopathies, neuropathies, and metabolic disorders like mucopolysaccharidosis. Children with static neurologic diagnoses generally improve in their OPD with developmental progress. Children with progressive neurologic conditions demonstrate early improvement but eventually lose these skills.

The most common neurologic condition encountered in children with OPD is CP. CP affects volitional oral movements and the involuntary reflexes (LARs) and compromises the neurologically dependent reflexive pharyngeal swallow. The situation is worsened by poor coordination of the suck-swallow-breathe sequence as infants.[12] CP patients frequently have a weak gag reflex and are prone to silent aspiration.[31] Volitional movements are affected when there is cortical injury or periventricular leukomalacia whereas reflex inhibition suggests subcortical injury involving brainstem and basal ganglia. Although it is hard to predict the incidence of OPD in CP patients, 85% to 90% of patients with CP are affected by dysphagia.[2] Chronic aspiration may be further complicated by the presence of gastroesophageal reflux disease (GERD) and drooling, which are present in more than 50% of cases.[32,33] Drooling is secondary to impaired volitional movements whereas posterior salivation causes recurrent aspiration and subsequent pulmonary infections.[34]

Other common static conditions include Arnold-Chiari and central arteriovenous malformations, which may be present with only subtle clinical evidence of OPD. A high index of suspicion for OPD is necessary in these patients. Greenlee and colleagues[35] reported that children with a Chiari malformation type 1 (CM-I) were most likely to present with OPD under 3 years of age. After evaluating the signs and symptoms of CM-I in children younger than 6 years of age, Albert and colleagues[36] also determined that 77.8% presented with OPD between 0 and 2 years of age. Indirect neurologic signs, such as a hoarse cry, delayed milestones, unsteady gait, and worsening OPD on VFSS, also may be present and should prompt an early brain MR imaging or neurology consult. This approach has been recommended in neurologically intact children with worsening or persistent OPD after 2 years of age. In a child with new onset of OPD, CNS neoplasms should also be ruled out using MR imaging.

O'Neill and colleagues[37] demonstrated that more than 50% of children with Down syndrome had evidence of persistent OPD. The mean age at diagnosis of OPD was 1.6 years. Resolution rates of OPD were also poor (15%) in this population, especially in patients with significant neurologic delay and prior tracheostomies. They suspected that inherent hypotonia and poor pharyngeal reflexes in the Down syndrome children contributed to the swallowing results found in their study. Moreover, procedures aimed at reducing upper airway obstruction had no effect on the resolution rates of OPD in their study.

Anatomic Contributors to OPD

Poor coordination of the suck-swallow-breath sequence may be observed in infants with upper airway obstruction. Similarly, in older infants and children, upper airway obstruction complicates swallowing by limiting normal respiration; this is particularly true in patients when OPD is multifactorial. Conditions associated with airway obstruction may contribute to OPD and include both congenital and acquired entities (**Box 2**).

Nasal or nasopharyngeal obstruction in an infant can complicate coordination of the suck-swallow-breathing rhythm. This is because neonates up to 3 months of age are obligate nasal breathers. Bilateral choanal atresia often causes respiration difficulty and swallowing dysfunction. Choanal stenosis patients typically fatigue and take short breaks during feeding, making coordination difficult. In older infants and children, nasal obstruction may be a result of allergic rhinitis, turbinate hypertrophy, adenoid hypertrophy, sinusitis, pyriform aperture stenosis, or nasopharyngeal or nasal congenital masses, such as glioma, meningocele, and nasal dermoid. It is important to document an appropriate patency of the nasopharyngeal airway in the evaluation of OPD. This is

---

Box 2
Anatomic correlates contributing to OPD in infants and children

Infants	*Older children*
• Laryngomalacia	• Sinusitis
• Laryngeal cleft	• Allergic rhinitis
• Tracheoesophageal fistula	• Adenoidal hypertrophy
• Esophageal atresia	• Adenotonsillar hypertrophy
• Vascular rings	• Narrow piriform aperture
• Vocal cord paralysis	• Cricopharyngeal achalasia
• Bilateral choanal atresia	
• Gliomas/meneingocele	
• Cleft palate/cleft lip	
• Congenital cysts	

particularly relevant in late infancy and the early second year of life when adenoid hypertrophy is a primary source of obstruction. Anecdotal evidence suggests that chronic rhinitis and nasal obstruction affect VFSS results and complicate weaning off a modified diet in young children with OPD.

Development of normal oral and oropharyngeal anatomy is important for natural suckling in neonates and the preparatory phases of swallowing in children. Craniofacial dysmorphisms and cleft lip or cleft palate have an impact on normal oral intake. Some children, as seen in Beckwith-Wiedemann syndrome, have a disproportionately large tongue that interferes with early oral preparation and oropharyngeal function.

Laryngeal elevation propels the food bolus whereas protective reflexes in the hypopharynx and larynx aid in the coordination of breathing and swallowing and at the same time offer laryngeal protection. Anatomic abnormalities of the hyphopharynx and larynx can result in OPD. These include vocal fold paralysis, vallecular cysts, laryngotracheal clefts, glottic webs, laryngomalacia, and subglottic stenosis. Laryngotracheal reconstruction, with alteration of normal laryngeal anatomy, can contribute to temporary or long-term OPD.[38] Vocal fold paralysis with the loss of recurrent laryngeal nerve function increases the chance of aspiration owing to reduced vocal fold adduction, an open posterior glottis, and potentially the loss of sensation associated with superior laryngeal nerve weakness. Airway obstruction due to webs or subglottic stenosis with difficulties in ventilation cause early fatigue of respiration and swallowing, leading to OPD. Deep laryngeal clefts (Benjamin-Inglis types 2–4) allow for passage of food contents directly into the larynx below the level of the vocal folds. The diagnosis and management of the less obvious type 1 laryngeal clefts can be challenging with late diagnosis and persistent OPD. These laryngoesophageal defects may often be associated with esophageal dysmotility and complicated by GERD.

Laryngomalacia is the most common cause of stridor in newborns and infants due to redundancy and/or weakness of the supraglottic larynx. Airway symptoms are secondary to dynamic inspiratory collapse of the supraglottic structures and redundant mucosa. Laryngomalacia is associated with OPD in more than 50% of patients.[22] Airway obstruction may interfere with the suck-swallow-breathing rhythm pattern and increases dysphagia and GERD, which in turn can reduce laryngeal sensation and exacerbate laryngeal edema. Management of GERD can improve the respiratory pattern and dysphagia and result in improved weight gain in these patients.[39] Laryngomalacia is associated with reduced laryngeal sensitivity, which enhances the risk of silent aspiration.[40] Increased diameter and surface area of the nerve endings have been reported in supra-arytenoid specimens harvested from laryngomalacia patients that may represent an autocrine enhancement of dysfunctional nervous system due to laryngomalacia.[41]

Cervical and distal esophageal anatomic anomalies may also contribute to persistent OPD, including esophageal atresia, tracheoesophageal fistula (TEF), and cricopharyngeal achalasia.

Dysphagia can be a persistent issue after repair of both esophageal atresia and TEF owing to disrupted upper esophageal neuromuscular control and chronic GERD. Patients may be on a modified diet (liquid thickeners) for many years after the repair. It is important to rule out an associated laryngeal cleft because this may also be present in a significant number of patients with distal esophageal anatomic anomalies.

The cricopharyngeus muscle is a striated muscle that is contracted at rest, thus keeping the esophagus closed during respiration. Cricopharyngeal achalasia is thought to involve spasm or incomplete relaxation of the cricopharyngeus muscle. This is uncommon in children but can be diagnosed by identification of a prominent bar on VFSS, with OPD found in approximately 50% of cases. Increased pressures proximal to the muscle can also be demonstrated on manometry[42] and confirmed by electromyography.[43] Management with cricopharyngeus myotomy or dilatation has been reported useful in relieving symptoms of affected patients.[42,44,45]

Inflammatory Conditions

Gastroesophageal reflux (GER) is a normal physiologic phenomenon known to occur in all healthy infants. Actual repeated expulsion of gastroesophageal contents from the oral cavity in GER is reported to occur in approximately 40% of infants.[46] On the other hand, the prevalence of symptomatic or pathologic GER or GERD is estimated to occur in 10% to 20% of infants in North America.[47] Some children are at higher risk of GERD, including those with neurologic impairment, obesity, esophageal achalasia, hiatal hernia, prematurity, bronchopulmonary dyplasia, and esophageal atresia.[48] GERD can contribute to persistent OPD by reducing mucosal sensation and laryngeal reactivity (LAR) during the pharyngeal phase of swallowing owing to mucosal injury by caustic reflex contents. Reduced laryngeal sensation has been demonstrated in the setting of chronic reflux in both animals and infants.[49] In view of the prevalence of GERD, treatment has become an important part of OPD management in children.[50]

Eosinophilic esophagitis (EoE) is a chronic immune-mediated condition characterized by clinical symptoms secondary to esophageal dysfunction and histologically by eosinophilic infiltration of the esophagus.[51,52] Feeding difficulties are the most common symptoms in infants and toddlers, with vomiting and retrosternal pain in children and adolescents. The main histologic feature of EoE is striking eosinophilia of esophageal mucosa with microabcesses and basal zone hyperplasia. The relationship to EoE to OPD is unclear. EoE is associated, however, with GERD and food allergies, both of which are thought to contribute to chronic inflammation and reduced sensitivity of the larynx.[53,54] Such a reaction to cow milk protein has been described[55] and careful history with radioallergosorbent (RAST) testing may be useful to help identify the cause quickly.

Esophageal biopsies and histology usually confirms the diagnosis of EoE and the management consists of dietary modification and reflux therapy. Three diet forms are commonly prescribed: an elemental diet that is a liquid formula based on amino acids and free of all allergens,[56] a 6-food elimination diet that removes commonly identified allergens,[57] or a targeted elimination diet[58] that eliminates food identified as allergic to patient after testing. Swallowed corticosteroids are also effective in treating acute exacerbations of EoE but the disease often relapses after discontinuation.

EVALUATION OF PEDIATRIC OROPHARYNGEAL DYSPHAGIA
History and Physical Examination

Slow feeding, blue spells, frequent respiratory pauses, or wheeze and/or cough during the feed suggests OPD in an infant. Wet respirations (biphasic washing machine sound) with a wet cry or voice suggest silent aspiration and OPD in both infants and children. The importance of detecting a postprandial wet voice by itself is not considered diagnostic but is likely useful in identifying those with dysphagia related to laryngeal dysfunction.[59] Airway symptoms, such as breathlessness, stridor, and wheeze, may mask silent aspiration and a high index of suspicion for OPD in these patients is well served. Weight gain is an important predictor of health and nutrition in children with OPD and should be followed closely. Discussion of perinatal events and gestational age help tease out the cause of OPD in otherwise normal children. Parents should also be asked about potential neurologic, inflammatory, and anatomic sources of OPD (discussed previously). A history of recurrent and chronic lower respiratory tract infections, reactive airway disease, and pneumonia, especially if severe enough to warrant hospitalization, is an important symptom of pediatric OPD. In less severe cases, infants may sound congested due to chronic respiratory secretions and bronchitis from chronic microaspiration. Delays in speech and gait may also indicate subtle central pathology in older children.

A complete and thorough otolaryngology examination is essential in the diagnosis of OPD and exploration of potential etiology. Syndromic facial characteristics should be searched for. Auscultation for wheezing, course breath sounds, and wet voice/cry or respiration before and after eating is essential. This is best performed by an SLP who can observe subtle symptoms of OPD during oral intake and postprandially. Nasal patency and identification of upper aerodigestive tract obstruction are essential components of the examination.[50]

Flexible fiberoptic nasolaryngoscopy should be performed as routine part of the examination in patients with OPD. This provides anatomic detail of the nasal cavity, nasopharynx, oropharynx, hypopharynx, and larynx while identifying evidence of chronic mucosal inflammation of these sites, which may be secondary to rhinitis, postnasal drip, and GERD. Low lying tonsils, laryngomalacia, laryngeal clefts, and evidence of hypopharyngeal residue can be seen with this examination.

In all cases of suspected OPD it is important to involve SLP early in the process of evaluation. Clinical bedside evaluation or clinical feeding evaluation can be easily performed (**Box 3**). Evaluation using 3-oz water challenge[60] has been described. With this brief study, a child is observed during and after oral consumption of up to 3 oz of water. OPD can manifest with coughing, choking, or tearing occurring during or shortly after the test. Suiter and colleagues[61] reported their results in children between

---

Box 3
Clinical bedside evaluation for a patient with suspected oropharyngeal dysphagia

History

Medical history: obtain thorough medical history from caregivers about child

Feeding history: obtain past feeding history and current feeding schedule for child

Examination

Inspection: make observations regarding child's oral sensorimotor (OM) skills at rest, such as open-mouth posture, drooling, low tone, facial symmetry, etc.

Palpation: with babies, used gloved finger to feel inside child's mouth to assess tongue mobility, restrictive frenulum, status of palate

Observe feeding ability

1. Bottle—child's ability to latch on to bottle nipple, child's efficiency in expressing liquid from the bottle, anterior liquid loss

2. Sippy cup/straw drinking—OM skills

3. Spoon feeding—ability to close lips on spoon, remove bolus, etc.

4. Solid ingestion—ability to manipulate/chew solid prior to swallow

Observe for signs of aspiration

Distress/increased work of breathing/stridor/gagging/gulping/choking/coughing during feed. Increased congestion (nasal or chest) or wet vocal quality or wheezing during or directly after feed

2 and 18 years of age. Compared with FEES, the investigators concluded that the 3-oz challenge had high sensitivity but a low specificity, indicating a high false-positive rate, suggesting that normal children who cleared this test may be safely given thin liquids. It is not a good screening tool for children at high risk of aspiration, however, and is not a good indicator of silent aspiration.

Chest Radiograph

A chest radiograph (CXR) is a good initial screening tool in children with suspect OPD but is not necessary in all. In the setting of fever, a CXR may be useful to identify an active pulmonary process. CXRs in chronic cases of OPD show bronchial thickening, hyperinflation, and segmental or subsegmental infiltrates. The infiltrates in OPD follow discreet patterns and settle in dependent areas, such as the posterior aspects of the lower lobes. Unfortunately, CXR is largely insensitive to early pulmonary injury related to chronic microaspiration.[62]

High-Resolution CT Scan

High-resolution CT (HRCT) is recommended when CXRs show evidence of chronic aspiration–related pulmonary injury and in cases where the severity of injury is not known. HRCT is sensitive compared with a plain CXR in detecting and delineating aspiration-related parenchymal injury. HRCT can detect bronchiectasis, centrilobular opacities (tree-in-bud), air trapping, and bronchial thickening.[63] Although not specific to aspiration, these findings are consistent with chronic aspiration.

MR imaging Scan of Head and Cervical Spine

MR imaging scan of the head and cervical spine is recommended to delineate intra-cranial pathology in selected cases of OPD. A diagnosis of Chiari I malformation using MR imaging can be made easily in younger patients, even those with minimal or no neurologic symptoms.[64] MR imaging scan is not routinely performed in all cases of OPD but should be considered in cases associated with even mild developmental delays or neurologic deficits because they are identified with increasing age of the child. An infant or child with progressively worsening OPD should undergo early MR imaging because this may be a sign of a potential central cause. This is also true for the neurologically intact and developmentally normal children who continue to have OPD beyond the age of 2.5 years. MR imaging scan may help in detection of minor cerebellar infarcts, Chiari malformations, vascular anomalies, or tumors affecting the swallow center in the medulla.[36]

Lipid-Laden Macrophage Index

The lipid-laden macrophage index (LLMI) can be used to help diagnose aspiration. Gastric contents often contain lipid material that can be taken up by the pulmonary macrophages after aspiration. For the LLMI as described by Colombo and Hallberg,[65] the macrophages are graded 0–4 based on the amount of lipid in the cytoplasm of each macrophage. A total of 100 macrophages is usually studied; hence, indices could range between 0 and 400. Furuya and colleagues[66] studied 41 children with pulmonary pathology and suspicion of aspiration and reported that an LLMI greater than 165 had a 98.6% sensitivity, 78% specificity, and 87.8% overall accuracy as a diagnostic test for aspiration. Kieran and colleagues[67] reported significantly higher LLMI in patients undergoing surgery for type 1 and type 2 laryngeal clefts and proposed measuring LLMI in cleft patients as an indicator of pulmonary injury. Although the LLMI may be increased in aspiration, it is not very specific. Other comorbidities seen in aspirators, such as asthma, GERD, and recurrent pneumonia, may also contribute to LLMI elevation.[68] Thus, LLMI is not routinely performed to assess aspiration, but it may be helpful in cases like chronic cough, where no other reason is found.

Microlaryngobronchoscopy and Esophagoscopy

A complete microlaryngobronchoscopy (MLB) is performed in cases of suspected anatomic sources of OPD, for example, a patient with history suggesting a laryngeal cleft or subglottic pathology. MLB should also be considered in a normal child with more than 2 years of age, who has objective evidence (VFSS/FEES) of aspiration, to rule out undetected laryngotracheal anomalies contributing to OPD. MLB may be also be required when office based flexible provides evidence of laryngeal anomalies contributing to OPD (laryngomalacia most commonly) that may require surgical management. MLB should be performed with patients breathing spontaneously to observe laryngeal function. Palpation is the best way to identify a type 1 cleft that may otherwise be missed. MLB is often performed with a planned esophagoscopy or vice versa. Esophagoscopy allows assessment and, if necessary, biopsies to identify GERD and EoE. The number of esophageal biopsies required remains unclear; however, 2 biopsies at the proximal, mid, and distal esphagous should be able to capture evidence of inflammation if present.

Instrumental Evaluations of Swallowing

VFSSs and FEES are the most commonly used tests in the evaluation of aspiration in infants and children. FEES may also be used with sensitivity testing. Both techniques have advantages and disadvantages, as outlined in **Table 1**, but are extremely useful in providing objective evidence of OPD. Although considered gold standard, these tests are confounded by a poor intrarater and inter-rater reliability because normative data for standardization are not available.[69]

Table 1
VFSS and FEES comparison

VFSS	FEES
Allows real-time view of oral preparatory; oral, pharyngeal, and cervical esophageal phases of swallow; and how structures interact during bolus transit	Oral phase is not visible; only before and after the swallow can be viewed; view is obstructed during the swallow by epiglottic inversion
Swallowing structures are visible only via videofluoroscopy	The anatomy of the nasopharyx, the supraglottic structures, and the true vocal cords are visible
Detects aspiration	Trace aspiration may be missed
Radiation exposure	No radiation exposure
Sample of swallows may be small due to time constraints and to attempts to limit radiation exposure	Multiple swallows of different consistencies may be viewed
Expensive procedure and requires appointment in radiology department	May be performed during outpatient clinic visit with otolaryngologist and SLP
Requires patient participation	Nasopharyngoscope may be invasive/uncomfortable for patient and thus lead to decreased cooperation
Study must be performed in radiology suite and patient must sit in swallow study chair	FEES can be performed at beside; may be more appropriate for medically complex children who are not mobile

Videofluoroscopic swallow study

The VFSS is the primary tool for formal dysphagia evaluation. The VFSS is performed by a team of professionals, including a radiologist and an SLP with extensive training in feeding and swallowing assessment and management.[70] In some institutions, an OT along with a radiologist may evaluate a child's swallowing function. VFSS may be warranted if a child demonstrates consistent signs and symptoms of aspiration during or immediately after a feeding. Other symptoms may include increased feeding times and poor weight gain. Prior to scheduling a swallow study, a child should be clinically evaluated by a physician and an SLP. During the clinical evaluation, the SLP obtains the child's pertinent medical history and observes the child clinically during a feeding.[71] In situations where a child's feeding cannot be observed by the SLP prior to the study, a thorough medical and feeding history for the child should be obtained.

For the study, the infant or younger child sits in a booster or tumbleform seat (Ability One Company, Bolingbrook, IL, USA) in the swallow study chair. Videofluoroscopy is used to capture the various stages of the swallow in real time. The lateral view is most common, although, in some cases, anterior-posterior view may be useful if asymmetry is suspected. Preferably, the caregiver stands in front of the child and helps the child during the feeding. The SLP, however, may also perform the feeding.[71] The initial consistency and manner of intake chosen depends on what liquids/solids the child is currently taking by mouth, the medical history of the child, and what information the SLP expects to gain from the study.

Information about the oral preparatory and oral, pharyngeal, and esophageal phases of the swallow may be obtained during VFSS. During the study, the SLP monitors a child's feeding. Reduced oral motor skills may be observed for several reasons, including prematurity, developmental delay, upper airway obstruction, and neurologic impairment.[72]

Delayed initiation of the swallow may lead to pooling of the barium in the valleculae or pyriform sinuses. Supraglottic penetration may be documented during the study, including a description of when, how deep, and how often these penetrations occur (**Fig. 2**). Shallow or midlevel penetration may be viewed without the presence of other swallowing dysfunction. Frequent, deep penetration, however, is often an indicator that the child is at a higher risk of aspiration with that consistency, flow, and manner of intake.[73] Transglottic aspiration may occur before, during, or after the swallow.

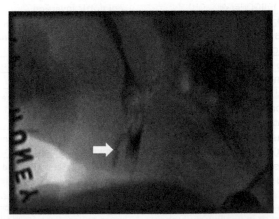

Fig. 2. VFSS image showing aspiration during the pharyngeal phase of swallow in a child. The aspirate is denoted by arrow.

Aspiration before the swallow indicates delayed initiation of the pharyngeal swallow. Aspiration during the swallow indicates incompetent or delayed pharyngoglottal reflex or true vocal cord dysfunction, and aspiration after the swallow occurs with pharyngeal residue. The SLP should note whether or not the child had any response to the aspiration event (absent cough, immediate cough, and delayed cough). Silent aspiration is frequently noted on VFSS in neurologically impaired children, children with developmental delays, and premature infants.[74,75] If pharyngeal residue is observed after the swallow, the amount and location of the residue should be noted. Pharyngeal residue may indicate reduced tongue base retraction and/or reduced pharyngeal contraction.[71]

The cause of a child's dysphagia may be better understood after VFSS if there is an adequate sample obtained and if the child participated well. Results of the study and feeding recommendations for the child are then made to the caregivers. Recommendations may include position changes during feeding, altering the flow of the liquid with a slower manner of intake, or thickening of feeds to aid in oral and/or pharyngeal control of the bolus. These recommendations, especially regarding thickening of liquids, should be approved by a child's managing physician.

Fibreoptic endoscopic evaluation of swallowing
The FEES was initially described in adults but is now commonly used in infants and children to further assess swallowing patterns.[76,77] Although initially not widely used for dysphagia assessment,[62] the practice of FEES has gained acceptance as a useful diagnostic and therapeutic tool for pediatric dysphagia assessment and management.[78,79] FEES may be indicated if the child is not appropriate for an initial or follow-up VFSS or if further evaluation of the anatomic structures of swallowing is warranted. FEES provides the SLP more opportunities to view various consistencies and compensatory swallowing strategies during feeding without detrimental radiation exposure. For a child who is not an oral feeder, information may be gained by observing the child's management of secretions, sometimes with the use of dye.[79]

FEES is usually performed together by an otolaryngologist and SLP. The flexible nasolaryngoscope is positioned by the physician as the SLP administers feeding. Interpretation of the examination is performed by both team members. A qualified SLP[80] can also place the scope but requires another participant to assist with feeding. A nurse is often required to help hold a young child undergoing the examination. During FEES, the nasopharynx, oropharynx, hypopharynx, supraglottis, and true vocal folds are visible. Food contents in this study do not have to be mixed with barium. Food dye may be necessary, however, to provide better visualization of the bolus during transit. Epiglottic inversion, as a result of pharyngeal constriction and hypolaryngeal excursion, prevents viewing of bolus transit during part of the pharyngeal phase. Delayed initiation of the swallow, supraglottic penetration, frank aspiration, and/or pharyngeal residue, however, after the swallow are best determined by FEES.

In studies comparing adult VFSS and FEES results, FEES has been noted as sensitive in the detection of delayed initiation of the swallow, penetration, aspiration, and pharyngeal residue.[76,81] In the pediatric population, a study by Leder and Karas[79] in 2000 reported 100% agreement in 7 patients who underwent both VFSS and FEES in recognition of penetration and aspiration occurrence. Research continues regarding the sensitivity and specificity of FEES in the pediatric population.

Deciding which instrumental examination is most appropriate for a child depends on several factors. For some children, obtaining both VFSS and FEES is ideal to obtain a more comprehensive picture of the anatomy and swallowing mechanism. FEES provides for a detailed anatomic assessment of the pharynx and larynx along with swallowing function data. VFSS shows all phases of the swallow, which is helpful in some children. Children between ages 1.5 years and 4 years have difficulty participating in FEES and following directions. Thus, FEES is more commonly used in infants and older children after a previous VFSS to follow their OPD course without radiation.

MANAGEMENT OF PEDIATRIC OROPHARYNGEAL DYSPHAGIA

Once identified, OPD in children follows a protracted course compared with other medical issues treated by an otolaryngologist. Fortunately, nutrition for most infants and children with OPD can be maintained using a modified feeding program with liquid thickeners. Early and open discussions with the family regarding the duration from diagnosis to final OPD resolution should occur at the time of diagnosis. Evidence suggests that infants diagnosed with OPD may take 2 to 3 years to be ultimately weaned from their diet modification to normal thin consistencies.[82] This delay is related to both the interval between the diagnosis and identification of the cause and the weaning period to safely graduate to each subsequent thinner consistency. Currently, a well-established management protocol for OPD does not exist. A multidisciplinary effort is necessary to help identify the source and optimize gastrointestinal and pulmonary health. Periodic visits, endoscopies, surgical procedures, and instrumental evaluations of swallowing are required during the course of pediatric OPD management.

Initial Management

When OPD is suspected, the initial physician visit consists of establishing the diagnosis, exploring potential contributors, and determining the patient's safe alimentation. A stepwise algorithm, used by the authors' institution, is provided (**Fig. 3**) on the first physician visit. Early SLP consultation provides detailed information regarding feeding habits, overall safety, and need of a VFSS or FEES (see **Box 3**). The families' working relationship with the SLP is fundamental in establishing an appropriate feeding paradigm for the child.

Important information gathered for infants with suspected OPD includes nipple flow, length of feeding time, and signs/symptoms of aspiration during or after a feed. From this information, early interventions (**Box 4**) may be a change to slower flow nipples, implementation of pacing during the feed, and altering a child's feeding position. These early interventions should always be practiced prior to introducing a thickening agent. Empiric thickening of liquid intake, however, may also help slow flow and reduce GERD. This can enhance laryngeal protection until a formal instrumental evaluation can take place. Other compensatory feeding strategies include small volumes, reducing the interval between feeds, and changing the formula or bottles used. For babies with reflux-associated OPD, empiric thickening with rice cereal may control mild symptoms and the patient can be followed in clinic periodically for signs of improvement. Many of these children have subtle evidence of mild laryngomalacia (periodic stridor with feeds and shortened aryepiglottic folds). Breastfed children in this scenario may continue their diet, with reflux precautions, because breast milk is not caustic to the pulmonary system. If an infant continues to have feeding difficulties and associated respiratory illnesses, a formal swallowing evaluation is warranted. Patients with severe GERD with regurgitation should be referred for gastroenterology evaluation.

Pulmonary consultation should be performed in cases in which pulmonary medical therapy (inhaled steroids) is required, patients with moderate to severe aspiration, and patients with unusually persistent OPD. These include infants with OPD requiring

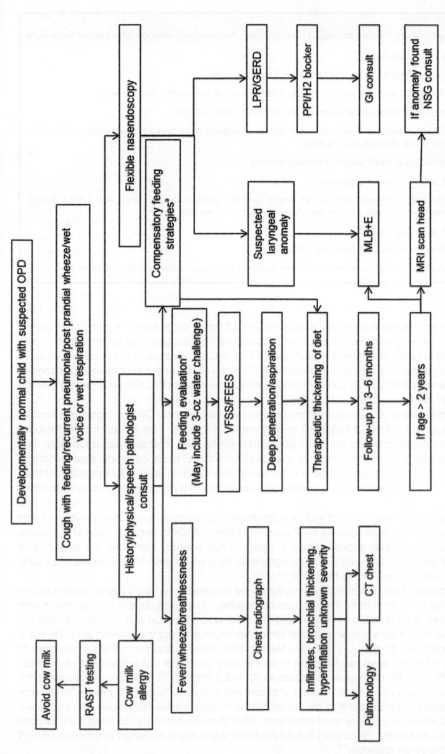

Fig. 3. Initial evaluation of a child with OPD. [a] Some patients with OPD may need just a bedside evaluation with compensatory feeding strategies without thickening of feed. Although SLP do not routinely include 3-oz water challenge, it may be used as a screening tool (for pros are cons please refer to the text). GI, gastroenterologist; H2 blocker, histamine H2 receptor antagonist; MLB+/−E, MLB with or without esophagoscopy; NSG, neuro surgery; RAST, radio allergo sorbent test.

Box 4
Compensatory feeding strategies recommended for a patient with oropharyngeal dysphagia

With bottle feeding

1. Change nipple shape and/or change flow of nipple
2. Implement external pacing to help with suck-swallow-breathe coordination
3. Feed in semiupright position or possibly side-lying position
4. Thicken liquids, if in spite of above measures patient continues to have feeding difficulties and is not efficient during feed
5. Patient may need ongoing feeding therapy

With sippy cup/open cup/straw

1. Introduce different manner of intake to help child with efficiency and safety during feeding—may need to thicken, feeding treatment may be helpful

With spoon and solids

1. Work on lip closure (feeding therapy)
2. Work on oral sensorimotor skills and learning to manipulate/chew (feeding therapy)

---

thickener greater than honey consistency or children older than 2.5 year still requiring honey-thick consistency. Instrumental swallowing evaluation may be necessary in this setting to help determine the severity of OPD. A CXR is valuable in the early investigation of pulmonary function and status. A CT scan of the chest is reserved for cases of concerning findings on CXR or those in which the impact of OPD on a patient's lungs cannot be assessed.

Investigation of an anatomic problem associated with the OPD or significant laryngopharyngeal reflux (LPR)/GERD is performed in infants. This is conducted for both neurologically affected and normal children by flexible fiberoptic laryngoscopy. Evidence suggests that prematurity and GERD are the 2 most common contributors to reduced laryngeal protective mechanisms and OPD in a developmentally normal child.[83] LPR management is recommended in the setting of signs and symptoms of reflux and OPD.

First-line therapy for LPR includes histamine H2 receptor antagonists (HRAs) at 6 to 10 mg/kg. The peak plasma level concentrations of HRAs are achieved at 2.5 hours and continue until approximately 6 hours. They should, therefore, be provided in 2 to 3 divided doses per day. Tachyphylaxis may occur with HRA 6 weeks after initiation and may limit long-term use.

In cases of persistent symptoms, it may be necessary to add a nightly proton pump inhibitor (PPI) or shift to this regimen completely. Tachyphalaxis is not observed with PPIs that are also able to inhibit meal-induced acid secretion and maintain gastric pH greater than 4 for a longer period of time. Maximum efficacy is achieved when PPIs are administered 30 minutes before a feed.[84] PPIs have a shorter half-life in children.[85] Thus, a higher dose per kilogram or twice-daily dosing is recommended—lansoprazole (0.73–1.66 mg/kg) or omeprazole (0.3–3.5 mg/kg).[86] PPIs are recommend for GERD in patients 1 year or older and are not proved effective in infants.[87] Caution has been advised regarding the use of PPIs in infants, particularly those with increased risk of lower respiratory tract infections, after a multicentric randomized trial demonstrated that lower respiratory tract infections were more common in children on PPI than those on placebo.[88]

Infants and children with suspected or confirmed OPD are followed every 1 to 3 months after the initial visit depending on the severity of dysphagia and LPR. Observation for and early control of inflammatory mediators of OPD and periodic assessment of developmental milestones and subtle delays are important components of clinical follow-up. When obvious laryngeal or other anatomic anomalies are detected (laryngeal cleft or severe laryngomalacia), an MLB is warranted for early corrective surgery and airway surveillance. Esophagoscopy with biopsies can be added to provide complete assessment of the entire aerodigestive tract under the same anesthetic.

Introducing Safe Alimentation

Safe alimentation entails a diet that can be negotiated during the pharyngeal phase with minimum risk of laryngeal penetration and aspiration into the trachea. This requires the use of an agent that is safe for dietary consumption and adequately thickens liquids to slow the pace at which they pass through the UES. The resultant and subtle delay during the pharyngeal phase of swallowing allows time for laryngeal closure and the LAR to protect the airway. In essence, the thicker the consistency, the more time (in milliseconds) available for the afferent-efferent reflex loop to complete laryngeal closure.[89]

The diet is therapeutically thickened to a consistency based on the findings on VFSS or FEES. Because these results are only a brief picture of a child's swallowing efficiency, they must be interpreted in the context of clinical data. A patient's clinical response and symptoms with a particular consistency take precedence in determining the appropriate degree of thickening. It is also important that the multidisciplinary members, including otolaryngologist, pulmonologist, gastroenterologist, dietician, and SLP, confer on the modified feeding regimen. Each discipline perceives the relative safety of the diet from a unique perspective.

In the absence of a multidisciplinary team, the general rule for a safe thickened diet is one level higher than the consistency deeply penetrating the larynx or aspirated. As long as this is tolerated, patients can be maintained on this consistency until symptoms resolve, they are asymptomatic during a clinical feeding evaluation, or an instrumental evaluation demonstrates safety (no aspiration) at lower levels of thickener. A weaning process from the thickener is then used (discussed later).

By increasing the viscosity of a child's liquid alimentation, the slower flowing fluid provides more time for oral and pharyngeal control of the bolus.[89] Various consistency levels are referred to when discussing swallowing dysfunction. Unthickened formulas, liquids, and breast milk are considered thin liquids. Nectar and honey refer to the degree of consistency obtained with specific recipes using thickening agents. These 2 consistencies can be further divided into thin or stiff (ie, thin nectar and stiff honey), demarcating a one-half step change in the degree of thickener. Dysphagia severity is often determined based on the results of a formal VFSS or FEES and the recommended feeding regimen. Penetration of thin liquids may be classified as mild pharyngeal dysphagia whereas transglottic aspiration of liquids may translate to moderate or severe dysphagia. This depends on the circumstances of the aspiration and a child's overall swallowing function.

Various commercial, artificial thickening agents exist for thickening liquids, like SimplyThick (SimplyThick, St Louis, MO, USA) and Thick-It (Kent Precision Foods Group, St Louis, MO, USA). Caution should be exercised when recommending use of thickening agents, especially in children with a history of prematurity, because thickening products may cause adverse gastrointestinal issues or exacerbate feeding difficulties. Infants and children need to be monitored for constipation or diarrhea secondary to thickener use. If present, consultation with gastroenterology is warranted.

Other patients may have prolonged feeding times and, in turn, poor oral intake, if feeding fatigue or incomplete intake results when a thickener is introduced.[90,91] Nutritional experts and speech therapy should assist when these issues arise. Currently, SimplyThick, whose product contains xanthan gum, does not recommend use of SimplyThick thickener in term or preterm infants 12 months and under. This warning extends to children under the age of 12 years with a history of necrotizing enterocolitis (http://www.simplythick.com/). Only gum-based thickening agents have been shown to successfully thicken expressed breast milk (EBM) and for the EBM to maintain this thicker consistency. EBM cannot maintain a thicker consistency when rice cereal or corn starch-based thickening agents are used, because inherent enzymes (amylase) denude rice and cornstarch.[92,93] EBM is, however, relatively safe to the pediatric pulmonary tree. Thus, an infant drinking EBM may continue in the presence of OPD when strict compensatory feeding strategies to reduce aspiration risk are also implemented.

OPD Follow-Up

The first follow-up visit for OPD, after compensatory feeding strategies with or without therapeutic thickener have been used, should be after 4 to 6 weeks. New feeding concerns, reflux control, pulmonary status, and gastrointestinal complaints secondary to a thickener agent, uncontrolled OPD or airway symptoms, and compliance should be addressed. An instrumental evaluation may be scheduled at this time if not previously performed. For stable infants with mild OPD (laryngeal penetration on nectar consistency), a 3 to 4 months' follow-up is often adequate. Once a safe and tolerable feeding regimen is implemented and confirmed, then periodic visits from 3 to 6 months should be sufficient, especially in those requiring higher levels of consistency. Children who are initiated on a thickened diet honey-thick or of greater thickness, frequently take months to years to improve. Periodic monitoring for weight gain, lower respiratory tract infections, developmental milestones, or worsening symptoms is also important.

Fortunately, in the majority of infants and children who are neurologically normal, OPD is associated with prematurity or LPR/GERD. These patients tend to improve or resolve their OPD by 2 to 3 years of age if no other new contributors arise.[94] Most patients improve with observation as neuromuscular maturity occurs and reflux subsides with increasing age. Severe dysphagia (requiring stiff honey), worsening symptoms, or failed improvement should prompt further investigation and testing of inflammatory, anatomic, and subtle neurologic contributors. In the setting of gradually worsening symptoms and poor achievement of physical milestones, including a newly weak or hoarse cry or gait instability, a neurology consult and MR imaging of the head is recommended to rule out CNS or dynamic neuromuscular causes.

Follow-up visits should include a thorough clinical history and examination and possible beside speech evaluation. Repeat flexible nasolaryngoscopy may be required in an older child with persistent OPD in which a FEES examination can also be conducted. It is the author's experience that once children are diagnosed and treated for OPD, they are more sensitive to the multiple anatomic and inflammatory factors that may contribute to the condition. For example, a reflux-associated OPD infant who persists into childhood may not resolve until intervention for cow's milk protein allergy, low-riding tonsillar hypertrophy, a shallow laryngeal cleft, or subtle cricopharyngeal achalasia.

A revised algorithm for management of this type of patient is provided in **Fig. 4**. In essence, potentially subtle sources of OPD need to be explored.[50] These include the use of a head MR imaging scan to rule out CM-I (or other CNS causes) and MLB with esophagoscopy for laryngeal sources (late-onset/persistent laryngomalacia and type 1 laryngeal clefts) and inflammatory contributors (EoE and GERD) to OPD. These

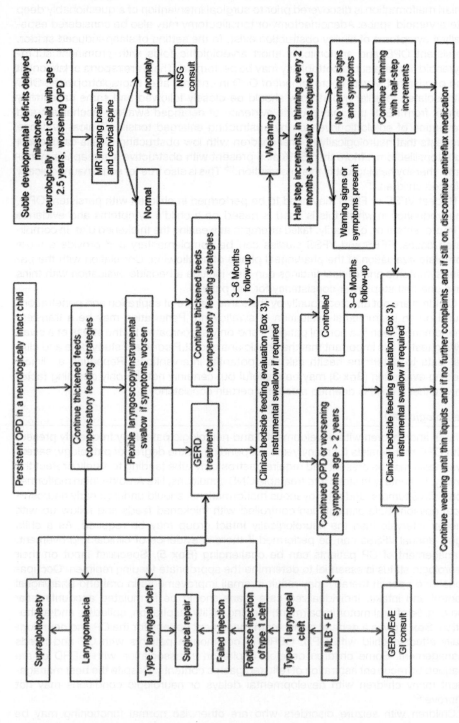

Fig. 4. Management algorithm for persistent OPD in neurologically normal child. Weaning priniciples. GI, gastroenterologist; MLB+E, MLB with or without esophagoscopy.

procedures can be used under the same anesthetic as the MR imaging first so that a Chiari malformation is discovered prior to surgical intervention of a questionably deep interarytenoid space. Adenoidectomy or tonsillectomy may also be considered especially if symptoms of airway obstruction exist. In the setting of sleep-induced stridor, persistent OPD and anatomically short aryepiglottic folds with prominent supra-arytenoid tissue, a supraglottoplasty may be performed. There are reports of late onset and persistent LM with improvement of OPD in children after supraglottoplasty. OPD with isolated tonsillar hypertrophy should be closely followed and some cases may benefit from FEES that may provide evidence of deranged swallow mechanism and prevention of epiglottic inversion by obstructing enlarged tonsils. Clinical evidence suggests that neurologically normal children with low obstructing tonsils can benefit from tonsillectomy. More than 50% also present with obstructive sleep apnea symptoms, thereby helping justify this intervention.[95] This is also true for some neurologically affected children.[18]

Repeat VFSS or FEES may need to be performed in children with persistent OPD. The frequency in which this is used is based on a child's symptoms and evidence of improvement or, contrarily, failed attempts at weaning the thickened diet. In complicated cases, FEES and VFSS studies can be complementary and provide a more complete evaluation of the pharyngeal phase of swallowing. Correlation with the patient symptoms and clinical findings can also include a bedside evaluation with thins (or a one-half step lower consistency for the patient).

Children are not affected equally by the same degree of aspiration and penetration[7] found on an instrumental evaluation of swallowing. Penetration may be a transient phenomenon seen in a normal patient[96] and only exacerbated by the stress of a swallowing test.[50] It is important that the physicians and SLP correlate study data and clinical data to determine health risk and potential interventions. Repeating a clinical feeding evaluation (**Box 3**) may be a useful but certainly not the only deciding factor on whether a child is deemed safe for a certain consistency.

Neurologic OPD

Infants and children with developmental and neurologic pathology frequently present with OPD that persists for many years. Depending on the degree of pathology, severe dysphagia may be present and require gastrostomy tube feeding to safely protect the airway. Patients with static and treatable CNS conditions, like Arnold-Chiari malformations, CNS tumors, and arteriovenous malformations, should undergo early neurosurgical opinion. Safe alimentation controlled with thickened feeds and follow-up with shorter intervals than the neurologically intact group may be required. As a child ages, annual VFSSs can be performed if there is evidence of clinical improvement. Management of CP patients can be challenging (**Box 5**). Specialist input on their neurologic status is essential to determine the appropriate feeding regimen. Occupational and speech therapy may result in small improvements in oral and pharyngeal control and intake. Individualized care plans should be formulated accounting for the degree of oral motor impairment, feeding ability, aspiration, epilepsy, and ambulation. **Box 5** gives a general outline of management options for the CP and neurologically affected child with OPD. GERD is common in patients with CP and needs management. Some children develop aspiration in association with GERD or are plagued by recurrent aspiration of refluxed gastric contents. Despite the best management many children with developmental delays or neurologic conditions may not improve.[37]

Children with seizure disorders who are otherwise normal functioning may be affected by OPD. Subtle disturbances in neuromuscular control and consciousness

---

Box 5

Assessment and management of oropharyngeal dysphagia in patients with neurologic pathology

History

Oral hygiene; occlusion; and assess drooling, gag reflex, ensure seizure control; rule out side effects of antiepileptic drugs

Volitional control of oral phase: sucking as neonate, oral-feeding habits

Developmental milestones, speech

History regarding aspiration: choking, postprandial tachypnea, wet voice, wet breathing

Examination

Rule out airway obstruction, dental examination

Oral sensorimotor examination (tongue lateralization, sensation, tone, strength, pathologic reactions)

Oropharyngeal stage of swallowing during eating and drinking (swallow on demand, oral control, frequency/efficiency/safety), 3-oz water challenge, VFSS

Speech (dysarthria/dyspraxia) and communication skills

Chest: assess for aspiration CXR—pulmonary consult

Assess: dental opinion/neurology opinion/physiotherapy/occupational therapy

Management

Thickener: as appropriate

GER: antireflux medication

Drooling: consider drooling treatment glycopyrrolate oral suspension (40–100 µg/kg/d with a maximum of 175 µg/kg/d), dosage given once daily

If no response, consider intense behavior therapy/surgical management: consider gastrostomy tube if failure to thrive, poor feeding with weight loss, recurrent pneumonias despite thickener, lack of progress and development

Speech pathologist

> Objective: modify food bolus, such as consistency, size, and texture; positioning of the patient; examining compensatory swallow maneuvers; posture and head control; mouth closure; lip seal; oral sensorimotor therapy for drooling

---

can affect normal swallowing by disrupting central midbrain processes. Some antiepileptics and neuroleptic drugs can contribute to neural blunting and subsequent OPD.

After excision of CNS neoplasms, patients may show improvement in dysphagia. Arnold-Chiari type 1–associated OPD usually resolves completely after posterior fossa decompression.[36] Those with progressive neurologic disorders, like mucopolysacharidoses and muscular dystrophy, show normal development initially but deteriorate rapidly and may need support for feeding and ventilation in later stages. Patients with CP show variable progress with some showing no improvement and others showing improving skills.

Clinical Course

Dysphagia in a neurologically normal child associated with prematurity and LPR tends to improve with time. This improvement is gradual with advanced neuromuscular coordination with age. These children can be managed expectantly with the diet that is deemed safe. Parents should be made aware of the need for watchfulness, however, regarding worsening symptoms.

Sheikh and colleagues[6] reported on a group of neurologically intact infants born at term without GER who had chronic aspiration due to dysphagia that resolved within 3 to 9 months. Research suggests that the average time to return to normal diet in the developmentally normal child with OPD is 3.2 years. In patients with an obvious laryngeal anomaly, the associated symptoms improve more quickly, but dysphagia improves slowly and gradually. Richter and colleagues[97] have noted a median interval of 3.8 months between supraglottoplasty for laryngomalacia and improvement of aspiration in infants. Durvasula and colleagues[22] reported 93.4% improvement of dysphagia at 6 months after supraglottoplasty in a cohort of 136 patients with laryngomalacia with no associated comorbidities. Preterm infants with gestation age less than 32 weeks at birth and laryngomalacia, however, had significantly high rates with 50% of patients still showing evidence of dysphagia 6 months after supraglottoplasty. The investigators thus concluded that prematurity has an independent role to play in dysphagia.

Similarly, Bakthavachalam and colleagues[98] reported in a case series of type 1 laryngeal clefts that the average time to resolution of aspiration was 7.8 months for the group managed surgically and 13.6 months for the nonsurgical group. They also reported that the average age of resolution of aspiration in patients with laryngeal cleft diagnosed before 2 years was significantly better than those who were diagnosed after 2 years. Repair of type 1 and type 2 clefts should be reserved for patients with persistent aspiration that is not improving with age, infants with cleft and recurrent pneumonia, those with worsening pulmonary status, and those with other severe comorbidities contributing to dysphagia. Endoscopic surgical repair is usually curative, but recently, augmentation of the cleft by injection of Radiesse (Merz Aesthetics, Franksville, WI, USA) in the interarytenoid notch has been reported with complete resolution of symptoms in 56%[99] and 72%.[100] Although concerns regarding long-term results of interarytenoid injection exist, it is prudent to try injection as a first step and reserving endoscopic repair for failures and relapses.

Weaning and Precautions

Signs and symptoms are the best predictors of successful weaning and return to normal swallowing. Dietary weaning is proposed when the signs and symptoms have improved for at least 6 months or when evident on VFSS or FEES. For example, improvement is declared in a patient who was aspirating honey but now only aspirates nectar. Despite VFSS evidence of improvement, weaning the thickener is recommended in a gradual manner with thinning trials of half-step increments in consistency. A patient on honey may be weaned to stiff nectar and observed for at least 2 to 3 months before proceeding to nectar consistency. Such a gradual approach is usually more successful and less stressful for the parent. The parents should be warned, however, that the original consistency should be on standby in case any signs and symptoms should recur or OPD should worsen. A comfortably feeding child is a good sign, but watering eyes, tachypnea, and wet respiration suggest poor swallow and silent aspiration. Bronchopulmonary events, like worsening asthma, increased need for respiratory medications, and lower respiratory tract infections, indicate aspiration. Parents should also be warned about transient worsening of swallowing, especially when there is an upper respiratory tract infection or fever that may improve once the acute condition has subsided. At this stage, the patient may be followed up once in 4 to 6 months. Medication for GERD should continue until the patient is on near-normal consistency.

Repeat VFSS is often performed in OPD cases once in 10 to 12 months. A repeat VFSS is not necessary, however, in cases showing clinical improvement and/or a VFSS showing no deep penetration or aspiration, unless symptoms worsen. In an infant, a repeat VFSS may be performed sooner due to the relatively quicker dynamic growth and functional improvement of the infant (ie, 6 months). Patients treated for laryngeal anomalies should have a repeat VFSS at 4 months after surgery to confirm their OPD status before weaning. Aspiration of thin fluids has shown increased risk of pneumonia, although similar risk was not noted on aspiration with puree consistency.[75,101] More caution should be in place, however, while introducing thinner consistencies.

There is variation in approach among physicians regarding interpretation of deep penetration on VFSS. Although some practitioners manage deep penetration as normal, others tend to be more careful and may continue a thickened diet. Friedman and Frazier in 2000[73] studied a group of 125 patients with dysphagia and reported that 85% of children with deep laryngeal penetration aspirated and suggested a strong correlation between the two. Emphasis on clinical history in such cases is important. Deep penetration in patients with recurrent pneumonias or neurologically impaired children should be considered higher risk and be treated like aspiration. A modified approach to radiation exposure has been used by the authors' team: the use of VFSSs is curtailed in infants and children who do not aspirate on prior studies and monitoring clinical symptoms during weaning proceeds.

SUMMARY

The incidence of OPD is on the rise due to increased awareness in neurologically normal children and increasing life expectancy of infants with prematurity and complex medical issues. Although a 3-oz water challenge test is a good clinical test for diagnosing OPD, VFSSs and FEES remain gold standard tests for diagnosing aspiration. Management is best accomplished by a multidisciplinary team with experience and training in pediatric OPD. Identification of subtle pathologies that can contribute to persistent OPD and appropriate medical and/or surgical management may expedite improvement in some patients. Most patients require modification of diet and medical management of GER. Repeat clinic assessment and slow weaning strategies are required, because neuromuscular control of the pharyngeal phase of swallowing requires time to improve.

REFERENCES

1. Miller CK, Willging JP. Advances in the evaluation and management of pediatric dysphagia. Curr Opin Otolaryngol Head Neck Surg 2003;11(6):442–6.
2. Lefton-Greif MA, Arvedson JC. Schoolchildren with dysphagia associated with medically complex conditions. Lang Speech Hear Serv Sch 2008;39(2):237–48.
3. Martin JA, Hamilton BE, Ventura SJ, et al. Births: final data for 2009. Natl Vital Stat Rep 2011;60(1):1–70.
4. Rommel N, De Meyer AM, Feenstra L, et al. The complexity of feeding problems in 700 infants and young children presenting to a tertiary care institution. J Pediatr Gastroenterol Nutr 2003;37(1):75–84.
5. Seddon PC, Khan Y. Respiratory problems in children with neurological impairment. Arch Dis Child 2003;88(1):75–8.
6. Sheikh S, Allen E, Shell R, et al. Chronic aspiration without gastroesophageal reflux as a cause of chronic respiratory symptoms in neurologically normal infants. Chest 2001;120(4):1190–5.

7. Hewetson R, Singh S. The lived experience of mothers of children with chronic feeding and/or swallowing difficulties. Dysphagia 2009;24(3):322–32.
8. Sleigh G. Mothers' voice: a qualitative study on feeding children with cerebral palsy. Child Care Health Dev 2005;31(4):373–83.
9. Jadcherla SR, Gupta A, Wang M, et al. Definition and implications of novel pharyngo-glottal reflex in human infants using concurrent manometry ultrasonography. Am J Gastroenterol 2009;104(10):2572–82.
10. Pereira NA, Motta AR, Vicente LC. Swallowing reflex: analysis of the efficiency of different stimuli on healthy young individuals. Pro Fono 2008;20(3):159–64.
11. Ulualp S, Brown A, Sanghavi R, et al. Assessment of laryngopharyngeal sensation in children with dysphagia. Laryngoscope 2013;123(9):2291–5.
12. Rempel G, Moussavi Z. The effect of viscosity on the breath-swallow pattern of young people with cerebral palsy. Dysphagia 2005;20(2):108–12.
13. Timms BJ, DiFiore JM, Martin RJ, et al. Increased respiratory drive as an inhibitor of oral feeding of preterm infants. J Pediatr 1993;123(1):127–31.
14. Kramer SS. Special swallowing problems in children. Gastrointest Radiol 1985; 10(3):241–50.
15. Harding R. Perinatal development of laryngeal function. J Dev Physiol 1984;6(3): 249–58.
16. Harding R. Function of the larynx in the fetus and newborn. Annu Rev Physiol 1984;46:645–59.
17. Lau C, Smith EO, Schanler RJ. Coordination of suck-swallow and swallow respiration in preterm infants. Acta Paediatr 2003;92(6):721–7.
18. Conley SF, Beecher RB, Delaney AL, et al. Outcomes of tonsillectomy in neurologically impaired children. Laryngoscope 2009;119(11):2231–41.
19. Sheppard JJ, Mysak ED. Ontogeny of infantile oral reflexes and emerging chewing. Child Dev 1984;55(3):831–43.
20. Stolovitz P, Gisel EG. Circumoral movements in response to three different food textures in children 6 months to 2 years of age. Dysphagia 1991;6(1):17–25.
21. Byars KC, Burklow KA, Ferguson K, et al. A multicomponent behavioral program for oral aversion in children dependent on gastrostomy feedings. J Pediatr Gastroenterol Nutr 2003;37(4):473–80.
22. Durvasula VS, Lawson BR, Bower CM, et al. Supraglottoplasty in premature infants with laryngomalacia: does gestation age at birth influence outcomes? Otolaryngol Head Neck Surg 2014;150(2):292–9.
23. Rommel N, van Wijk M, Boets B, et al. Development of pharyngo-esophageal physiology during swallowing in the preterm infant. Neurogastroenterol Motil 2011;23(10):e401–8.
24. Uhm KE, Yi SH, Chang HJ, et al. Videofluoroscopic swallowing study findings in full-term and preterm infants with Dysphagia. Ann Rehabil Med 2013;37(2): 175–82.
25. Derkay CS, Schechter GL. Anatomy and physiology of pediatric swallowing disorders. Otolaryngol Clin North Am 1998;31(3):397–404.
26. Medoff-Cooper B, McGrath JM, Bilker W. Nutritive sucking and neurobehavioral development in preterm infants from 34 weeks PCA to term. MCN Am J Matern Child Nurs 2000;25:64–70.
27. Hack M, Estabrook MM, Robertson SS. Development of sucking rhythm in preterm infants. Early Hum Dev 1985;11:133–40.
28. Medoff-Cooper B, McGrath JM, Shults J. Feeding patterns of full-term and preterm infants at forty weeks postconceptional age. J Dev Behav Pediatr 2002;23:231–6.

29. Ancel PY, Livinec F, Larroque B, et al. Cerebral palsy among very preterm children in relation to gestational age and neonatal ultrasound abnormalities: the EPIPAGE cohort study. Pediatrics 2006;117(3):828–35.
30. Rotschild A, Dison PJ, Chitayat D, et al. Mid-facial hypoplasia associated with long-term intubation for bronchopulmonary dysplasia. Am J Dis Child 1990; 144:1302–6.
31. Rogers B, Arvedson J, Buck G, et al. Characteristics of dysphagia in children with cerebral palsy. Dysphagia 1994;9(1):69–73.
32. Spiroglou K, Xinias I, Karatzas N, et al. Gastric emptying in children with cerebral palsy and gastroesophageal reflux. Pediatr Neurol 2004;31(3):177–82.
33. Tahmassebi JF, Curzon ME. Prevalence of drooling in children with cerebral palsy attending special schools. Dev Med Child Neurol 2003;45(9):613–7.
34. Tahmassebi JF, Curzon ME. The cause of drooling in children with cerebral palsy - hypersalivation or swallowing defect? Dev Med Child Neurol 1993; 35(4):285–97.
35. Greenlee JD, Donovan KA, Hasan DM, et al. Chiari I malformation in the very young child: the spectrum of presentations and experience in 31 children under age 6 years. Pediatrics 2002;110(6):1212–9.
36. Albert GW, Menezes AH, Hansen DR, et al. Chiari malformation Type I in children younger than age 6 years: presentation and surgical outcome. J Neurosurg Pediatr 2010;5(6):554–61.
37. O'Neill AC, Richter GT. Pharyngeal dysphagia in children with Down syndrome. Otolaryngol Head Neck Surg 2013;149(1):146–50.
38. Smith ME, Mortelliti AJ, Cotton RT, et al. Phonation and swallowing considerations in pediatric laryngotracheal reconstruction. Ann Otol Rhinol Laryngol 1992;101(9):731–8.
39. Thompson DM. Abnormal sensorimotor integrative function of the larynx in congenital laryngomalacia: a new theory of etiology. Laryngoscope 2007; 117(6 Pt 2 Suppl 114):1–33.
40. Link DT, Willging JP, Miller CK, et al. Pediatric laryngopharyngeal sensory testing during flexible endoscopic evaluation of swallowing: feasible and correlative. Head Neck Surg 2013;149(1):146–50.
41. Munson PD, Saad AG, El-Jamal SM, et al. Submucosal nerve hypertrophy in congenital laryngomalacia. Laryngoscope 2011;121:627–9.
42. Goyal RK, Martin SB, Shapiro J, et al. The role of cricopharyngeus muscle in pharyngoesophageal disorders. Dysphagia 1993;8(3):252–8.
43. Elidan J, Shochina M, Gonen B, et al. Electromyography of the inferior constrictor and cricopharyngeal muscles during swallowing. Ann Otol Rhinol Laryngol 1990;99(6 Pt 1):466–9.
44. Chun R, Sitton M, Tipnis NA, et al. Endoscopic cricopharyngeal myotomy for management of cricopharyngeal achalasia (CA) in an 18-month-old child. Laryngoscope 2013;123(3):797–800.
45. Dinari G, Danziger Y, Mimouni M, et al. Cricopharyngeal dysfunction in childhood: treatment by dilatations. J Pediatr Gastroenterol Nutr 1987;6(2): 212–6.
46. Dent J, El-Serag HB, Wallander MA, et al. Epidemiology of gastro-oesophageal reflux disease: a systematic review. Gut 2005;54(5):710–7.
47. Martin AJ, Pratt N, Kennedy JD, et al. Natural history and familial relationships of infant spilling to 9 years of age. Pediatrics 2002;109(6):1061–7.
48. Hassall E. Endoscopy in children with GERD: "the way we were" and the way we should be. Am J Gastroenterol 2002;97(7):1583–6.

49. Aviv JE, Liu H, Parides M, et al. Laryngopharyngeal sensory deficits in patients with laryngopharyngeal reflux and dysphagia. Ann Otol Rhinol Laryngol 2000; 109(11):1000–6.

50. Richter GT. Management of oropharyngeal dysphagia in the neurologically intact and developmentally normal child. Curr Opin Otolaryngol Head Neck Surg 2010;18(6):554–63.

51. Liacouras CA, Furuta GT, Hirano I, et al. Eosinophilic esophagitis: updated consensus recommendations for children and adults. J Allergy Clin Immunol 2011;128(1):3–20.

52. Dellon ES, Gonsalves N, Hirano I, et al, American College of Gastroenterology. ACG clinical guideline: evidenced based approach to the diagnosis and management of esophageal eosinophilia and eosinophilic esophagitis (EoE). Am J Gastroenterol 2013;108(5):679–92.

53. Dauer EH, Freese DK, El-Youssef M, et al. Clinical characteristics of eosinophilic esophagitis in children. Ann Otol Rhinol Laryngol 2005;114(11):827–33.

54. Dauer EH, Ponikau JU, Smyrk TC, et al. Airway manifestations of pediatric eosinophilic esophagitis: a clinical and histopathologic report of an emerging association. Ann Otol Rhinol Laryngol 2006;115(7):507–17.

55. Garcia-Careaga M Jr, Kerner JA Jr. Gastrointestinal manifestations of food allergies in pediatric patients. Nutr Clin Pract 2005;20(5):526–35.

56. Markowitz JE, Spergel JM, Ruchelli E, et al. Elemental diet is an effective treatment for eosinophilic esophagitis in children and adolescents. Am J Gastroenterol 2003;98(4):777–82.

57. Kagalwalla AF, Sentongo TA, Ritz S, et al. Effect of six-food elimination diet on clinical and histologic outcomes in eosinophilic esophagitis. Clin Gastroenterol Hepatol 2006;4(9):1097–102.

58. Furuta GT, Liacouras CA, Collins MH, et al, First International Gastrointestinal Eosinophil Research Symposium (FIGERS) Subcommittees. Eosinophilic esophagitis in children and adults: a systematic review and consensus recommendations for diagnosis and treatment. Gastroenterology 2007;133(4):1342–63.

59. Warms T, Richards J. "Wet Voice" as a predictor of penetration and aspiration in oropharyngeal dysphagia. Dysphagia 2000;15(2):84–8.

60. De Pippo KL, Holas MA, Reding MJ. Validation of the 3-ounce water swallow test for aspiration. Arch Neurol 1992;49(12):1259–61.

61. Suiter DM, Leder SB, Karas DB. The 3-ounce (90-cc) water swallow challenge: a screening test for children with suspected oropharyngeal dysphagia. Otolaryngol Head Neck Surg 2009;140(2):187–90.

62. Boesch RP, Daines C, Wilging JP, et al. Advances in the diagnosis and management of chronic pulmonary aspiration in children. Eur Respir J 2006;28(4):847–61.

63. de Benedictis FM, Carnielli VP, de Benedictis D. Aspiration lung disease. Pediatr Clin North Am 2009;56(1):173–90.

64. Steinbok P. Clinical features of Chiari I malformations. Childs Nerv Syst 2004; 20(5):329–31.

65. Colombo JL, Hallberg TK. Recurrent aspiration in children: lipid-laden alveolar macrophage quantitation. Pediatr Pulmonol 1987;3(2):86–9.

66. Furuya ME, Moreno-Cordova V, Ramirez-Figueroa JL, et al. Cutoff value of lipid-laden alveolar macrophages for diagnosing aspiration in infants and children. Pediatr Pulmonol 2007;42(5):452–7.

67. Kieran SM, Katz E, Rosen R, et al. The lipid laden macrophage index as a marker of aspiration in patients with type I and II laryngeal clefts. Int J Pediatr Otorhinolaryngol 2010;74(7):743–6.

68. Knauer-Fischer S, Ratjen F. Lipid-laden macrophages in bronchoalveolar lavage fluid as a marker for pulmonary aspiration. Pediatr Pulmonol 1999; 27(6):419–22.
69. Stoeckli SJ, Huisman TA, Seifert B, et al. Interrater reliability of videofluoroscopic swallow evaluation. Dysphagia 2003;18(1):53–7.
70. Logemann JA. The role of the speech language pathologist in the management of dysphagia. Otolaryngol Clin North Am 1988;21(4):783–8.
71. Arvedson JC. Assessment of pediatric dysphagia and feeding disorders: clinical and instrumental approaches. Dev Disabil Res Rev 2008;14(2):118–27.
72. Miller CK, Willging JP. The implications of upper airway obstruction on successful infant feeding. Semin Speech Lang 2007;28(3):190–203.
73. Friedman B, Frazier JB. Deep laryngeal penetration as a predictor of aspiration. Dysphagia 2000;15:153–8.
74. Newman LA, Keckley C, Petersen MC, et al. Swallowing function and medical diagnoses in infants suspected of dysphagia. Pediatrics 2001;108:E106.
75. Weir KA, McMahon S, Taylor S, et al. Oropharyngeal aspiration and silent aspiration in children. Chest 2011;140:589–97.
76. Langmore SE, Schatz K, Olsen N. Fiberoptic endoscopic examination of swallowing safety: a new procedure. Dysphagia 1988;2:216–9.
77. Willging JP. Endoscopic evaluation of swallowing in children. Int J Pediatr Otorhinolaryngol 1995;32(Suppl):S107–8.
78. Hartnick C, Hartley BE, Miller C, et al. Pediatric fiberoptic endoscopic evaluation of swallowing. Ann Otol Rhinol Laryngol 2000;109:996–9.
79. Leder SB, Karas DE. Fiberoptic endoscopic evaluation of swallowing in the pediatric population. Laryngoscope 2000;110:1132–6.
80. American Speech-Language-Hearing Association. Role of the speech-language pathologist in the performance and interpretation of endoscopic evaluation of swallowing. ASHA Position Statement. 2005. http://dx.doi.org/10.1044/policy. PS2005-00112. Available at: www.ASHA.org.
81. Miller CK, Willging JP, Strife JL, et al. Fiberoptic endoscopic examination of swallowing in infants and children with feeding disorders. Dysphagia 1994;9:266.
82. Lefton-Greif MA, Carroll JL, Loughlin GM. Long-term follow-up of oropharyngeal dysphagia in children without apparent risk factors. Pediatr Pulmonol 2006; 41(11):1040–8.
83. Giambra BK, Meinzen-Derr J. Exploration of the relationships among medical health history variables and aspiration. Int J Pediatr Otorhinolaryngol 2010; 74(4):387–92.
84. Rudolph CD, Mazur LJ, Liptak GS, et al, North American Society for Pediatric Gastroenterology and Nutrition. Guidelines for evaluation and treatment of gastroesophageal reflux in infants and children: recommendations of the North American Society for Pediatric Gastroenterology and Nutrition. J Pediatr Gastroenterol Nutr 2001;32(Suppl 2):S1–31.
85. Litalien C, Theoret Y, Faure C. Pharmacokinetics of proton pump inhibitors in children. Clin Pharmacokinet 2005;44(5):441–66.
86. Gibbons TE, Gold BD. The use of proton pump inhibitors in children: a comprehensive review. Paediatr Drugs 2003;5(1):25–40.
87. van der Pol RJ, Smits MJ, van Wijk MP, et al. Efficacy of proton-pump inhibitors in children with gastroesophageal reflux disease: a systematic review. Pediatrics 2011;127(5):925–35.
88. Orenstein SR, Hassall E, Furmaga-Jablonska W, et al. Multicenter, double-blind, randomized, placebo-controlled trial assessing the efficacy and safety of proton

pump Inhibitor lansoprazole in infants with symptoms of gastroesophageal reflux disease. J Pediatr 2009;154(4):514–20.e4.

89. Miller CK. Aspiration and swallowing dysfunction in pediatric patients. Infant Child Adolesc Nutr 2011;3:336–43.

90. Gosa MS, Schooling T, Coleman J. Thickened liquids as a treatment for children with dysphagia and associated adverse effects: a systematic review. Infant Child Adolesc Nutr 2011;3:344–50.

91. McCallum S. Addressing nutrient density in the context of the use of thickened liquids in dysphagia treatment. Infant Child Adolesc Nutr 2011;3:351–60.

92. Cichero JA, Nicholson TM, September C. Thickened milk for the management of feeding and swallowing issues in infants: a call for interdisciplinary professional guidelines. J Hum Lact 2013;29(2):132–5.

93. Almeida MB, Almeida JA, Moreira ME, et al. Adequacy of human milk viscosity to respond to infants with dysphagia: experimental study. J Appl Oral Sci 2011; 19(6):554–9.

94. Montero M, Bower CM, Richter GT. Oropharyngeal dysphagia in neurologically normal children. Chicago: American Society of Pediatric Otolaryngology; 2011.

95. Friedman AB, O'Neill AC, Bower CM, et al. Impact of tonsillectomy on aspiration in neurologically normal children. Presented at Society of Ear Nose and Throat Advancement in Children Meeting. Kansas City, December 4–5, 2011.

96. Allen JE, White CJ, Leonard RJ, et al. Prevalence of penetration and aspiration on videofluoroscopy in normal individuals without dysphagia. Otolaryngol Head Neck Surg 2010;142(2):208–13.

97. Richter GT, Wootten CT, Rutter MJ, et al. Impact of supraglottoplasty on aspiration in severe laryngomalacia. Ann Otol Rhinol Laryngol 2009;118:259–66.

98. Bakthavachalam S, Schroeder JW Jr, Holinger LD. Diagnosis and management of type I posterior laryngeal clefts. Ann Otol Rhinol Laryngol 2010;119(4): 239–48.

99. Cohen MS, Zhuang L, Simons JP, et al. Injection laryngoplasty for type 1 laryngeal cleft in children. Otolaryngol Head Neck Surg 2011;144(5):789–93.

100. Mangat HS, El-Hakim H. Injection augmentation of type I laryngeal clefts. Otolaryngol Head Neck Surg 2012;146(5):764–8.

101. Weir K, McMahon S, Barry L, et al. Oropharyngeal aspiration and pneumonia in children. Pediatr Pulmonol 2007;42(11):1024–31.

Pediatric Cervical Lymphadenopathy

Tara L. Rosenberg, MD, Abby R. Nolder, MD*

KEYWORDS

- Cervical lymphadenopathy • Pediatric • Neck mass • Differential diagnosis
- Infectious

KEY POINTS

- The differential diagnosis for cervical lymphadenopathy in a pediatric patient is broad, but the most common cause is infectious.
- Thorough history and physical examination are essential to identify the correct diagnosis.
- Ultrasound is the initial imaging modality of choice for most pediatric patients who require further evaluation of cervical lymphadenopathy.
- Fine-needle aspiration biopsy (FNAB) may be used as the initial biopsy method in selected pediatric patients with cervical lymphadenopathy, possibly obviating the need for open biopsy in some cases.
- Clinical judgment should guide the clinician to open biopsy in the setting of negative FNAB and suspected malignancy.

INTRODUCTION

Cervical lymphadenopathy is common in the pediatric population, with estimates of 38% to 45% of otherwise healthy children having palpable lymphadenopathy.[1] Park[2] reported that 90% of children between the ages of 4 and 8 years have lymphadenopathy. In the head and neck, most providers consider nodes greater than 1 cm enlarged, except for anterior deep cervical (jugulodigastric) nodes, which may reach 1.5 cm before they are considered enlarged.[3,4] Most cases represent benign lymphadenopathy and are self-limited.[5,6] The differential diagnosis for cervical lymphadenopathy in children is broad, and a thorough history and physical examination are important in identifying the correct diagnosis. Infection is the most common cause of pediatric cervical lymphadenopathy and is the emphasis of the current discussion. The management of pediatric cervical lymphadenopathy is also discussed, including when imaging and biopsy should be considered.

Disclosures: No conflicts of interest.
Department of Otolaryngology/Head and Neck Surgery, Arkansas Children's Hospital, University of Arkansas for Medical Sciences, 1 Children's Way, Slot 836, Little Rock, AR 72202, USA
* Corresponding author.
E-mail address: nolderabbyr@uams.edu

ANATOMIC AND PHYSIOLOGIC CONSIDERATIONS

The neck is often considered in several anatomic subsites (**Fig. 1**), including the submental, submandibular, anterior cervical, posterior cervical, supraclavicular, and parotid (preauricular) sites. Anterior cervical nodes are located anterior to the posterior border of the sternocleidomastoid muscle (ie, in the anterior triangle of the neck) and are often divided into upper, middle, and lower groups. They may further be divided into superficial and deep nodes relative to their location along the external or internal jugular veins, respectively.[7] Posterior cervical nodes are posterior to the posterior border of the sternocleidomastoid muscle (ie, in the posterior triangle of the neck). This basic subsite classification of cervical lymph nodes established by Hajek and colleagues[8] has been reported to be the most reproducible classification scheme on neck ultrasound, which is an important imaging study in the pediatric population. Mastoid (postauricular) and suboccipital locations may also be included as anatomic subsites of cervical lymph nodes.[7]

CLINICAL PRESENTATION AND PHYSICAL EXAMINATION

A thorough history and physical examination are paramount in accurately diagnosing cervical lymphadenopathy in pediatric patients. Important historical questions should be asked to help narrow the differential diagnosis. The onset and duration of the neck mass, changes in mass size or character, recent illnesses, fever, anorexia, weight loss, night sweats, fatigue, recent travel, animal exposure, treatment (such as antibiotics), and response to treatment should all be addressed. During physical examination, mass locations (including laterality), size, mobility, tenderness, and characteristics on palpation (soft, rubbery, fluctuant, firm, warm), and overlying skin changes should be noted.[6,7,9]

Key historical information and physical examination findings may indicate a benign versus malignant origin. Benign reactive lymphadenopathy with infectious origin may

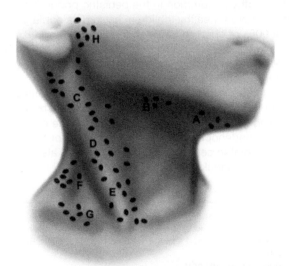

Fig. 1. Cervical lymph node subsites in the pediatric patient. (A) Submental; (B) submandibular; (C) upper, (D) middle, (E) lower anterior cervical; (F) posterior cervical; (G) supraclavicular; (H) parotid. (*Courtesy of* Dawn Rosenberg Davis, Yazoo City, MS.)

be suggested by an associated illness (viral or bacterial), such as an upper respiratory infection, pharyngitis, tonsillitis, or otitis media. Viral-associated cervical lymphadenopathy is often soft, small, bilateral, mobile, nontender, and without overlying skin changes, although this general rule may not be true with some of the more subacute and chronic viral infections, such as Epstein-Barr virus (EBV) and cytomegalovirus.[6,7]

Bacterial-associated cervical lymphadenopathy is usually of acute onset and unilateral. Bacterial lymphadenitis develops more commonly in submandibular (50%–60%) or upper cervical (25%–30%) regions compared with other cervical lymph node subsites.[7] Up to 25% of patients with acute bacterial lymphadenitis will demonstrate fluctuance on physical examination, and this is especially true with *Staphylococcus aureus* lymphadenitis.[7]

Concerning findings that may suggest malignancy include nodes that are rapidly enlarging, firm, nontender, and fixed to the skin or underlying structures. Also, generalized lymphadenopathy, supraclavicular nodes regardless of size, lower cervical nodes, increased patient age (≥8 years), lymph nodes greater than 2 to 3 cm, and hepatosplenomegaly are associated with increased risk of malignancy.[1,10,11] Associated systemic symptoms, such as weight loss, night sweats, unexplained fever, or fatigue, should initiate further workup for possible malignancy or chronic inflammatory conditions.[12,13] Lymphadenopathy present for greater than 6 months is much less likely to be malignant.[13]

DIFFERENTIAL DIAGNOSIS

The differential diagnosis for a pediatric patient with cervical lymphadenopathy is broad and should include benign and malignant causes (**Box 1**). In a study of 126 children initially diagnosed with lymphadenopathy, Yaris and colleagues[10] reported that 22.2% actually had another disease process, such as a congenital neck mass; 76.6% of the patients had lymphadenopathy associated with benign disease; and 23.4% had malignancy. The current discussion focuses on the most common etiologies of pediatric cervical lymphadenopathy, which are infectious in nature (**Box 2**). These are divided into acute, subacute, and chronic causes. Cases in the subacute and chronic categories are often a greater challenge to diagnose and manage.[5,9]

Acute lymphadenopathy is defined as lymphadenopathy that is present for fewer than 3 weeks.[3] Causes of acute cervical lymphadenopathy include bacterial and viral infections, and overall these are the most common causes of cervical lymphadenopathy in children. In cases of cervical lymphadenitis, thorough history and physical examination are usually sufficient for diagnosis, preventing the need for unnecessary biopsy.[11,14] Among these acute causes, viral upper respiratory tract infection is the most common cause of pediatric cervical lymphadenopathy.[15] This lymphadenopathy is self-limited and will improve with resolution of the inciting viral illness.

Acute bacterial lymphadenitis is most commonly caused by *S aureus* in the neonate and in children up to age 4 years. Group B streptococcus infection should also be considered in the neonatal age group. In children aged 1 to 4 years, Group A β-hemolytic streptococcus infections become more prevalent, though *S aureus* is still the most common isolate in this age group. Anaerobic infections should be considered in older children and adolescents, especially in the setting of poor dentition or periodontal disease.[6,7] Treatment should include antibiotic therapy targeted at the suspected pathogens, with a solo agent (such as clindamycin) usually sufficient for adequate empiric coverage for *S aureus* and *Streptococcus pyogenes*. Local resistance patterns of methicillin resistant *S aureus* should be examined when making this antibiotic selection. Other oral antibiotic options include amoxicillin/clavulanate,

---

Box 1
Differential diagnosis of pediatric cervical lymphadenopathy

Congenital

- Branchial cleft cyst
- Thyroglossal duct cyst
- Dermoid cyst
- Vascular malformation (eg, lymphatic malformation, venous malformation, arteriovenous malformation)
- Vascular tumor (eg, hemangioma)
- Sternocleidomastoid tumor

Malignancy

- Lymphoma (eg, Hodgkin/Non-Hodgkin)
- Leukemia
- Thyroid cancer
- Rhabdomyosarcoma
- Nasopharyngeal carcinoma
- Parotid tumor
- Neuroblastoma
- Metastatic disease

Other

- Kawasaki disease
- Sarcoidosis
- Drug-induced (eg, phenytoin, isoniazid, pyrimethamine)
- Vaccination-induced (eg, after diphtheria, tetanus, pertussis vaccine)

Data from Rajasekaran K, Krakovitz P. Enlarged neck lymph nodes in children. Pediatr Clin North Am 2013;60(4):923–36; and Kelly CS, Kelly RE. Lymphadenopathy in children. Pediatr Clin North Am 1998;45(4):875–88.

---

trimethoprim/sulfamethoxazole, cephalosporins, or macrolides. Intravenous antibiotic options include clindamycin alone, clindamycin and ceftriaxone, and vancomycin among others. When abscess formation is clinically suspected or noted on examination or imaging, incision and drainage is indicated for complete treatment in addition to antibiotic therapy. Cultures from the abscess contents should be obtained for targeted antibiotic therapy.[16] Subacute lymphadenopathy is defined as lymphadenopathy present for 2 to 6 weeks, whereas chronic lymphadenopathy persists for greater than 6 weeks. Possible infectious causes of subacute and chronic cervical lymphadenopathy include cat-scratch disease (*Bartonella henselae*), mycobacterial infections (tuberculosis vs atypical mycobacterium), EBV, toxoplasmosis, cytomegalovirus, and HIV.[5,17]

Cat-scratch disease is a granulomatous infection caused by *B henselae*. It is usually transmitted by a cat scratch or bite in the skin of a child. Lymphadenopathy may develop weeks after exposure and persist for months before resolving. Fewer than half of infected patients demonstrate systemic symptoms. Serologic testing (*B henselae* titers) can confirm the diagnosis of cat scratch disease, and excisional biopsy is

> **Box 2**
> **Infectious causes of pediatric cervical lymphadenopathy**
>
> - Viral causes
>   - Upper respiratory tract infection (eg, rhinovirus, adenovirus, influenza virus)
>   - Epstein-Barr virus
>   - Cytomegalovirus
>   - HIV
>   - Herpes simplex virus
>   - Measles
>   - Mumps
>   - Rubella
> - Bacterial causes
>   - Streptococcal infection
>   - Staphylococcal infection
>   - Anaerobic bacterial infection
>   - Mycobacterial infection
>   - Cat-scratch disease
> - Other
>   - Toxoplasmosis
>   - Histoplasmosis
>
> *Data from* Rajasekaran K, Krakovitz P. Enlarged neck lymph nodes in children. Pediatr Clin North Am 2013;60(4):923–36; and Kelly CS, Kelly RE. Lymphadenopathy in children. Pediatr Clin North Am 1998;45(4):875–88.

rarely indicated. Most patients will have spontaneous resolution of symptoms without medical or surgical treatment; however, antibiotics may hasten resolution of lymphadenopathy.[9,15] First-line treatment is once-daily azithromycin for 5 days, but other antibiotic options include clarithromycin, rifampin, ciprofloxacin, and sulfamethoxazole/trimethoprim. Surgical management is indicated only when there is a need for confirmation of diagnosis, or when the lymph node is complicated by an enlarging violaceous skin mass or chronic draining sinus, or to improve cosmesis.[18,19] Surgical management has a high probability of success in these situations.

Atypical mycobacterial infection (most commonly *Mycobacterium avium-intracellulare* and *M scrofulaceum*) typically presents with gradual onset, chronic cervical lymphadenitis in young children and should be suspected if lymphadenopathy persists despite routine antibiotic therapy. Upper anterior cervical and submandibular nodes are most commonly affected; however, preauricular and parotid nodes may also be involved. The affected nodes may become enlarged, indurated, or tender, and, in late stages of infection, often develop overlying violaceous skin discoloration and fragility (**Fig. 2**). Approximately half of patients develop fluctuance in the involved node, and approximately 10% will develop a spontaneous draining tract if not adequately treated.[20] Purified protein derivative (PPD) tuberculin skin testing may be performed but is usually negative or only weakly positive. Definitive diagnosis is made on histology showing noncaseating granulomatous inflammation, acid-fast

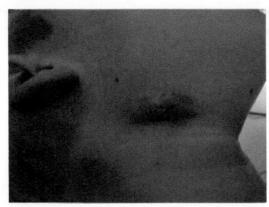

Fig. 2. Atypical mycobacterial infection involving right submandibular lymph node in a pediatric patient. (*Courtesy* of Dr Charles M. Bower, Little Rock, AR.)

bacilli, or positive cultures of the mycobacterial species from the lymph node material. Treatment ideally involves complete surgical excision of the affected node; however, curettage may be considered if there is high risk of facial nerve injury with complete excision. Postoperative antibiotic therapy should be considered to treat residual disease and usually involves combination drug therapy, such as azithromycin and rifampin.[7,9] Infectious disease consultation may be considered for medical management of these patients.

M tuberculosis cervical lymphadenitis, or scrofula, is uncommon, but may occur in individuals in the urban setting with prior exposure to tuberculosis. Cervical lymphadenitis may arise from paratracheal node extension or from direct spread of an apical lung lesion into supraclavicular nodes. It is difficult to clinically distinguish atypical mycobacterial infection from *M tuberculosis* infection based on symptoms alone. However, 28% to 71% of individuals with *M tuberculosis* lymphadenitis will have abnormal chest radiograph findings. Purified protein derivative skin test positivity is also highly suggestive of *M tuberculosis* infection.[7] Treatment includes infectious disease consultation and prolonged administration of systemic antibiotics.

Infectious mononucleosis is associated with primary EBV infection and involves pharyngitis, fever, and acute cervical lymphadenopathy, often posterior cervical in location. Fatigue is a commonly associated symptom, but patients may also demonstrate a skin rash, palatal petechiae, palpebral edema, or splenomegaly. Diagnosis is confirmed with positive results of a heterophile antibody test (Monospot). In children younger than 12 years, elevated antibodies against the viral capsid antigen is diagnostic, because approximately 25% to 50% of children in this age group demonstrate a false-negative Monospot test.[21,22] Treatment is supportive care.

Toxoplasmosis is a parasitic infection caused by *Toxoplasma gondii*, a protozoan that may infect humans because of its possible presence in cat feces or raw pork meat. This disease may present in a variety of ways depending on the immune status of the person infected. Except for those with congenital toxoplasmosis, which is not discussed in this article, most immunocompetent children who are exposed to *T gondii* are asymptomatic. Cervical or occipital lymphadenopathy is the most typical clinical manifestation. The associated lymphadenopathy is usually discrete, nontender, and nonsuppurative, and resolves by 4 to 6 weeks after onset. Diagnosis may be performed using multiple direct or indirect methods, with indirect detection of serum antibodies to *T gondii* the most commonly used method in immunocompetent individuals.[23]

Cytomegalovirus infection causes an illness similar to that seen with EBV infection. Cervical lymphadenopathy is a prominent feature, with posterior cervical nodes being the most commonly enlarged, similar to EBV. Compared with EBV, cytomegalovirus causes more frequent hepatosplenomegaly, rash, and upper airway obstruction. Pharyngitis and sore throat are comparatively more common in EBV. Cytomegalovirus infection is diagnosed through serologic assay.[7]

HIV may present in a multitude of ways. One possible presentation is with chronic cervical lymphadenopathy. When the cause of chronic cervical lymphadenopathy is unknown or when HIV infection is suspected, serologic testing for the presence of HIV should be performed.[9]

DIAGNOSTIC MODALITIES

Thorough history and physical examination are key to identifying the correct diagnosis. However, when indicated, laboratory tests and imaging may be helpful in this process. Yaris and colleagues[10] reported that 61.2% of diagnoses in their pediatric study population were obtained through history and physical examination and laboratory testing alone. The remaining 38.8% of diagnoses were obtained after biopsy.

Laboratory tests that a provider should consider (when clinically indicated) are complete blood cell count with differential, erythrocyte sedimentation rate (ESR), rapid strep test, and lactate dehydrogenase (LDH). Yaris and colleagues[10] also reported that in their cohort of patients the only laboratory test result that was significantly associated with malignancy was for elevated levels of LDH. Other laboratory tests are available and should be performed when specific infectious causes are suspected. Serologic testing is available for *Bartonella*, EBV, cytomegalovirus, toxoplasmosis, and HIV. In addition, if tuberculosis is suspected, intradermal skin testing Is performed using PPD antigen.[5,10,14]

Most children presenting with cervical lymphadenopathy will not require imaging for accurate diagnosis. However, when the diagnosis is still unclear despite a thorough history and physical examination and other diagnostic workup, imaging may be helpful. In addition, if a concerning condition is suspected, imaging may provide further characterization of the mass or assist in surgical planning if indicated. In children, ultrasound is the recommended initial imaging modality for cervical lymphadenopathy. Ultrasound has multiple benefits in that it avoids radiation exposure, usually has no need for sedation or general anesthesia, is rapidly obtained and interpreted, and is usually less costly than some other forms of neck imaging (eg, computerized tomography or magnetic resonance imaging [MRI]).[3,5,12,14,24]

High-resolution and color Doppler ultrasound can help differentiate between benign reactive nodes, infected or inflamed nodes, and those suspicious for malignancy.[1] An oval shape with minimal hilar vascularity and echogenic fatty hilum characterizes benign or reactive lymph nodes. Infected or inflamed lymph nodes may have increased vascularity, central necrosis, and inflammation of adjacent soft tissues. An absent or eccentric hilum, aggregation of nodes into a mass, irregular borders, cystic necrosis, irregular capsular blood flow pattern, and displacement of hilar vasculature are all concerning findings on ultrasound that may indicate malignancy.[1,12,25,26]

Computerized tomography or MRI should be considered when further anatomic characterization of lymphadenopathy is required for diagnosis or surgical planning. Chest radiography should be considered in the setting of suspected malignancy. Yaris and colleagues[10] reported a significant association between enlarged mediastinal lymph nodes and malignancy in their patient population.

FINE-NEEDLE ASPIRATION BIOPSY

Fine-needle aspiration biopsy (FNAB) may be helpful in the diagnosis of select patients with persistent cervical lymphadenopathy. Benign reactive lymphoid hyperplasia is the most common finding on FNAB, which is consistent with results from open biopsy. Anne and colleagues[27] and Handa and colleagues[28] supported FNAB as a minimally invasive and reliable diagnostic method with no complications in the pediatric study population. van de Schoot and colleagues[29] showed FNAB results of 86% sensitivity and 96% specificity in 39 pediatric patients with lymphadenopathy. Most (61%) patients in their study required only FNAB for diagnosis, obviating the need for further surgical intervention.

Fine-needle aspiration biopsy has several limitations in the pediatric population. For high-yield specimens and accurate interpretation of results, an experienced pediatric cytopathologist is necessary and may not be available at all institutions. Sedation or general anesthesia is often required to perform FNAB in young children. The possibility exists for more diagnostic inaccuracy with FNAB when compared with open biopsy, with some studies reporting up to 20% of FNAB samples as nondiagnostic.[9] In the setting of negative FNAB and suspected malignancy, open biopsy should be considered for definitive diagnosis, and clinical judgment should be used in these cases.[5,27]

INDICATIONS FOR OPEN BIOPSY

Despite the potential benefits of FNAB, open biopsy remains the gold standard for histologic diagnosis of cervical lymphadenopathy in the pediatric population.[1] When open biopsy is indicated, the largest node should be completely excised, with the capsule intact to preserve tissue architecture.[9,16]

In general, treatment depends on the underlying cause, allowing for directed therapy. Most cervical lymphadenopathy in the pediatric population is benign and self-limited. Therefore, clinical observation is appropriate in most of these patients. Some cases require biopsy for definitive diagnosis. Currently, no formal published guidelines indicate when pediatric cervical lymphadenopathy should be biopsied. However, multiple parameters can be used to help guide the provider in this decision-making process (**Box 3**).[5,6,14] In the general population seen by primary care providers, biopsy is required in a small minority of cases (3.2%), of which only 1.1% had malignancy in some reports.[30] In other reports, biopsy results of

---

Box 3
Parameters indicating possible need for biopsy of cervical lymphadenopathy

- Suspicion of malignancy.
- Lymphadenopathy of unknown cause that persists for greater than 4 to 6 weeks, despite a trial of antibiotics.
- Lymphadenopathy increasing in size over 2 weeks.
- Lymphadenopathy greater than 2.0 cm.
- Supraclavicular lymphadenopathy.
- Abnormal chest radiograph.
- Systemic signs/symptoms suggesting malignancy: weight loss, hepatosplenomegaly, fever, and arthralgia.

Data from Refs.[5,6,14]

approximately 15% of cervical lymph nodes in children show malignancy.[10,31] These numbers increase significantly in the patient population seen in referral centers and pediatric oncology-hematology departments, where 28% to 38% of cases require biopsy, of which 23% to 30% are malignant.[10,32,33] When lymphadenopathy is persistent for greater than 4 to 6 weeks or increases in size despite appropriate treatment, biopsy should be considered. Biopsy should also be obtained if malignancy is suspected.[10,16] A multidisciplinary approach before a biopsy is performed may be beneficial in patients whose diagnosis is unclear, because some studies have shown decreased need for biopsy performance due to better diagnosis with multispecialty physician assessment.[34]

SUMMARY

Cervical lymphadenopathy is common in the pediatric population. A thorough history and physical examination are critical for accurately diagnosing this condition. The pediatric population has an increased incidence of infectious processes as the cause of lymphadenopathy compared with adults, but neoplasms should also be considered. Judicious use of imaging studies, namely ultrasound, can provide valuable information for accurate diagnosis. Surgical intervention is rarely indicated for evaluation, but when biopsy is necessary, FNAB may provide accurate diagnostic material, possibly obviating the need for open biopsy in some patients. If malignancy is suspected, open biopsy should be performed.

ACKNOWLEDGMENTS

The authors would like to thank Dawn Rosenberg Davis for her skill and creativity in making the figure of pediatric cervical lymph node subsites.

REFERENCES

1. Larsson LO, Bentzon MW, Berg K, et al. Palpable lymph nodes in the neck in Swedish schoolchildren. Acta Paediatr 1994;83:1092–4.
2. Park YW. Evaluation of neck masses in children. Am Fam Physician 1995;51(8): 1904–12.
3. Restrepo R, Oneto J, Lopez K, et al. Head and neck lymph nodes in children: the spectrum from normal to abnormal. Pediatr Radiol 2009;39:836–46.
4. Knight PJ, Hamoudi AB, Vassy LE. The diagnosis and treatment of midline neck masses in children. Surgery 1983;93:603–11.
5. Nolder AR. Paediatric cervical lymphadenopathy: when to biopsy. Curr Opin Otolaryngol Head Neck Surg 2013;21(6):567–70.
6. Rajasekaran K, Krakovitz P. Enlarged neck lymph nodes in children. Pediatr Clin North Am 2013;60(4):923–36.
7. Kelly CS, Kelly RE. Lymphadenopathy in children. Pediatr Clin North Am 1998; 45(4):875–88.
8. Hajek PC, Salomonowitz E, Turk R, et al. Lymph nodes of the neck: evaluation with US. Radiology 1986;158:739–42.
9. Twist CJ, Link MP. Assessment of lymphadenopathy in children. Pediatr Clin North Am 2002;49:1009–25.
10. Yaris N, Cakir M, Sozen E, et al. Analysis of children with peripheral lymphadenopathy. Clin Pediatr 2006;45:544–9.
11. Soldes OS, Younger JG, Hirschl RB. Predictors of malignancy in childhood peripheral lymphadenopathy. J Pediatr Surg 1999;34:1447–52.

12. Niedzielska G, Kotowski M, Niedzielski A, et al. Cervical lymphadenopathy in children: incidence and diagnostic management. Int J Pediatr Otorhinolaryngol 2007;71:51–6.
13. Knight JP, Mulne AF, Vassy LE. When is lymph node biopsy indicated in children with enlarged peripheral nodes? Pediatrics 1982;69:391–6.
14. Nield LS, Kamat D. Lymphadenopathy in children: when and how to evaluate. Clin Pediatr 2004;43:25–33.
15. Peters TR, Edwards KM. Cervical lymphadenopathy and adenitis. Pediatr Rev 2000;21:399–405.
16. Neff L, Newland JG, Sykes KJ, et al. Microbiology and antimicrobial treatment of pediatric cervical lymphadenitis requiring surgical intervention. Int J Pediatr Otorhinolaryngol 2013;77:817–20.
17. Leung AK, Robson WL. Childhood cervical lymphadenopathy. J Pediatr Health Care 2004;18:3–7.
18. Munson PD, Boyce TG, Salomao DR, et al. Cat-scratch disease of the head and neck in a pediatric population: surgical indications and outcomes. Otolaryngol Head Neck Surg 2008;139:358–63.
19. Conrad DA. Treatment of cat-scratch disease. Curr Opin Pediatr 2001;13:56–9.
20. Chesney PJ. Cervical lymphadenitis and neck infections. In: Long SS, Pickering LK, Prober CG, editors. Principles and practice of pediatric infectious diseases. New York: Churchill Livingstone; 1997. p. 188.
21. Abdel-Aziz M, El-Hoshy H, Rashed M, et al. Epstein-Barr virus infection as a cause of cervical lymphadenopathy in children. Int J Pediatr Otorhinolaryngol 2011;75:564–7.
22. Luzuriaga K, Sullivan JL. Infectious mononucleosis. N Engl J Med 2010;362(21):1993–2000.
23. Montoya JG, Liesenfeld O. Toxoplasmosis. Lancet 2004;363:1965–76.
24. Friedman ER, John SD. Imaging of pediatric neck masses. Radiol Clin North Am 2011;49:617–32.
25. Fraser LF, O'Neill K, Locke R, et al. Standardising reporting of cervical lymphadenopathy in paediatric neck ultrasound: a pilot study using an evidence-based reporting protocol. Int J Pediatr Otorhinolaryngol 2013;77:1248–51.
26. Ludwig BJ, Wang J, Nadgir RN, et al. Imaging of cervical lymphadenopathy in children and young adults. AJR Am J Roentgenol 2012;199:1105–13.
27. Anne S, Teot LA, Mandell DL. Fine needle aspiration biopsy: role in diagnosis of pediatric head and neck masses. Int J Pediatr Otorhinolaryngol 2008;72:1547–53.
28. Handa U, Mohan H, Bal A. Role of fine needle aspiration cytology in evaluation of pediatric lymphadenopathy. Cytopathology 2003;14:66–9.
29. van de Schoot L, Aronson DC, Behrendt H, et al. The role of fine-needle aspiration cytology in children with persistent or suspicious lymphadenopathy. J Pediatr Surg 2001;36:7–11.
30. Karadeniz C, Ezer U, Ozturk G, et al. The etiology of peripheral lymphadenopathy in children. Pediatr Hematol Oncol 1999;16:525–31.
31. Fitjen GH, Blijham GH. Unexplained lymphadenopathy in family practice: an evaluation of probability of malignant causes and effectiveness of physicians' workup. J Fam Pract 1985;20:449–58.
32. Moussatos GH, Baffes TG. Cervical masses in infants and children. Pediatrics 1963;32:251–6.

33. Kumral A, Olgun N, Uysal KM, et al. Assessment of peripheral lymphadenopathies: experience at a pediatric hematology oncology department in Turkey. Pediatr Hematol Oncol 2002;19:211–8.
34. Srouji IA, Okpala N, Nilssen E, et al. Diagnostic cervical lymphadenectomy in children: a case for multidisciplinary assessment and formal management guidelines. Int J Pediatr Otorhinolaryngol 2004;68:551–6.

82. Karadeniz C, Oğuz A, Ünal E, et al. Assessment of pediatric lymphadenopathy after experience at a pediatric hematology oncology department in Turkey. Pediatr Hematol Oncol 2005;19:211-6.

83. Yaris N, Cakir M, Ozturk F, et al. Diagnostic value of lymph node biopsy in children: analysis of 134 cases and review of the literature. Turk J Pediatr 2006;48:50-5.

Pediatric Rhinosinusitis

Anthony Magit, MD, MPH

KEYWORDS

- Rhinosinusitis • Topical therapy for sinusitis • Paranasal sinus imaging
- Adenoidectomy • Complications of sinusitis • Endoscopic sinus surgery
- Nasal irrigations

KEY POINTS

- The diagnosis of rhinosinusitis is primarily a clinical diagnosis based on the duration of illness and complex of signs and symptoms.
- Imaging of the paranasal sinuses is indicated for suspected or confirmed complications of sinusitis or when a surgical intervention is being considered for chronic rhinosinusitis.
- Topical and systemic steroids have been demonstrated to have efficacy in treating chronic rhinosinusitis.
- Nasal saline irrigations, with and without antibiotics, may yield benefits for treating chronic rhinosinusitis.
- Surgical therapy for chronic rhinosinusitis should be implemented using a stepwise approach after medical therapy fails.

Abbreviations	
ARS	Acute rhinosinusitis
BCD	Balloon catheter dilation
CF	Cystic fibrosis
CRS	Chronic rhinosinusitis
CT	Computed tomography
GER	Gastroesophageal reflux
MRI	Magnetic resonance imaging
URI	Upper respiratory infection

OVERVIEW

Pediatric rhinosinusitis represents a spectrum of disease that consumes a vast amount of health care resources with an estimated $1.8 billion spent on treating

Disclosures: The author has no actual or potential conflicts of interest, including employment, consultancies, stock ownership, patent applications/registrations, grants or other funding.
Department of Surgery, Rady Children's Hospital, University of California San Diego School of Medicine, 3030 Children's Way, Suite 402, San Diego, CA 92123, USA
E-mail address: amagit@rchsd.org

Otolaryngol Clin N Am 47 (2014) 733–746
http://dx.doi.org/10.1016/j.otc.2014.06.003
0030-6665/14/$ – see front matter © 2014 Elsevier Inc. All rights reserved.

sinusitis in children under the age 12 years in 1996.[1] Managing pediatric rhinosinusitis requires a systematic approach given the difficulty in diagnosis, multiple contributing factors, and various outcome measures (**Table 1**).[2] Additionally, the wide array of diagnostic and treatment options creates challenging clinical situations when deciding on the timing and type of therapeutic interventions. Pediatric rhinosinusitis is typically categorized as acute, subacute, or chronic, with acute sinusitis considered lasting between 10 and 30 days, subacute sinusitis between 30 days and 12 weeks, and chronic sinusitis lasting longer than 12 weeks. These 3 conditions represent a spectrum of disease based on the length of illness, with each category associated with different diagnostic and therapeutic approaches. In addition to these 3 categories, specific situations warrant further consideration, including complications of sinusitis, sinusitis in the immunologically compromised host, fungal sinusitis, sinusitis in patients with cystic fibrosis (CF), and sinusitis in patients with primary ciliary abnormalities.

PATHOPHYSIOLOGY

The paranasal sinuses are air-containing spaces aligned around the nasal cavity with ventilation achieved through natural openings or ostia. Sinuses are lined by respiratory epithelium possessing cilia that serve to function in a coordinated fashion to clear secretions and maintain a sterile environment.[2] The sinuses demonstrate progressive development with the paired maxillary and ethmoid sinuses present at birth, the sphenoid sinuses showing evidence of pneumatization at approximately 9 months of age, and the frontal sinuses usually appearing between 7 and 8 years of age. The frontal sinuses continue to enlarge throughout adolescence.[3]

Sinusitis denotes an inflammatory condition that may or not be associated with an infectious process. The intimate relationship, both anatomically and pathophysiologically, between the nose and paranasal sinuses has expanded the approach to sinus disease as evidenced by the term rhinosinusitis. The path to developing bacterial sinusitis often begins with a viral respiratory infection with concomitant mucosal inflammation, resulting in obstruction of the sinus ostia with diminished aeration of the sinuses, impaired ciliary function, and stasis of secretions within the sinuses. The usually sterile sinuses then become secondarily infected by bacteria residing within the nose and nasopharynx.

Biofilms and bacterial exotoxins have also been implicated in the pathogenesis of sinusitis. Biofilms describe bacteria aggregating on surfaces within a matrix of polysaccharides, nucleic acids, and proteins.[4] Biofilms provide a protected environment for pathogens, and may be responsible for persistent disease and decreasing efficacy of antimicrobials. This explanation for the development of bacterial sinusitis may

Table 1
Contributing factors for chronic rhinosinusitis

Local	Inflammatory	Systemic
Sinus obstruction	Upper respiratory infection	Cystic fibrosis
Septal deviation	Bacterial infection	Primary ciliary dyskinesia
Nasal polyps	Allergy	Immune deficiency
Trauma	Gastroesophageal reflux	
Foreign body	Tobacco smoke	

From Rose AS, Thorp BD, Zanation AM, et al. Chronic rhinosinusitis in children. Pediatr Clin North Am 2013;60:981; with permission.

account for the fact that 0.5% to 10% of upper respiratory infections (URIs) in children evolve into bacterial sinusitis.[5,6]

ACUTE RHINOSINUSITIS
Diagnosis

Acute rhinosinusitis (ARS) is a clinical diagnosis with the primary difficulty being distinguishing ARS from an uncomplicated viral URI or a "cold." Although the signs and symptoms of an uncomplicated URI and ARS overlap, an uncomplicated URI typically begins to show evidence of improvement 7 to 12 days into the illness. ARS is diagnosed by the presence of 2 major, or 1 major and 2 or more minor criteria, which persist for more than 10 days (**Table 2**).[7] Acute sinusitis may have 3 patterns of illness: Onset with persistent symptoms, onset with severe symptoms, or worsening after initial improvement (**Table 3**).[7–10] Pediatric patients with ARS may be less likely than adults to complain of headache and fatigue; behavioral problems, such as irritability, are a more common finding.[11]

The physical examination is not specific for ACR; findings including rhinorrhea and turbinate swelling, as well as edema and erythema of the nasal mucosa. Color and viscosity of the nasal secretions do not distinguish between a bacterial or viral illness.

Radiographic imaging is not indicated for the evaluation of ARS unless complications are suspected or confirmed.[10] According to DeMuri and Wald,[10] symptoms or signs suggesting complications of sinusitis include severe headache, seizures, focal neurologic deficits, periorbital edema or abnormal extraocular muscle function. Computed tomography (CT) is not helpful in diagnosing ARS because more than 80% of patients with an uncomplicated URI in 1 study had abnormal CT findings.[12] Ultrasonography has been used for evaluating ARS with the maxillary sinuses being the primary focus of imaging. Ultrasonography may have a role in identifying the presence of fluid within a maxillary sinus with acceptable sensitivity and specificity when the 3 findings of mucosal thickening, an air–fluid level, and opacification are grouped together; however, ultrasonography has a high error rate with regard to mucosal thickening.[13] The European position paper on rhinosinusitis and nasal polyps concluded that ultrasonography had limited usefulness for the diagnosis of rhinosinusitis.[14]

Magnetic resonance imaging (MRI) is a highly sensitive means of detecting mucosal edema; however, the role of MRI for evaluating ARS even in a research setting is not clear. In a recent study, 60 children with symptoms of an acute URI were imaged with

Table 2	
Major and minor criteria for bacterial sinusitis	
Major Criteria	**Minor Criteria**
Facial pain or pressure (second major criteria necessary)	Headaches
Facial congestion or fullness	Fever (subacute and chronic sinusitis)
Nasal congestion or obstruction	Halitosis
Nasal discharge, purulence, or discolored postnasal discharge	Fatigue
Hyposmia or anosmia	Dental pain
Fever (for acute sinusitis, requires a second major criterion)	Cough
Purulence on intranasal examination	Ear pain, pressure, or fullness

From Brook I. Acute sinusitis in children. Pediatr Clin North Am 2013;60:410; with permission.

Table 3	
Acute sinusitis patterns of illness	
Symptoms	**Description**
Persistent symptoms	Symptoms continue beyond 10 d without improvement. Rhinorrhea can be of any quality
Severe symptoms at onset of illness	High fever ($\geq$38.5°C) of $\geq$3–4 d with purulent rhinorrhea
Worsening symptoms after initial improvement ("biphasic illness")	Symptoms appear approximately 1 wk after onset of illness (includes new fever, increased nasal discharge and/or daytime cough)

From DeMuri GP, Wald ER. Clinical practice. Acute bacterial sinusitis in children. N Engl J Med 2012;367:1130.

MRI. Twenty-six of these children with abnormal MRIs underwent a second MRI 2 weeks after the initial symptoms of a URI. Despite clinical improvement, 69% of the subjects continued to have major MRI abnormalities.[15]

Treatment

Observation for up to 3 days after the diagnosis of ARS has been suggested as an acceptable approach for management based on rates of spontaneous improvement.[16] Antibiotic therapy is the mainstay of medical therapy for ARS with the major challenge being the choice and duration of specific antibiotics. The choice of antibiotic should be based on the microbiology of ARS with awareness of local patterns of antibiotic resistance. A systematic review of the management of ARS identified 4 randomized, double-blind, placebo-controlled studies of antibiotic therapy for ARS.[17] Placebo groups had a range of clinical improvement from 14% to 79%, whereas the treatment groups demonstrated clinical improvement from 50% to 81%. The difficulty in applying the results of this review stems from the heterogeneity of the methodology of these studies as well as the change in antibiotic resistance patterns noted over the years in which these studies were completed. There has not been conclusive evidence of the superiority of 1 antimicrobial over another; however, owing to current resistance trends, specific antibiotics are not recommended for the treatment of ARS, these being trimethoprim, clarithromycin and azithromycin.[10]

Empiric antimicrobial therapy without identifying specific bacteria is a standard approach for ARS, given the invasive nature of obtaining culture material from a paranasal sinus. Studies in adult patients have shown a correlation between culture results from the middle meatus and the content of the maxillary sinus; however, similar studies have not been performed in children. One confounding factor with middle meatus cultures in children is that the middle meatus in asymptomatic children is often colonized with *Streptococcus pneumonia*, *Haemophilus influenzae*, or *Moraxella catarrhalis*. In addition, no recent studies of maxillary sinus aspirates have determined whether the microbiology of acute bacterial sinusitis has changed over the past 3 decades.[10] The primary source of information about the prevalence of specific bacteria and resistance rates in the local community is extrapolated from middle ear cultures from patients with acute otitis media, because these cultures are more commonly obtained as part of surveillance programs. The introduction of the conjugated pneumococcal vaccine has been associated with a relative increase in the percentage of episodes of acute otitis media containing *H influenza* with a decrease in *S pneumonia*. These changes are likely to be similar for ARS and will impact recommendations for empiric antibiotic therapy.

Recommended first-line treatment for uncomplicated ARS is amoxicillin or amoxicillin–clavulanate.[10] The standard dose of amoxicillin is appropriate unless there is a high prevalence of nonsusceptible pneumococcus in the community leading to a recommendation for starting with a higher dose of amoxicillin (90–100 mg/kg per day). Individual risk factors for resistant pneumococcus include daycare attendance, age less than 2 years, and having received an antibiotic within the past 30 days. An increased prevalence of beta-lactamase–producing organisms in the community supports the initial use of a broader spectrum antibiotic. For children who are more ill or younger than 2 years of age, the broader spectrum amoxicillin–clavulanate is recommended. Other antibiotic choices should be considered for patients with penicillin sensitivity. Published studies suggest that patients with type 1 sensitivity to penicillin can be safely treated with second- and third-generation cephalosporins.

The duration of antimicrobial therapy for ARS ranges from 10 to 28 days with 1 recommendation being to treat patients for 7 days beyond the resolution of symptoms. Persistent symptoms after 72 hours warrant a change in medical management. Antimicrobial treatment for ARS has not been shown to reduce the rate of complications associated with ARS.[16]

Side effects from antimicrobial therapy must be a consideration; 1 investigator determined that approximately one half of patients on antibiotic therapy developed adverse effects, with 20% to 22% experiencing diarrhea.[18]

Adjuvant therapies for ARS include antihistamines, decongestants, nasal irrigations, nasal steroids, mucolytic agents, humidification, nasal saline sprays, spicy food, and hot air. A systematic review of antihistamines and decongestants for ARS found no evidence to support the use of these medications for treating ARS.[19] Although there may be transient improvement in symptoms with antihistamines and/or decongestants, there does not seem to be a positive impact on the duration of the illness. Additionally, adverse side effects from these interventions may offset any positive benefits. Corticosteroids may reduce cough and nasal drainage; outcomes 2 weeks after initiating treatment showed no differences when assessing outcomes at 3 weeks.[7,20] Nasal irrigations have been associated with a reduction in symptoms and improved quality of life for acute sinusitis.[21]

CHRONIC RHINOSINUSITIS
Diagnosis

The diagnosis of chronic rhinosinusitis (CRS) in children is based on symptoms persisting for more than 12 weeks with associated endoscopic or radiographic findings.[11] The major and minor criteria used to diagnosis CRS are the same as those utilized for diagnosing ARS. The symptom complex for children includes cough, nasal congestion, and rhinorrhea. Children are less likely to articulate the presence of a headache and may present with irritability or a behavior disorder. The nasal examination can be accomplished with anterior rhinoscopy using an otoscope or a flexible endoscope because rigid endoscopy may be not tolerated by a young patient and could result in significant discomfort or injury with movement during the examination.

Plain radiographs may possess the sensitivity and specificity necessary to diagnose CRS with 1 study showing that a plain Water's view had a sensitivity of 84.2% and a specificity of 76.6% when using nasal endoscopy as the reference standard.[22] One challenge with plain radiographs is the inability to differentiate between a mass, polyp, infection, or mucosal disease in an opacified sinus.[3] CT is now the preferred method for imaging the paranasal sinuses owing to its greater ability to demonstrate complex anatomy with superior resolution of both bone and soft tissue.[14] A high false-positive rate of abnormalities requires careful correlation with clinical findings and history. Utilizing a CT scoring system, such as the Lund–McKay score increases the predictive value of CT imaging. Whereas adults without sinus disease should have a score of 0, children without active sinus disease may have a score of up to 3, with 5 being the cutoff for being consistent with sinus disease.[23,24] The opacification/development ratio is a more recently developed scoring system and takes into account the developing sinuses of a pediatric patient and has been shown to have good correlation with the Lund–McKay score.[25]

Concerns about radiation exposure have led to developing imaging protocols specifically designed to reduce radiation exposure. A higher threshold for obtaining a CT scan with greater reliance on a clinical diagnosis is also favored owing to concerns about radiation exposure.

MRI provides superior imaging of soft tissue compared with CT scans, with inferior imaging of bone.[3] Soft tissue lesions, complications of sinusitis, and extension of disease beyond the paranasal sinuses are visualized well with MRI; however, the lack of information regarding bone makes MRI inadequate for surgical planning or intraoperative image guidance for sinus surgery.

Ultrasonography is a fourth imaging modality that has been used in evaluating CRS. The lack of radiation and wide availability of ultrasonography are attractive features; however, there is a high error rate with regard to mucosal thickening and relatively low sensitivity and specificity when comparing ultrasonography with antral lavage. These shortcomings led to the European position paper on rhinosinusitis and polyps to state that ultrasonography has limited usefulness in the diagnosis of CRS and, more globally, that the diagnosis of CRS does not require imaging.[3]

Treatment

The primary treatment for CRS is medical therapy with long-term antibiotics being the primary type of medication. The recommended duration of therapy ranges from 3 to 6 weeks.[11] The choice of antimicrobial is driven by knowledge of the microbiology of CRS. Bacteria associated with chronic CRS include S pneumonia, M catarrhalis, nontypeable H influenza, Staphylococcus aureus, Pseudomonas, and anaerobes.[2] A broad-spectrum antibiotic should be chosen for first-line therapy, with similar antibiotics as used for ARS.[26] Most patient are treated empirically with a broad spectrum antimicrobial because specific cultures of the sinuses are not routinely obtained before initiating treatment given the invasive procedures needed to obtain culture material. Fungal infections as contributing factors to pediatric CRS are not well described and the use of antifungal therapy for pediatric CRS is not prevalent.

The role of aerosolized topical antibiotic therapy for pediatric CRS has not been systematically evaluated.

Obtaining culture material to guide antibiotic therapy for CRS has been investigated using maxillary sinus aspiration to guide 1 to 4 weeks of intravenous therapy. Don and colleagues,[27] reported on 70 patients treated with maxillary sinus aspiration, intravenous antibiotic therapy, and selected adenoidectomy with 62 (89%) having complete symptom relief. Several adverse events were noted in the study, including superficial thrombophlebitis, serum sickness, pseudomembranous colitis, and drug fevers.

Deckard and colleagues[28] compared maxillary sinus irrigation and culture to endoscopic-guided middle meatus cultures and antral biopsy for patients also having an adenoidectomy. Patients received an extended course of 2 antibiotics after the procedures. The endoscopic-guided middle meatus cultures group had a shorter time to the resolution of nasal symptoms than the maxillary sinus irrigation group (mean, 4.9 vs 8.8 weeks; $P = .01$).

Adjuvant medical therapy consisting of antihistamines and decongestants for pediatric CRS has been used extensively with unproven benefit. Systemic antihistamines and decongestants may provide symptomatic improvement; however, the overall duration of the illness may not be affected. In addition, the effects of antihistamines and decongestants on mucosa and secretions may adversely affect the inherent physiologic mechanisms of the nose and sinuses to manage inflammation and infection.[26]

Topical and systemic steroids are routinely used in combination with antimicrobial agents. Evidence suggests that topical steroids may hasten the resolution of symptoms of CRS when assessed in the short term, although ultimate resolution of CRS may be not be improved.[2] Including steroids in the management of CRS may be influenced by suspected or proven allergic disease. Specifically, nasal steroids should be continued when an allergic patient is being treated for CRS.

Ozturk and colleagues,[29] in a prospective, randomized study comparing amoxicillin–clavulanate with and without methylprednisolone, investigated the benefit of adding systemic steroids to oral antibiotics for the treatment of CRS. Both treatment arms showed improvement compared with baseline with the steroid treatment being significantly more effective with regard to reducing CT scores and total rhinosinusitis symptoms, as well as individual symptoms of nasal obstruction, postnasal drainage, and cough.

Intranasal irrigations with saline solutions are widely used for treating acute and chronic nasal conditions. Pediatric patients are capable of using nasal saline irrigations with various degrees of adult assistance. Few studies have assessed outcomes using saline irrigations, with the literature suggesting that, for pediatric patients without an underlying systemic disease, the addition of an antibiotic to the saline solution does not improve outcomes.[30] This study reported that subjects had 95% compliance with irrigations. Evidence does suggest that using saline nasal irrigations is beneficial; however, no prospective, placebo-controlled studies provide definitive information regarding the benefit of nasal saline irrigations for pediatric CRS. In a study of 6 weeks of nasal saline irrigations for CRS, only 11 of 91 patients were recommended for endoscopic sinus surgery after treatment as an indication of treatment failure. The addition of an antibiotic or antifungal to the saline irrigation does not seem to improve outcomes.[31,32]

GASTROESOPHAGEAL REFLUX

For a subgroup of pediatric patients, CRS may be more of an inflammatory condition than a primary infectious process. The extraesophageal manifestations of gastroesophageal reflux (GER) have been implicated in chronic laryngeal conditions, otitis media, and rhinosinusitis. The incidence of GER as determined by distal esophageal biopsies was determined to be approximately 40% in a review of 63 children diagnosed with CRS (J. Nation, personal communication, 2013) A study of 28 patients treated for GER after referral for a gastroesophageal evaluation with the primary diagnosis of CRS reported that 25 of 28 patients avoided surgery after being treated for GER with a 68% reduction in symptoms.[33] Management initially consisted of diet modification with medical therapy for refractory cases including ranitidine or omeprazole combined with cisapride. This medical management is no longer possible with the elimination of cisapride from general use. Factors predicting a positive response to treatment for GER included daycare attendance and a positive pH probe.

SURGERY FOR CRS

An array of operative interventions may be used to treat CRS. Maxillary sinus lavage to direct long-term parenteral antibiotic treatment has been investigated with evidence of improvement. Negative aspects of this management approach include risks associated with the prolonged use of parenteral antibiotics and complications related to an indwelling venous catheter.

Adenoidectomy is a commonly performed procedure used for treating chronic upper respiratory conditions, including otitis media, nasal obstruction, and rhinosinusitis. Overlap in the signs and symptoms of chronic adenoid disease (hypertrophic adenoid tissue resulting in nasal obstruction or chronic adenoiditis) and CRS pose a challenge in evaluating the benefit of adenoidectomy in treating pediatric CRS.

A metaanalysis and systematic review of adenoidectomy concludes that approximately 50% to 80% children with CRS improve after an adenoidectomy. This study was based on studies of medically refractory patients with a mean age of 5.9 years with a follow-up of 1 to 9 months. The authors noted that there was marked heterogeneity among the studies, including inclusion criteria and surgical technique.[34]

The transition from external to endoscopic approaches for sinus surgery has seemingly lowered the threshold for performing sinus surgery in pediatric patients with CRS. Various retrospective studies assessing endoscopic sinus surgery in pediatric patients provide evidence that endoscopic sinus surgery can be performed in children with minimal morbidity and without a clinically significant impact on facial growth.[35]

The long-term utility of endoscopic sinus surgery for CRS has not been thoroughly evaluated in prospective, randomized studies. One study with a 10-year follow-up for patients having undergone endoscopic sinus surgery between 2 and 5 years of age reported no difference in the severity of 6 nasal and sinus symptoms.[36] Parental satisfaction and use of antibiotics favored the surgical group. The surgical and medical groups were statistically different with regard to age at the time of surgery and severity of sinus disease.

Rosenfeld[37] published a pilot study of a stepped protocol for CRS or recurrent rhinosinusitis beginning with a minimum of 3 weeks of antimicrobial therapy with refractory cases subsequently treated with an adenoidectomy and ultimately by functional endoscopic sinus surgery for adenoidectomy failures. Subjects were excluded if they had obstructive symptoms. Resolution of all symptoms was achieved in only 27% of cases with there being a 65% to 95% chance of meeting caregiver expectations. Subjects undergoing functional endoscopic sinus surgery were more likely to be allergic, have a greater number of symptoms, or have more frequent infections.

Balloon catheter dilation (BCD) of the maxillary and frontal sinuses has recently been introduced as another surgical approach to managing CRS. The proposed benefits of BCD compared with endoscopic sinus surgery include BCD being a tissue preservation technique and resulting in less postoperative debris and inflammation. A nonrandomized study of patients treated with BCD for persistent symptoms after an adenoidectomy reported 81% of patients being treated successfully based on a comparison of pre- and postdilation SN-5 symptom scores. Postoperative imaging was not performed and 4 of the patients had an ethmoidectomy performed.[38]

BCD combined with functional endoscopic sinus surgery was compared with standard functional endoscopic sinus surgery in a retrospective review of 31 patients with a mean age of 9.3 years. There was no difference in overall improvement between the 2 groups. Significant differences favoring the BCD group included the subsequent use of antibiotics, sinus congestion, and headache.[39]

Literature assessing the efficacy of functional endoscopic sinus surgery in children is limited. A review of functional endoscopic sinus surgery in children did not identify any randomized, controlled trials.[40] Eleven studies were evaluated, consisting of 3 prospective and 8 retrospective studies. The reported rate of complications was 1.4% of a combined 440 cases with no reports of major orbital complications or cerebrospinal fluid leak. Overall success for patients having failed medical therapy was 82% to 100%. Only 1 study had an objective outcome, this being the CT scan score. Another systematic analysis of functional endoscopic sinus surgery resulted in similar conclusions with positive outcomes reported in 71% to 100% of children having had surgery.[41] Five of the studies included in the analysis specifically evaluated quality of life and reported significant improvement. This study reported a major complication rate of 0.6%, consisting of bleeding, cerebrospinal fluid leak, and meningitis.

SUBPERIOSTEAL ABSCESS OF THE ORBIT

Chandler and co-workers[42] based a classification system for complications of sinusitis on the location and type of inflammatory or infectious process related to the complication (**Table 4**). Orbital complications account for the majority of complications of sinusitis with 1 study reporting 91% of complications involving the orbit. A subperiosteal abscess of the orbit secondary to acute ethmoid sinusitis may present with proptosis, chemosis, restricted extraocular movements or periorbital edema. Therapeutic options include antibiotic therapy and surgery (functional endoscopic sinus surgery with abscess drainage), with nonsurgical therapy appropriate for a subgroup of patients. Oxford and McClay[43] published a series of 43 patients with subperiosteal abscesses and proposed criteria for medical management (**Box 1**). The authors commented that, in contrast with other smaller studies, their study supported the use of medical management in older children (ages 9 to 17 years) when utilizing specific clinical criteria. A review of medical versus surgical management of pediatric orbital subperiosteal abscesses supports the opinion that select patients can be treated medically using strict criteria and close monitoring, with surgery recommended when patients fail to improve after 48 hours of medical therapy.[44]

EVALUATION OF THE PATIENT WITH CRS

Multiple factors likely contribute to pediatric patients developing CRS. Establishing a systematic approach to evaluating the patient with CRS is intended to avoid obtaining unnecessary laboratory tests or imaging studies. The prevalence of environmental allergies in a patient with CRS is difficult to determine given discrepancies in the literature. Some authors report that approximately 70% of patients with CRS have allergies, whereas others determine that the prevalence of sensitization to aeroallergens in children with CRS is the same as that of the general population.[45–47] Identifying allergies in the patient with CRS may be done through various means. The type of allergy assessment is determined by the expertise of the physician evaluating the patient as well as access to ancillary services and allergists.

Table 4	
Chandler classification of complications in acute sinusitis	
Grade	**Symptoms**
1	Inflammatory edema: affects eyelids with or without edema of the orbit
2	Orbital cellulitis
3	Subperiosteal abscess: collection of pus between periorbital and bony wall of the orbit
4	Orbital abscess
5	Cavernous sinus thrombosis

From Chandler JR, Langenbrunner DJ, Stevens ER. The pathogenesis of orbital complications in acute sinusitis. Laryngoscope 1970;80:1418–20; with permission.

> **Box 1**
> **Criteria for medical management of medial subperiosteal abscess**
>
> 1. Normal vision, pupil, and retina
>
> 2. No ophthalmoplegia in 1 or more directions of gaze
>
> 3. Intraocular pressure less than 20 mm Hg
>
> 4. Proptosis of 5 mm or less
>
> 5. Width of 4 mm or less on computed tomography
>
> *From* Oxford LE, McClay J. Medical and surgical management of subperiosteal orbital abscess secondary to acute sinusitis in children. Int J Pediatric Otorhinolaryngol 2006;70:1859; with permission.

Immune deficiencies as a factor in CRS should be considered when a patient presents with a history of having been treated for multiple infections beyond the paranasal sinuses, including acute otitis media and pneumonia. Initial evaluation may include quantitative immunoglobulins as well as immunoglobulin subclasses. Before the universal implementation of the conjugated pneumococcal vaccine for young children, pre- and post-pneumococcal vaccination titers provided some assessment of active immunity. Pneumococcal titers may still be helpful in the young patient when including valences in the conjugated vaccine or for the older child who would be expected to respond to the polyvalent, nonconjugated vaccine.

Impaired ciliary function can be transient or permanent. Patients with primary ciliary abnormalities are likely to have chronic middle ear disease owing to the deleterious impact on clearance through the Eustachian tube. Cilia can be sampled from the inferior aspect of the inferior turbinate or by a biopsy of the tracheal mucosa. Having a pathologist available to evaluate ciliary movement from a nasal biopsy with light microscopy will obviate the need for electron microscopy if normal ciliary movement is detected. Impaired ciliary movement may be the result of an acute infectious process or a primary disorder of the cilia.

Evaluating a patient with CRS for CF despite the absence of polyps is warranted given that 1 series of patients with CF reported that only 23 of 126 (18.3%) had nasal polyps.[48] There is significant heterogeneity of clinical presentations for patients with CF with noted associations for specific genotypes. Despite the availability of genetic tests for CF and more than 1500 mutations having been identified, the sweat chloride test remains the gold standard laboratory test for CF.[49] Because the sweat chloride test is not 100% specific, the diagnosis of CF is based on the presence of 1 or more clinical features of CF plus evidence of an abnormality in the CF transmembrane conductance regulator gene or protein. The finding of expansion of the paranasal sinuses (especially the maxillary sinuses), without evidence of bone erosion on CT scan, is a strong radiographic indicator of CF (**Fig. 1**).

SURGERY FOR CF

Decisions regarding performing sinus surgery in patients with CF should be based on the specific desired clinical outcomes. Inflammation of sinus and nasal mucosa is nearly universal in patients with CF.[48] Indications for sinus surgery in CF patients have included preparation for lung transplantation and declining pulmonary function tests, as well as signs and symptoms of nasal and sinus disease, including cough, nasal congestion, headache, and rhinorrhea. A systematic review of endoscopic sinus surgery in patients with CF concludes that nasal obstruction, facial pain, headaches,

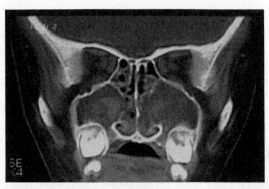

Fig. 1. Coronal computed tomography demonstrates nonerosive expansion of maxillary sinuses and ostia in a patient with cystic fibrosis.

rhinorrhea, and olfaction are improved by endoscopic sinus surgery, although pulmonary function is not consistently affected.[50] Another systematic review of clinical outcomes and quality of life related to sinus surgery concluded that functional endoscopic sinus surgery in CF patients with nasal polyps improves quality of life and sinus symptoms; however, the duration of improvement is less than that for children without CF.[41]

ALLERGIC FUNGAL SINUSITIS

Allergic fungal sinusitis is caused by a hypersensitivity to fungi and is estimated to occur in 5% to 10% of adults with chronic sinusitis who require surgery.[51] Children with allergic fungal sinusitis may present with proptosis and polyposis.[52] Therapy consists of sinus surgery to remove inflammatory tissue, polyps, and fungus. Immunotherapy, steroids, and topical therapy may provide benefit; however, strong evidence does not exist for these interventions despite their common use to manage these patients. A high index of suspicion must exist to make the diagnosis of allergic fungal sinusitis. A typical radiographic finding with allergic fungal sinusitis is unilateral sinus opacification with nonerosive expansion of the sinuses (**Fig. 2**).

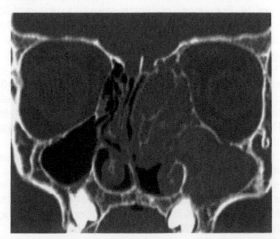

Fig. 2. Coronal computed tomography with unilateral left sided sinus opacification with expansion of sinuses characteristic of a patient with allergic fungal sinusitis.

SUMMARY

Rhinosinusitis in children is a challenging entity to diagnose and treat given the significant overlap with simple URIs and noninfectious conditions, primarily allergic disease and extraesophageal manifestations of GER. Possible contributing factors for ARS and CRS continue to be elucidated as evidenced by the identification of biofilms and their possible role in refractory sinusitis.

The diagnosis of ARS and CRS relies on recognition of a constellation of signs and symptoms while noting the duration of these clinical features. Radiographic imaging is primarily indicated for evaluating complications of sinusitis or when surgical intervention is being considered. Despite concern about the degree of radiation exposure, CT scanning remains the primary modality for imaging paranasal sinus disease.

Treatment of ARS primarily relies on antibiotic therapy with the choice, dose, and duration of antimicrobial therapy based on the local bacterial milieu and response to treatment. Management of CRS relies on antimicrobial therapy with evidence supporting the use of nasal saline irrigations and topical or systemic steroids.

A range of nonrandomized studies of surgical therapy for CRS indicates that multiple surgical interventions are available, including adenoidectomy, maxillary lavage, endoscopic sinus surgery, and most recently BCD. The level of evidence regarding the variety of surgical interventions suggests that a staged approach to CRS is appropriate with endoscopic sinus surgery being reserved for persistent disease after adenoidectomy, in the majority of patients.

REFERENCES

1. Ray NF, Baraniuk JN, Thamer M, et al. Healthcare expenditures for sinusitis in 1996: contributions of asthma, rhinitis, and other airway disorders. J Allergy Clin Immunol 1999;103:408–14.
2. Rose AS, Thorp BD, Zanation AM, et al. Chronic rhinosinusitis in children. Pediatr Clin North Am 2013;60:979–91.
3. Leo G, Triulzi F, Incorvaia C. Sinus imaging for diagnosis of chronic rhinosinusitis in children. Curr Allergy Asthma Rep 2012;12:136–43.
4. Sanclement JA, Webster P, Thomas J, et al. Bacterial biofilms in surgical specimens of patients with chronic rhinosinusitis. Laryngoscope 2005;115:578–82.
5. Aitken M, Taylor JA. Prevalence of clinical sinusitis in young children followed up by primary care pediatricians. Arch Pediatr Adolesc Med 1998;152:244–8.
6. Revai K, Dobbs LA, Nair S, et al. Incidence of acute otitis media and sinusitis complicating upper respiratory tract infection: the effect of age. Pediatrics 2007;119:e1408–12.
7. Brook I. Acute sinusitis in children. Pediatr Clin North Am 2013;60:409–24.
8. Meltzer EO, Hamilos DL, Hadley JA, et al. Rhinosinusitis: developing guidance for clinical trials. Otolaryngol Head Neck Surg 2006;135:S31–80.
9. Rosenfeld RM, Andes D, Bhattacharyya N, et al. Clinical practice guideline: adult sinusitis. Otolaryngol Head Neck Surg 2007;137:S1–31.
10. DeMuri GP, Wald ER. Clinical practice. Acute bacterial sinusitis in children. N Engl J Med 2012;367:1128–34.
11. Wu AW, Shapiro NL, Bhattacharyya N. Chronic rhinosinusitis in children: what are the treatment options? Immunol Allergy Clin North Am 2009;29:705–17.
12. Gwaltney JM Jr, Phillips CD, Miller RD, et al. Computed tomographic study of the common cold. N Engl J Med 1994;330:25–30.
13. Fufezan O, Asavoaie C, Chereches Panta P, et al. The role of ultrasonography in the evaluation of maxillary sinusitis in pediatrics. Med Ultrason 2010;12:4–11.

14. Fokkens W, Lund V, Mullol J. EP3OS 2007: European position paper on rhinosinusitis and nasal polyps 2007. A summary for otorhinolaryngologists. Rhinology 2007;45:97–101.
15. Kristo A, Uhari M, Luotonen J, et al. Paranasal sinus findings in children during respiratory infection evaluated with magnetic resonance imaging. Pediatrics 2003;111:e586–9.
16. Wald ER, Applegate KE, Bordley C, et al. Clinical practice guideline for the diagnosis and management of acute bacterial sinusitis in children aged 1 to 18 years. Pediatrics 2013;132:e262–80.
17. Smith MJ. Evidence for the diagnosis and treatment of acute uncomplicated sinusitis in children: a systematic review. Pediatrics 2013;132:e284–96.
18. Garbutt JM, Goldstein M, Gellman E, et al. A randomized, placebo-controlled trial of antimicrobial treatment for children with clinically diagnosed acute sinusitis. Pediatrics 2001;107:619–25.
19. Shaikh N, Wald ER, Pi M. Decongestants, antihistamines and nasal irrigation for acute sinusitis in children. Cochrane Database Syst Rev 2012;(9):CD007909.
20. Barlan IB, Erkan E, Bakir M, et al. Intranasal budesonide spray as an adjunct to oral antibiotic therapy for acute sinusitis in children. Ann Allergy Asthma Immunol 1997;78:598–601.
21. Wang YH, Yang CP, Ku MS, et al. Efficacy of nasal irrigation in the treatment of acute sinusitis in children. Int J Pediatr Otorhinolaryngol 2009;73:1696–701.
22. Leo G, Triulzi F, Consonni D, et al. Reappraising the role of radiography in the diagnosis of chronic rhinosinusitis. Rhinology 2009;47:271–4.
23. Bhattacharyya N, Jones DT, Hill M, et al. The diagnostic accuracy of computed tomography in pediatric chronic rhinosinusitis. Arch Otolaryngol Head Neck Surg 2004;130:1029–32.
24. Hill M, Bhattacharyya N, Hall TR, et al. Incidental paranasal sinus imaging abnormalities and the normal Lund score in children. Otolaryngol Head Neck Surg 2004;130:171–5.
25. Araujo Neto SA, Baracat EC, Felipe LF. A new score for tomographic opacification of paranasal sinuses in children. Braz J Otorhinolaryngol 2010;76:491–8 [in English, Portuguese].
26. Novembre E, Mori F, Pucci N, et al. Systemic treatment of rhinosinusitis in children. Pediatr Allergy Immunol 2007;18(Suppl 18):56–61.
27. Don DM, Yellon RF, Casselbrant ML, et al. Efficacy of a stepwise protocol that includes intravenous antibiotic therapy for the management of chronic sinusitis in children and adolescents. Arch Otolaryngol Head Neck Surg 2001;127:1093–8.
28. Deckard NA, Kruper GJ, Bui T, et al. Comparison of two minimally invasive techniques for treating chronic rhinosinusitis in the pediatric population. Int J Pediatr Otorhinolaryngol 2011;75:1296–300.
29. Ozturk F, Bakirtas A, Ileri F, et al. Efficacy and tolerability of systemic methylprednisolone in children and adolescents with chronic rhinosinusitis: a double-blind, placebo-controlled randomized trial. J Allergy Clin Immunol 2011;128:348–52.
30. Wei JL, Sykes KJ, Johnson P, et al. Safety and efficacy of once-daily nasal irrigation for the treatment of pediatric chronic rhinosinusitis. Laryngoscope 2011;121:1989–2000.
31. Wei CC, Adappa ND, Cohen NA. Use of topical nasal therapies in the management of chronic rhinosinusitis. Laryngoscope 2013;123:2347–59.
32. Fiocchi A, Sarratud T, Bouygue GR, et al. Topical treatment of rhinosinusitis. Pediatr Allergy Immunol 2007;18(Suppl 18):62–7.

33. Bothwell MR, Parsons DS, Talbot A, et al. Outcome of reflux therapy on pediatric chronic sinusitis. Otolaryngol Head Neck Surg 1999;121:255–62.
34. Brietzke SE, Brigger MT. Adenoidectomy outcomes in pediatric rhinosinusitis: a meta-analysis. Int J Pediatr Otorhinolaryngol 2008;72:1541–5.
35. Bothwell MR, Piccirillo JF, Lusk RP, et al. Long-term outcome of facial growth after functional endoscopic sinus surgery. Otolaryngol Head Neck Surg 2002; 126:628–34.
36. Lusk RP, Bothwell MR, Piccirillo J. Long-term follow-up for children treated with surgical intervention for chronic rhinosinusitis. Laryngoscope 2006;116: 2099–107.
37. Rosenfeld RM. Pilot study of outcomes in pediatric rhinosinusitis. Arch Otolaryngol Head Neck Surg 1995;121:729–36.
38. Ramadan HH, Bueller H, Hester ST, et al. Sinus balloon catheter dilation after adenoidectomy failure for children with chronic rhinosinusitis. Arch Otolaryngol Head Neck Surg 2012;138:635–7.
39. Thottam PJ, Haupert M, Saraiya S, et al. Functional endoscopic sinus surgery (FESS) alone versus balloon catheter sinuplasty (BCS) and ethmoidectomy: a comparative outcome analysis in pediatric chronic rhinosinusitis. Int J Pediatr Otorhinolaryngol 2012;76:1355–60.
40. Makary CA, Ramadan HH. The role of sinus surgery in children. Laryngoscope 2013;123:1348–52.
41. Vlastarakos PV, Fetta M, Segas JV, et al. Functional endoscopic sinus surgery improves sinus-related symptoms and quality of life in children with chronic rhinosinusitis: a systematic analysis and meta-analysis of published interventional studies. Clin Pediatr 2013;52:1091–7.
42. Chandler JR, Langenbrunner DJ, Stevens ER. The pathogenesis of orbital complications in acute sinusitis. Laryngoscope 1970;80:1414–28.
43. Oxford LE, McClay J. Medical and surgical management of subperiosteal orbital abscess secondary to acute sinusitis in children. Int J Pediatr Otorhinolaryngol 2006;70:1853–61.
44. Bedwell JR, Choi SS. Medical versus surgical management of pediatric orbital subperiosteal abscesses. Laryngoscope 2013;123:2337–8.
45. Rachelefsky GS, Goldberg M, Katz RM, et al. Sinus disease in children with respiratory allergy. J Allergy Clin Immunol 1978;61:310–4.
46. Furukawa CT. The role of allergy in sinusitis in children. J Allergy Clin Immunol 1992;90:515–7.
47. Leo G, Piacentini E, Incorvaia C, et al. Chronic sinusitis and atopy: a cross-sectional study. Eur Ann Allergy Clin Immunol 2006;38:361–3.
48. Babinski D, Trawinska-Bartnicka M. Rhinosinusitis in cystic fibrosis: not a simple story. Int J Pediatr Otorhinolaryngol 2008;72:619–24.
49. Farrell PM, Rosenstein BJ, White TB, et al. Guidelines for diagnosis of cystic fibrosis in newborns through older adults: Cystic Fibrosis Foundation consensus report. J Pediatr 2008;153:S4–14.
50. Macdonald KI, Gipsman A, Magit A, et al. Endoscopic sinus surgery in patients with cystic fibrosis: a systematic review and meta-analysis of pulmonary function. Rhinology 2012;50:360–9.
51. Schubert MS. Medical treatment of allergic fungal sinusitis. Ann Allergy Asthma Immunol 2000;85:90–7 [quiz: 97–101].
52. Campbell JM, Graham M, Gray HC, et al. Allergic fungal sinusitis in children. Ann Allergy Asthma Immunol 2006;96:286–90.

Facial Fractures in Children

Jennings R. Boyette, MD

KEYWORDS

- Pediatric facial trauma • Maxillofacial trauma • Orbital fractures • Mandible fractures
- Facial growth

KEY POINTS

- The stages of facial growth and development often determine the fracture patterns seen for each age group.
- Children are more likely to sustain an intracranial injury in combination with a facial fracture.
- Extraocular muscle entrapment is more common in children and may present with a fairly normal-appearing eye.
- Most mandibular fractures can be treated with either soft diet or a closed reduction.
- Long-term follow-up to assess for growth disturbances is needed.

INTRODUCTION

Pediatric facial trauma can be especially disturbing to the family and to the physician faced with the task of reconstruction. The expectation and goal of complete resolution to the premorbid facial structure and appearance can be a daunting task. Fortunately, many advances in the diagnosis and treatment of maxillofacial trauma have helped bring the achievement of this goal closer. Although much of the understanding and experience in regards to maxillofacial trauma comes from the adult population, one must recognize that there are additional concerns in the growing facial skeleton and that the solution for an adult may be entirely different than the solution for a child. Nevertheless, the principles of a comprehensive initial evaluation, a correct diagnosis of the injury, and a patient-based treatment plan remain the same.

GROWTH AND DEVELOPMENT

Many of the unique features of pediatric facial trauma are directly related to the underdevelopment and continuing growth of the facial skeleton. Most of the bone of the

Disclosures: None.
Department of Otolaryngology – Head and Neck Surgery, Arkansas Children's Hospital, University of Arkansas for Medical Sciences, 4301 West Markham Street, Slot 543, Little Rock, AR 72205, USA
E-mail address: jrboyette@uams.edu

Otolaryngol Clin N Am 47 (2014) 747–761
http://dx.doi.org/10.1016/j.otc.2014.06.008
0030-6665/14/$ – see front matter © 2014 Elsevier Inc. All rights reserved.

oto.theclinics.com

craniofacial structure is derived from membranous ossification, although there are portions of the skull base and temporomandibular joints that undergo endochondral ossification.[1] The functional matrix concept of growth posits that the growth of the facial skeleton is directed by the overlying muscles acting on the bone.[2] This translates to the theory that scarring and contraction of the soft tissue envelope is responsible for growth disturbances secondary to trauma or surgery.[1]

One of the key factors that relates to the incidence of pediatric facial injuries is the ratio between cranial and facial volume, which is approximately 8:1 starting at birth. This small proportion of the midface in comparison with the cranium is thought to be responsible for the higher incidences of cranial injuries in young children.[3,4] Brain growth continues to expand the cranium to reach approximately 85% of adult size by the age of 5 years.[5,6] During the same time period the orbit is growing rapidly and reaches about 90% of its adult size by age 5.[7] However, mid and lower facial growth lag behind considerably. Midfacial growth proceeds in a vertical and anterior direction and nasal growth typically does not reach full adult size until the late teenage years.[8] The mandible reaches its adult width early, by about age 1 year; however, its height is not complete until the teenage years.[8]

The gradual pneumatization of the paranasal sinuses is also thought to contribute to the decreased frequency of facial fractures, because the bone is more solid. The paranasal sinuses grow at different rates. In the newborn period the ethmoid sinuses are present but the remainder of the paranasal sinuses is relatively underdeveloped. The maxillary sinus may begin to develop before 1 year of age, but significant growth may not be seen until 5 years.[9,10] The frontal sinus is the slowest to pneumatize, starting around 2 years of age, and may not even be identifiable radiologically until around 8 years of age.[11] The frontal sinus continues to grow past puberty to reach full size in young adulthood.[12]

The unerupted teeth in the maxilla and mandible are also thought to contribute to form more dense and stable bone thus increasing the force required to produce a fracture in pediatric patients.[13] Additionally, the prominent buccal fat pads in children are thought to help disperse the force of a blow to the midface region. The bone in this region is also considered more elastic and therefore less likely to completely fracture, but more likely to result in greenstick fracture patterns.

The variations seen in the types of facial injuries that occur between children and adults are related to these variations in the structural anatomy. Initially, children younger than age 2 have much more of the surface anatomy of their craniofacial skeleton centered on the cranium and are therefore more likely to experience more fronto-orbital injuries.[14] As children age and their facial structure begins to grow downward and outward their injury patterns begin to mirror those of adults. Therefore, by the teenage years the patterns of injury are very similar to adult patients.

EPIDEMIOLOGY

Despite advancements in child safety, trauma remains the most common cause of pediatric morbidity and mortality in this country.[15] It has been reported that facial trauma may comprise up to 11% of pediatric emergency department visits.[1] However, most of these visits are related to dentoalveolar and soft tissue injuries.[16,17] Imahara and colleagues[18] examined 277,008 pediatric trauma patients requiring admission and found facial fractures present in 4.6% of cases. In regard to the total population of maxillofacial fracture patients, children younger than age 17 comprise approximately 14.7% of patients.[19] However, a large number of these patients are teenagers, because the reported incidence of fractures in children younger than the age of 5 years ranges from less than 1% to 5%.[16,19] It has been reported that the risk of a child with facial trauma to sustain a fracture of the facial skeleton increases by 14% with every year of age.[13]

The cause of pediatric facial fractures also changes with age, but most are related to falls or recreational sports.[13,20] However, motor vehicle accidents are the most common cause of severe facial fractures or fractures in those children with multisystem injuries.[18] It should also be noted that craniofacial injuries are commonly seen in cases of child maltreatment.[21]

Male gender also increases the likelihood of facial trauma, with boys outnumbering girls almost 2 to 1.[13,22] It is thought that increased participation in sporting activities or a tendency toward dangerous activities may be responsible for this difference. Interpersonal violence, which is a common cause of maxillofacial fractures in adults, is less common; however, its incidence increases in the teenage population.[23]

The most common site of injury varies according the study population. Because most studies are conducted based on data from trauma databases or from patients seen at trauma centers, many minor, isolated fractures are likely underreported, such as dentoalveolar and nasal bone fractures. Imahara and colleagues[18] examined the National Trauma Data Bank and found the most common pediatric fractures to be mandible (32.7%), nasal bone (30.2%), and maxilla/zygoma (28.6%). Mandible fractures were found more commonly in teenagers.[18] Grunwaldt and colleagues[14] examined the frequency of fractures seen at their emergency room based on age group. In 0 to 5 year olds and in 6 to 11 year olds, orbital fractures were the most commonly seen fractures.[14] However, in 12 to 18 year olds mandible fractures were the most common.[14]

DIAGNOSIS AND INITIAL MANAGEMENT

The initial evaluation of a child sustaining facial trauma is to confirm and maintain adequate airway, breathing, and circulation, just as in an adult patient. However, a child's airway is much smaller and therefore can be more prone to airway compromise from swelling or bleeding. Furthermore, children have lower blood volumes and can quickly lose hemodynamic stability.

As with any trauma patient, once the patient is stabilized it is necessary to give priority to diagnosing and addressing life-threatening or high morbidity injuries before focusing on their facial injuries. Because of the previously mentioned small size of the face and its increased bony density, a pediatric facial fracture often indicates high-energy trauma and concomitant injuries to other organ systems must be evaluated. In fact, concomitant injuries have been reported in up to 55% of pediatric facial trauma patients.[14]

Among pediatric trauma service admissions, those with facial fractures have been reported to have almost double the mean Injury Severity Score, and much higher rates of cerebrovascular injuries.[18] In these children, facial fractures were associated with a 63% higher mortality rate.[18] Given the cranial to facial proportions in the growing patient, infants and toddlers have a significantly higher incidence of severe intracranial injuries, and 57% of children younger than 5 years of age with a facial fracture have been found to have a concomitant intracranial injury.[14,18] In contrast to adults, who may experience cervical spine injuries in around 10% of cases, children are less likely to suffer a concomitant cervical spine injury (0.9%–2.3%).[14,24,25] However, concomitant ocular injuries are just as common in children as in adults and because orbital fractures are more frequently seen in children, a thorough ophthalmic examination is crucial. Fifty percent of orbital fractures in children result in ocular injuries and 0.5% to 3% of these may be blinding.[14,26,27]

The assessment begins with a thorough history and physical examination. Fear and pain can make this evaluation especially challenging in children. Interviewing the parents or any witnesses to the trauma is likely necessary. The physical examination is commonly compromised by poor cooperation from the child, and therefore, should be approached gently and with as little trauma as possible. Caution is advised in regards to sedated examinations during the primary evaluation. A comprehensive orbital examination is indicated in all patients and should include pupil reactivity and size, visual acuity if possible, assessment for diplopia, and evaluation of extraocular muscle function. Assessment of extraocular movement is even more important in children because of the so-called "white eye" syndrome, in which the eye looks otherwise completely normal except for extraocular movement limitation. Because greenstick fractures are more common in children, orbital floor fractures causing a trapdoor effect and muscle impingement are more likely to be seen in the pediatric population. These patients may also have pain with eye movement, nausea, vomiting, and bradycardia that can mimic the symptoms of a closed head injury. Enophthalmos or hypoglobus should also be noted. The orbital rims can be palpated for bony step-offs but these are often difficult to feel in the pediatric patient. Presence of lateral subconjunctival hemorrhage is a good indicator of an underlying periorbital fracture. A cranial nerve examination can reveal numbness of the V2 or V3 distributions suggesting a fracture. Facial nerve function should also be documented initially because intervention for peripheral or temporal segment injuries may be indicated. Assessing the contour of the zygomatic arch and the symmetry of malar emminences may be difficult because of the increased fat distribution of this region in children. A good nasal examination focusing on symmetry and support of the nasal dorsum and assessing for a septal hematoma should also be part of the initial evaluation. Examination of the oral cavity includes assessing for dental trauma, trismus, malocclusion, and visible step-offs. Remember that the history and physical examination guides the use of further diagnostic testing, not the other way around—this is especially true in the pediatric population.

After suspicion is raised for a fracture a radiologic evaluation is indicated. Although there are many plain film options, these are notoriously unreliable in children because the undeveloped sinuses, unerupted tooth buds, propensity for greenstick fractures, and incompletely ossified areas make identifying fractures difficult.[28] However, panoramic radiography (panorex) continues to be useful in the evaluation of mandibular fractures. Ultimately, computed tomography (CT) remains the gold standard for assessing facial fractures in adult and pediatric patients. Coronal and sagittal formatting of the images allows for improved evaluation of displacement and volume changes around the midface and orbits. CT offers the distinct advantage of providing the operating surgeon with a visible conceptualization of the reconstruction needing to occur in the operating room; this is further aided by three-dimensional reformatting.

Recently there have been significant concerns regarding excess radiation exposure in children. The multiplanar techniques that allow for excellent, detailed images also incur a higher radiation dose.[28] As a result, many institutions have been exploring protocols that lower the dose of radiation with a sacrifice in image quality. This requires a certain balance between the ability to identify subtle greenstick fractures and the need to decrease radiation exposure. Unfortunately, there is insufficient data regarding the diagnostic sensitivity and specificity of these low-dose CT scans in pediatric maxillofacial trauma. However, because many nondisplaced pediatric facial fractures can be treated conservatively, these low-dose CT scans should be considered as a means to diagnose large disruptions in the facial skeleton that require operative intervention. Furthermore, additional postreduction scans are discouraged if the postoperative physical examination is normal. For postoperative evaluation of mandibular injuries, a panoramic radiograph is recommended instead of CT.

Fronto-Orbital Fractures

Because of the increased ratio of cranial vault to the facial skeleton, fractures of the frontal bone and superior orbital rim and roof are more common in children.[1,14] Thus, these fractures are more common in children younger than 5 years of age when the skull is at its largest.[14] Because the frontal sinus does not start to pneumatize substantially until age 6, these frontal bone fractures are more accurately cranial fractures, which may explain the increased frequency of intracranial injuries in the pediatric population. Without the "crumple zone" of the frontal sinus, forces to the frontal region may result more commonly in fractures of the supraorbital rim and the orbital roof. Because of this differential anatomy, orbital roof fractures are the most common orbital fractures seen in children younger than 10 years of age.[27,29] Although a fracture of the supraorbital rim can sometimes be palpated on physical examination, diagnosis of an orbital roof fracture can be difficult without CT imaging. However, a depressed fracture of the orbital roof can result in exophthalmos or muscle entrapment limiting extraocular movement. Superior orbital fissure syndrome is also possible in severe fracture patterns. These frontal and orbital roof fractures require a multidisciplinary effort with Neurosurgical and Ophthalmologic involvement. In general, orbital roof fractures rarely require surgical intervention, except for cases with muscle entrapment or when the defect is large-which may lead to orbital pulsations or a late encephalocele.[1,30] Frontal bone fractures that are displaced more than the full-thickness width of the bone are often repaired to reduce contour deformities.[1] This should be performed in concert with Neurosurgery to evacuate epidural hematomas, repair dural tears, and manage brain injuries. These patients need long-term follow-up because continued brain growth can push apart the fracture site and result in brain herniation that may require cranioplasty In the future.[31]

As children age and the frontal sinus develops, true frontal sinus fractures are more common and are similar to their adult counterparts. However, it has been reported that frontal sinus fractures in children are twice as likely to sustain posterior table injuries and to develop a cerebrospinal fluid leak.[32] The treatment of these injuries is essentially the same as their adult counterparts. Displacement of the posterior table more than the full-thickness width of the bone is a general indication of the possibility for dural injury and mucosal displacement, thus necessitating operative intervention in the form of cranialization.[1] Significant disruption of the nasofrontal duct is another indication for operative intervention. As in adults, there has been a shift away from frontal sinus obliteration and a move toward sinus preservation and delayed endoscopic sinus surgery if necessary. Therefore, follow-up clinic visits and imaging are needed at regular intervals.

Naso-Orbito-Ethmoid Fractures

Naso-orbito-ethmoid (NOE) fractures are often considered the most challenging facial fractures to repair. Fortunately, although reported incidences vary, they are considered relatively rare in children.[28,33] One of the problems with diagnosing NOE fractures in children is that children already tend to have a low nasal dorsum and an overrotated nasal tip. Therefore, it is necessary to palpate the nasal dorsum to assess whether it is impacted into the midface. This part of the examination can help distinguish between simple nasal bone fractures and NOE fractures needing CT imaging. In addition to a saddle nose deformity, NOE fractures can also result in telecanthus from bony displacement or from medial canthal tendon (MCT) disruption. Disruption at the

MCT can be assessed by pulling the eyelids laterally while palpating over the medial canthal region. Normally, the MCT creates an area of tautness (bowstring sign), which may still be present if the MCT is not completely avulsed from the bone. Therefore, bimanual palpation of the medial orbital wall using an intranasal instrument should be performed to test for mobility of the entire complex.

The management of NOE fractures is primarily surgical with open reduction and internal fixation. However, some authors advocate for closed reduction and extraction of the impacted nose if the reduced nasal pyramid feels stable.[1] Open reduction and internal fixation is commonly approached through existing brow lacerations or via a coronal approach. The primary goals are to restore nasal dorsal height and to restore medial canthal attachments and contour. However, bony fragments are often very small and not amenable to screw fixation. Transnasal wiring to stabilize the MCTs or MCT-bearing bone fragments may be necessary, along with cantilevered bone grafts for support at the nasal dorsum. The initial surgery is often the best chance to restore normal positioning, because revision NOE surgery is difficult.[34] The normal narrowing and convexity at the medial canthal region is difficult to re-establish; therefore, external bolsters are recommended to help coapt the overlying soft tissue and splint the underlying bony fragments. Typically these are made from petroleum gauze and secured with transnasal wires or sutures to be left in place for as long as possible (usually 4–6 weeks). Nguyen and colleagues[34] have shown excellent results after long-term bolsters caused ulceration that was allowed to heal secondarily. Stenting of the nasolacrimal system is generally not necessary during the immediate repair, and long-term complaints of epiphora are rare.[35] Ultimately, there are few long-term studies examining outcomes of NOE fracture repairs in children, but the need for revision surgery is common, especially in the growing child.[36]

Orbital Fractures

Orbital fractures are common in children, but treatment strategies remain controversial. It is important to again emphasize that greenstick "trapdoor" fractures with muscle entrapment are more common in children and to be aware of the "white eye" orbital fracture (**Fig. 1**). In general, after 5 years of age orbital floor fractures become more common than orbital roof fractures.[14] Ophthalmology evaluation is warranted in all cases of pediatric orbital injury. Traumatic optic neuropathy may be discovered, which

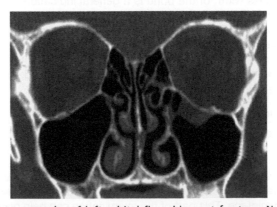

Fig. 1. Computed tomography of left orbital floor blowout fracture. Note the greenstick fracture pattern with entrapment of the inferior rectus muscle. (*From* Fraioli RE, Branstetter BF, Deleyiannis WB. Facial fractures: beyond Le Fort. Otolaryngol Clin N Am 2008;41:67; with permission.)

would warrant aggressive steroid therapy. If visual acuity does not respond or if bony fragments impinge on the optic canal, optic nerve decompression can be considered, although results have been mixed in pediatric trauma patients.[37,38]

Fractures of the orbital floor remain controversial in regard to which ones require repair. However, most surgeons agree on the criteria of large floor defects (>1 cm^2) or extraocular muscle entrapment.[1,39] Muscle entrapment is the most pressing cause for early repair, and those with an oculocardiac reflex require emergent repair. Children heal quickly; therefore, muscle entrapment in a child may result in fibrosis and shortening of the muscle within a couple days. As a result, diplopia can be present for months after the initial injury, or it may be permanent.[40] Fractures of the medial wall should also be considered. A transcaruncular approach can allow for access to place an implant to reduce the intraorbital volume; however, some surgeons prefer to compensate with augmentation of the orbital floor instead.[39]

Repair of an orbital floor fracture can be performed through a variety of approaches; however, the transconjunctival approach is favored from a cosmetic standpoint and also may reduce the incidence of postoperative ectropion.[41] A variety of implants can be used to reconstruct the orbital floor. Split calvarial bone grafts have classically been used, and some surgeons continue to advocate for their use in children younger than 7 years of age who may continue to undergo further orbital growth.[1] Otherwise, titanium and porous polyethylene are commonly used with significantly less donor site morbidity.

Nasal Fractures

Nasal bone fractures are suspected to be the most common facial bone fracture in children, because their true incidence is very likely underreported in the literature.[42] Because these fractures are often isolated and occur without concomitant injuries, they are more likely to be treated on an outpatient basis. These fractures can also remain undiagnosed if swelling obscures the assessment of nasal bone symmetry. An initial intranasal examination is key to diagnosing airway obstruction and to defining concomitant septal fracture or septal hematoma. Most nasal bone fractures can be diagnosed on physical examination alone, thus conserving radiologic examinations for those patients in whom the history or physical examination warrants further investigation. The finding of a septal hematoma should prompt urgent surgical evacuation to prevent cartilage necrosis and saddle nose deformity.

Long-term growth disturbance is a cause for concern. The septum is thought to harbor important growth zones, which if injured may result in a lack of nasal projection.[43] Because full growth of the nose is not achieved until age 16 to 18 years in girls and 18 to 20 years in boys, damage to these growth centers from either the initial trauma or from surgery can have long-lasting effects.

Early closed reduction of nasal bone fractures within a few days of the injury is usually recommended.[44,45] This can be accomplished under sedation or general anesthesia. However, the results of closed nasal reduction are often dissatisfying for the surgeon and the patient. Grymer and colleagues[46] examined the long-term results of nasal bone fractures treated in childhood, and found that by adulthood these patients tended to have a higher incidence of dorsal humps, saddle nose deformities, and deviations of the dorsum, despite most patients being satisfied with the outcomes after the initial closed reduction. Therefore, there is some indication that despite best efforts to correct these injuries, there may be deformities that develop gradually with growth. Parents should be counseled regarding this possibility.

Septal fractures can also be managed conservatively with a closed reduction technique. In those children with significant nasal airway obstruction, a limited, cartilage-sparing septoplasty can be performed, although the risk of growth impairment is always a concern. If the nasal obstruction is without secondary consequences then delay until the teenage years is recommended.

An unusual fracture pattern that is typically only seen in children is that of the "open book."[42] Direct frontal impact to the nose can cause blood to develop and spread apart the nasal bones centrally (**Fig. 2**). This is suspected to occur in children more readily because of incomplete fusion of the nasal bones at the midline. This type of injury has been treated in young children with the conservative technique of frequent bimanual compression in the clinic.[47]

Midface and Zygomaticomaxillary Fractures

Because of the aforementioned small paranasal sinuses and unerupted tooth buds in children, midface fractures of the classical Le Fort patterns are unusual. Therefore, they are usually the result of high-impact trauma, such as motor vehicle accidents.[48] Goals of repair are similar to those in adults, such as restoration of facial contour, height, and dental occlusion. Many fractures in children are nondisplaced and can be treated conservatively. Maxillomandibular fixation can be applied to stabilize many of these fractures. Despite concerns that subperiosteal elevation can cause long-term maxillary growth restriction, fractures resulting in significant displacement of the buttresses typically require open reduction and internal fixation.[49] Screw placement can injure the unerupted tooth follicles and should be used judiciously and as far away from the dentition as possible. In cases of severely comminuted fractures at the buttresses, primary bone grafting can be considered.[3] Because of growth concerns, some authors recommend removing titanium hardware at 3 to 4 months postoperatively.[50] Resorbable plating can also be effectively used to stabilize midface fractures, especially at the zygomaticomaxillary buttress where the elevated profile of the plates is less noticeable.

Indications for zygomaticomaxillary complex fracture repair in children are similar to adult indications: mainly cheek asymmetry and functional concerns related to the orbital component. Nondisplaced fractures can be observed, but comminuted fractures should be addressed with fixation. Minimally invasive approaches, such as the transconjunctival approach to the orbital rim, are recommended. In children, one-point fixation of noncomminuted zygomaticomaxillary complex fractures has been reported as sufficient.[39] Outcome studies of one- and two-point fixation have

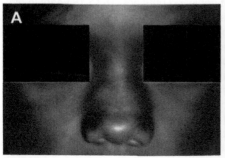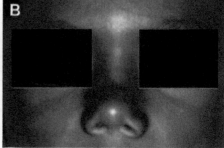

Fig. 2. "Open-book" nasal fracture pattern that can be encountered in pediatric patients. (*A*) Splayed appearance of the nasal bones on frontal view. (*B*) Treatment of splayed nasal bones with sequential manual compression in clinic and no surgical intervention. (*Courtesy* of Dr Frederick Stucker, Shreveport, LA.)

generally not included children, but given the rapid bone healing of children, the findings of these studies should translate well to the pediatric population.[51,52]

Mandibular Fractures

Mandible fractures are commonly reported as the most frequent facial fracture seen in children, and many more may go undiagnosed.[18,53,54] The management of pediatric mandibular fractures presents several challenges related to unerupted teeth, temporomandibular joint dysfunction, and facial growth disturbances. In children, not every fracture needs an open reduction and internal fixation. Instead, the surgeon must contemplate the interplay of fracture location to bony growth and dental development, and chose an intervention that lessens the potential for long-term impairment and deformity (**Fig. 3**). In contrast to adults, many pediatric mandibular fractures can be treated with conservative measures, such as soft diet alone.

The condyle is the most frequently injured portion of the mandible.[54] However, the location of the condylar fracture changes with age, because children younger than 5 years are more likely to sustain condylar head fractures, whereas older adolescents are more likely to sustain condylar neck fractures.[55,56] Symphaseal fractures are the second most commonly seen in all age groups.[57] However, as adolescents get older mandibular fracture patterns begin to resemble adult fractures and body and angle fractures can be encountered.[57]

In very young children, fractures that are nondisplaced and that do not affect dental occlusion can be treated with soft diet.[3,57] Noncompliance with diet restrictions is less of a problem in children than adults, since parents can control the child's diet. Many nondisplaced condylar fractures can therefore be treated with this conservative approach. However, displaced fractures of the condyle should undergo closed reduction.[1,22,57] Intermaxillary fixation can then be applied to further stabilize the fractured segments; however, only a brief period (7–10 days) of intermaxillary fixation is recommended because prolonged intermaxillary fixation can cause severe ankylosis in children.[1,3,57,58]

Generalized Algorithm for Management of Pediatric Mandible Fractures

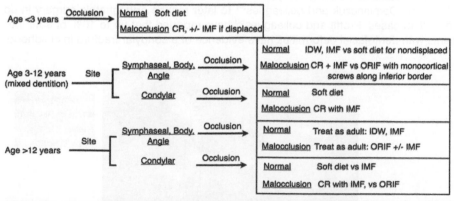

Fig. 3. Algorithm for the treatment of mandible fractures in children. These are general considerations and may not be appropriate for all patients. The degree of fracture displacement necessitates consideration of a more aggressive fixation approach. CR, closed reduction; IDW, interdental fixation; IMF, intermaxillary fixation; ORIF, open reduction internal fixation.

Displaced fractures of other regions of the mandible can be treated with closed reduction and dental stabilization or open reduction and internal fixation. In general, an attempt at a closed technique is recommended for younger children (<6 years of age), whereas teenagers can be treated with open reduction and internal fixation similar to adults. If closed reduction is successful, there are many methods to achieve stability including traditional arch bars, wire ligatures, or Risdon cables.[1] Acrylic splints fixated with circum-mandibular wires are also a good option if the deciduous dentition does not support wiring. However, the child must undergo general anesthesia up to three times because the mold must first be made, the splint wired in place, and then the splint removed. In general, these types of fixation can be removed after 3 weeks.[57]

Open reduction internal fixation is a viable and necessary option in many patients. In general, open reduction internal fixation is applied to displaced fractures of the tooth-bearing portion of the mandible that cannot be properly reduced or stabilized with closed techniques.[57] Multiple fracture sites or comminuted fractures are another indication.[59] As mentioned previously, if the patient has already reached skeletal and dental maturity, open reduction internal fixation can be applied similar to an adult patient. In a recent study, Smith and colleagues[59] report on using open reduction internal fixation on 75% of mandible fractures in children older than 12 years of age.

The use of internal fixation in younger children with developing dentition requires that screws be placed to avoid damaging the unerupted teeth (**Fig. 4**). Single mini-plate fixation is typically all that is necessary for stabilization in children.[57,60] Fixation at the inferior border of the mandible with monocortical screws avoids damaging the unerupted tooth buds. Additional stabilization to prevent rotation at the superior border can be obtained with an arch bar. Avoiding placement of permanent rigid fixation across the midline of the mandible in young children is recommended, because there is a potential for growth restriction.[61,62] Although some surgeons recommend hardware removal after a few months, this practice is controversial and objective evidence is lacking.[57,62,63]

However, long-term problems with mandibular growth are a major concern. Growth disturbance following mandibular fractures is more commonly encountered with fractures of the condyle because this area is considered the primary growth center.[53,58,64] Fractures sustained during the years of active vertical growth have been demonstrated by Demianczuk and colleagues[58] to later require orthognathic surgery in up to 24% of cases. Proffit and colleagues[53] have reported that up to 10% of adult patients with dentofacial deformities have evidence of a condylar fracture in childhood.

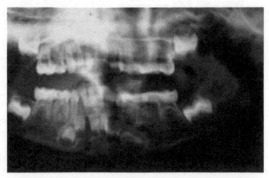

Fig. 4. Panorex radiograph demonstrating unerupted tooth buds of the pediatric mandible. Note the particularly low-lying position of the tooth buds in the parasymphaseal region.

Therefore, parents of children with condylar fractures should be counseled that growth disturbance and need for future orthognathic procedures may be needed. Additionally, there have been concerns about growth in the tooth-bearing portion of the mandible following rigid fixation, although recent animal studies have suggested no effect on growth.[65,66] Regardless, these concerns have stimulated interest in applying bioresorbable fixation to pediatric mandibular fractures.

RESORBABLE FIXATION

Perhaps the greatest area of current debate in the management of pediatric facial trauma is use of bioresorbable fixation hardware (**Fig. 5**). Its widespread use in cranial vault remodeling has spurred interest in applying it to maxillofacial fractures to address the same concerns about rigid titanium fixation causing growth disturbances. Features, such as less muscular load on the hardware and rapid bony healing, make resorbable plating ideal for the pediatric population. The downsides to resorbable hardware are that they have less inherent strength, the plates are more bulky, the screws require tapping, the plates have little memory to allow for overbending, and inflammatory reactions may occur.[57,62]

Resorbable hardware has been used successfully for maxillofacial fractures in children.[50,67] Most notably, Eppley[50] reported on its use in 44 pediatric patients younger than 10 years of age with no reported implant-related complications. However, the same advantages achieved in cranial vault surgery do not necessarily translate into the face, because titanium fixation is not typically placed in regions of such rapid growth or over bony suture lines. Pediatric facial fractures are also commonly managed with judicious use of fixation and closed techniques in very young patients. Therefore, the use of resorbable fixation in maxillofacial fractures has been questioned because there is not a significant amount of data indicating that titanium fixation results in maxillofacial growth restriction.[62,65,66] Furthermore, a recent Cochrane review questioned whether resorbable hardware was as effective as titanium hardware.[68] Therefore, although many surgeons are exploring the use of resorbable fixation hardware in pediatric facial fractures, definitive indications and recommendations for its use cannot be made at this time.

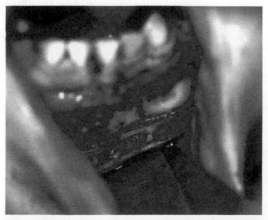

Fig. 5. Resorbable plate fixation used for a parasymphaseal mandibular fracture. (*From* Eppley BL. Use of resorbable plates and screws in pediatric facial fractures. J Oral Maxillofac Surg 2005;63(3):386; with permission.)

SUMMARY

Although maxillofacial fractures are not as common in children as in adults, the constantly growing facial skeleton adds several levels of complexity to the treatment of these injuries. Fortunately, children heal well and conservative techniques can frequently be used. Growth disturbances from the initial trauma and from the surgeon's interventions are difficult to predict, but avoiding aggressive dissection and extensive fixation is recommended. Long-term follow-up with a multidisciplinary team is often needed to manage the future changes in facial development that may occur with these injuries.

REFERENCES

1. Morris C, Kushner GM, Tiwana PS. Facial skeletal trauma in the growing patient. Oral Maxillofac Surg Clin North Am 2012;24(3):351–64.
2. Moss ML. The functional matrix hypothesis revisited. 1. The role of mechanotransduction. Am J Orthod Dentofacial Orthop 1997;112(1):8–11.
3. Cole P, Kaufman Y, Hollier LH Jr. Managing the pediatric facial fracture. Craniomaxillofac Trauma Reconstr 2009;2(2):77–83.
4. Gussack GS, Luterman A, Powell RW, et al. Pediatric maxillofacial trauma: unique features in diagnosis and treatment. Laryngoscope 1987;97(8 Pt 1): 925–30.
5. Sgouros S, Goldin JH, Hockley AD, et al. Intracranial volume change in childhood. J Neurosurg 1999;91(4):610–6.
6. Farkas LG, Posnick JC, Hreczko TM. Anthropometric growth study of the head. Cleft Palate Craniofac J 1992;29(4):303–8.
7. Farkas LG, Posnick JC, Hreczko TM, et al. Growth patterns in the orbital region: a morphometric study. Cleft Palate Craniofac J 1992;29(4):315–8.
8. Farkas LG, Posnick JC, Hreczko TM. Growth patterns of the face: a morphometric study. Cleft Palate Craniofac J 1992;29(4):308–15.
9. Shah RK, Dhingra JK, Carter BL, et al. Paranasal sinus development: a radiographic study. Laryngoscope 2003;113(2):205–9.
10. Wolf G, Anderhuber W, Kuhn F. Development of the paranasal sinuses in children: implications for paranasal sinus surgery. Ann Otol Rhinol Laryngol 1993; 102(9):705–11.
11. Yavuzer R, Sari A, Kelly CP, et al. Management of frontal sinus fractures. Plast Reconstr Surg 2005;115(6):79e–93e.
12. Brown WA, Molleson TI, Chinn S. Enlargement of the frontal sinus. Ann Hum Biol 1984;11(3):221–6.
13. Gassner R, Tuli T, Hachi O, et al. Craniomaxillofacial trauma in children: a review of 3,385 cases with 6,060 injuries in 10 years. J Oral Maxillofac Surg 2004;62(4): 399–407.
14. Grunwaldt L, Smith DM, Zuckerbaun NS, et al. Pediatric facial fractures: demographics, injury patterns, and associated injuries in 772 consecutive patients. Plast Reconstr Surg 2011;128(6):1263–71.
15. Heron M. Deaths: leading causes for 2009. Natl Vital Stat Rep 2012;61(7): 1–96.
16. Gassner R, Tuli T, Hachi O, et al. Cranio-maxillofacial trauma: a 10 year review of 9,543 cases with 21,067 injuries. J Craniomaxillofac Surg 2003;31(1):51–61.
17. Alvi A, Doherty T, Lewen G. Facial fractures and concomitant injuries in trauma patients. Laryngoscope 2003;113(1):102–6.

18. Imahara SD, Hopper RA, Wang J, et al. Patterns and outcomes of pediatric facial fractures in the United States: a survey of the National Trauma Data Bank. J Am Coll Surg 2008;207(5):710–6.
19. Vyas RM, Dickinson BP, Wasson KL, et al. Pediatric facial fractures: current national incidence, distribution, and health care resource use. J Craniofac Surg 2008;19(2):339–49.
20. Posnick JC. Management of facial fractures in children and adolescents. Ann Plast Surg 1994;33(4):442–57.
21. Horswell BB, Istfan S. Child maltreatment. Oral Maxillofac Surg Clin North Am 2012;24(3):511–7.
22. Posnick JC, Wells M, Pron GE. Pediatric facial fractures: evolving patterns of treatment. J Oral Maxillofac Surg 1993;51(8):836–44.
23. McGraw BL, Cole RR. Pediatric maxillofacial trauma. Age-related variations in injury. Arch Otolaryngol Head Neck Surg 1990;116(1):41–5.
24. Mithani SK, St-Hilaire H, Brooke BS, et al. Predictable patterns of intracranial and cervical spine injury in craniomaxillofacial trauma: analysis of 4786 patients. Plast Reconstr Surg 2009;123(4):1293–301.
25. Thoren H, Schaller B, Suominen AL, et al. Occurrence and severity of concomitant injuries in other areas than the face in children with mandibular and midfacial fractures. J Oral Maxillofac Surg 2012;70(1):92–6.
26. Holt GR, Holt JE. Incidence of eye injuries in facial fractures: an analysis of 727 cases. Otolaryngol Head Neck Surg 1983;91(3):276–9.
27. Hatton MP, Watkins LM, Rubin PA. Orbital fractures in children. Ophthal Plast Reconstr Surg 2001;17(3):174–9.
28. Alcala-Galiano A, Arribas-Garcia IJ, Martin-Perez MA, et al. Pediatric facial fractures: children are not just small adults. Radiographics 2008;28(2):441–61.
29. Koltai PJ, Amjad I, Meyer D, et al. Orbital fractures in children. Arch Otolaryngol Head Neck Surg 1995;121(12):1375–9.
30. Messinger A, Radkowski MA, Greenwald MJ, et al. Orbital roof fractures in the pediatric population. Plast Reconstr Surg 1989;84(2):213–6.
31. Dufresne CR, Manson PN. Pediatric craniofacial trauma: challenging pediatric cases-craniofacial trauma. Craniomaxillofac Trauma Reconstr 2011;4(2): 73–84.
32. Wright DL, Hoffman HT, Hoyt DB. Frontal sinus fractures in the pediatric population. Laryngoscope 1992;102(11):1215–9.
33. Liau JY, Woodlief J, van Aalst JA. Pediatric nasoorbitoethmoid fractures. J Craniofac Surg 2011;22(5):1834–8.
34. Nguyen M, Koshy JC, Hollier LH Jr. Pearls of nasoorbitoethmoid trauma management. Semin Plast Surg 2010;24(4):383–8.
35. Gruss JS, Hurwitz JJ, Nik NA, et al. The pattern and incidence of nasolacrimal injury in naso-orbital-ethmoid fractures: the role of delayed assessment and dacryocystorhinostomy. Br J Plast Surg 1985;38(1):116–21.
36. Singh DJ, Bartlett SP. Pediatric craniofacial fractures: long-term consequences. Clin Plast Surg 2004;31(3):499–518.
37. Goldenberg-Cohen N, Miller NR, Repka MX. Traumatic optic neuropathy in children and adolescents. J AAPOS 2004;8(1):20–7.
38. Gupta AK, Gupta AK, Gupta A, et al. Traumatic optic neuropathy in pediatric population: early intervention or delayed intervention? Int J Pediatr Otorhinolaryngol 2007;71(4):559–62.
39. Hatef DA, Cole PD, Hollier LH Jr. Contemporary management of pediatric facial trauma. Curr Opin Otolaryngol Head Neck Surg 2009;17(4):308–14.

40. Criden MR, Ellis FJ. Linear nondisplaced orbital fractures with muscle entrapment. J AAPOS 2007;11(2):142–7.

41. Ridgway EB, Chen C, Colakoglu S, et al. The incidence of lower eyelid malposition after facial fracture repair: a retrospective study and meta-analysis comparing subtarsal, subciliary, and transconjunctival incisions. Plast Reconstr Surg 2009;124(5):1578–86.

42. Wright RJ, Murakami CS, Ambro BT. Pediatric nasal injuries and management. Facial Plast Surg 2011;27(5):483–90.

43. Verwoerd CD, Verwoerd-Verhoef HL. Rhinosurgery in children: basic concepts. Facial Plast Surg 2007;23(4):219–30.

44. Yilmaz MS, Guven M, Kayabasoglu G, et al. Efficacy of closed reduction for nasal fractures in children. Br J Oral Maxillofac Surg 2013;51:e256–8.

45. Rohrich RJ, Adams WP Jr. Nasal fracture management: minimizing secondary nasal deformities. Plast Reconstr Surg 2000;106(2):266–73.

46. Grymer LF, Gutierrez C, Stoksted P. Nasal fractures in children: influence on the development of the nose. J Laryngol Otol 1985;99(8):735–9.

47. Stucker FJ, Bryarly RC, Shockley WW. Management of nasal trauma in children. Arch Otolaryngol 1984;110(3):190–2.

48. Iizuka T, Thoren H, Annino DJ Jr, et al. Midfacial fractures in pediatric patients. Frequency, characteristics, and causes. Arch Otolaryngol Head Neck Surg 1995;121(12):1366–71.

49. Wheeler J, Phillips J. Pediatric facial fractures and potential long-term growth disturbances. Craniomaxillofac Trauma Reconstr 2011;4(1):43–52.

50. Eppley BL. Use of resorbable plates and screws in pediatric facial fractures. J Oral Maxillofac Surg 2005;63(3):385–91.

51. Kim ST, Go DH, Jung JH, et al. Comparison of 1-point fixation with 2-point fixation in treating tripod fractures of the zygoma. J Oral Maxillofac Surg 2011; 69(11):2848–52.

52. Kim JH, Lee JH, Hong SM, et al. The effectiveness of 1-point fixation for zygomaticomaxillary complex fractures. Arch Otolaryngol Head Neck Surg 2012; 138(9):828–32.

53. Proffit WR, Vig KW, Turvey TA. Early fracture of the mandibular condyles: frequently an unsuspected cause of growth disturbances. Am J Orthod 1980; 78(1):1–24.

54. Ferreira PC, Amarante JM, Silva PN, et al. Retrospective study of 1251 maxillofacial fractures in children and adolescents. Plast Reconstr Surg 2005;115(6): 1500–8.

55. Thoren H, Iizuka T, Hallikainen D, et al. An epidemiological study of patterns of condylar fractures in children. Br J Oral Maxillofac Surg 1997;35(5):306–11.

56. Chao MT, Losee JE. Complications in pediatric facial fractures. Craniomaxillofac Trauma Reconstr 2009;2(2):103–12.

57. Goth S, Sawatari Y, Peleg M. Management of pediatric mandible fractures. J Craniofac Surg 2012;23(1):47–56.

58. Demianczuk AN, Verchere C, Phillips JH. The effect on facial growth of pediatric mandibular fractures. J Craniofac Surg 1999;10(4):323–8.

59. Smith DM, Bykowski MR, Cray JJ, et al. 215 mandible fractures in 120 children: demographics, treatment, outcomes, and early growth data. Plast Reconstr Surg 2013;131(6):1348–58.

60. Cole P, Kaufman Y, Izaddoost S, et al. Principles of pediatric mandibular fracture management. Plast Reconstr Surg 2009;123(3):1022–4.

61. Zimmermann CE, Troulis MJ, Kaban LB. Pediatric facial fractures: recent advances in prevention, diagnosis and management. Int J Oral Maxillofac Surg 2006;35(1):2–13.
62. Siy RW, Brown RH, Koshy JC, et al. General management considerations in pediatric facial fractures. J Craniofac Surg 2011;22(4):1190–5.
63. Smartt JM Jr, Low DW, Bartlett SP. The pediatric mandible: II. Management of traumatic injury or fracture. Plast Reconstr Surg 2005;116(2):28e–41e.
64. Smartt JM Jr, Low DW, Bartlett SP. The pediatric mandible: I. A primer on growth and development. Plast Reconstr Surg 2005;116(1):14e–23e.
65. Fernandez H, Osorio J, Russi MT, et al. Effects of internal rigid fixation on mandibular development in growing rabbits with mandibular fractures. J Oral Maxillofac Surg 2012;70(10):2368–74.
66. Bayram B, Yilmaz AC, Ersoz E, et al. Does the titanium plate fixation of symphaseal fracture affect mandibular growth? J Craniofac Surg 2012;23(6):e601–3.
67. Yerit KC, Hainich S, Enislidis G, et al. Biodegradable fixation of mandibular fractures in children: stability and early results. Oral Surg Oral Med Oral Pathol Oral Radiol Endod 2005;100(1):17–24.
68. Dorri M, Nasser M, Oliver R. Resorbable versus titanium plates for facial fractures. Cochrane Database Syst Rev 2009;(1):CD007158.

Pediatric Sialadenitis

Carrie L. Francis, MD[a,b,*], Christopher G. Larsen, MD[a,b]

KEYWORDS

- Pediatric sialadenitis • Salivary gland disease • Juvenile recurrent parotitis
- Submandibular sialadenitis • Salivary duct calculi • Sialolithiasis • Sialendoscopy
- Mumps

KEY POINTS

- Viral parotitis and juvenile recurrent parotitis (JRP) are the two most common etiologies of sialadenitis in children.
- Mumps should be distinguished from other causes of sialadenitis; however, the incidence of mumps has significantly declined as a result of vaccination efforts.
- Salivary stones are uncommon in children but may cause chronic obstructive sialadenitis.
- Sialendoscopy has emerged as the leading diagnostic and intervention technique for pediatric sialadenitis.

INTRODUCTION

Sialadenitis is defined as inflammation of the salivary glands. The saliva they produce is essential for the normal functioning and health of the mouth. Sialadenitis in the pediatric population accounts for up to 10% of all salivary gland disease.[1] Viral parotitis and juvenile recurrent parotitis (JRP) are the two most common causes.

Viral sialadenitis is most commonly caused by the paramyxovirus. Mumps should be distinguished from other causes of sialadenitis; however, the incidence has significantly declined as a result of vaccination. Infectious sialadenitis may also be the result of bacterial infections. Acute suppurative parotitis can develop from aerobic and anaerobic bacterial pathogens.[2] Both are likely the result of diminished salivary flow with ascending infection from the oral cavity or transitory bacteremia, where contact is made with the ductal epithelium.[2,3]

Less well characterized is obstructive and recurrent acute sialadenitis. JRP is the most commonly reported clinical entity.[1,4,5] JRP is the subject of an increasing amount

The authors have no financial disclosures.
[a] Department of Otolaryngology-Head and Neck Surgery, University of Kansas Medical Center, 3901 Rainbow Boulevard, Kansas City, KS 66160, USA; [b] Division of Pediatric Otolaryngology, Children's Mercy Hospitals and Clinics, 2401 Gillham Road, Kansas City, MO 64108, USA
* Corresponding author. Department of Otolaryngology-Head and Neck Surgery, University of Kansas Medical Center, 3901 Rainbow Boulevard, MS 3010, Kansas City, KS 66160.
E-mail address: cfrancis@kumc.edu

Otolaryngol Clin N Am 47 (2014) 763–778
http://dx.doi.org/10.1016/j.otc.2014.06.009
0030-6665/14/$ – see front matter © 2014 Elsevier Inc. All rights reserved.

of research to adequately characterize its cause and reach a consensus on treatment. A variety of factors are thought to cause JRP, including genetic, immune, infection, dehydration, allergy, ductal abnormalities, and ductal obstruction.[3,4,6–8] Presently, most authors favor a multifactorial cause. Salivary stones are the most common cause of chronic obstructive sialadenitis. Although common in the adult population, salivary stones are far less common in the pediatric population. Pediatric sialolithiasis is thought to occur in less than 5% of all reported cases.[9,10]

Other systemic processes, including immune deficiency (IgA), autoimmune disease (Sjögren syndrome), viral infection (HIV), genetic factors (HLA B-27), and allergy have all been suggested as predisposing factors in the development of a form of chronic sialadenitis. There are scattered case series and case reports, without formal investigations to substantiate a strong association.

In the last 20 years, there has been a paradigm shift in the management of sialadenitis. Historically, open surgical and gland excision procedures were the treatment of choice for conservative management failures. Transition to gland preservation techniques has advanced nonsurgical, minimally invasive interventions, alone or in combination with other surgical approaches. Sialendoscopy was first reported more than two decades ago and has become the leading diagnostic technique and intervention for pediatric sialadenitis.[11–13]

This article presents a comprehensive review of pathophysiology, clinical presentation, diagnosis, and treatment of pediatric sialadenitis.

ANATOMY AND PATHOPHYSIOLOGY

A review of the anatomy of the salivary gland network can aid in understanding the pathophysiology of sialadenitis. The function of the major salivary glands is to secrete saliva through a network of ducts. Saliva has numerous functions, including taste, digestion, lubrication, tooth integrity, and antibacterial activity, which maintain the health of the mouth.[14,15] The paired major salivary glands consist of the submandibular, parotid, and sublingual glands. There are numerous minor salivary glands scattered along the lips, tongue, buccal mucosa, palate, and pharynx.

The parotid glands are the largest of the salivary glands. Stensen duct travels parallel and approximately 1 cm below the zygoma to exit opposite the second upper molar. The length of Stensen duct is 4 to 6 cm.[15] The glossopharyngeal nerve provides autonomic innervation to the parotid gland for the secretion of saliva.

The submandibular glands are the second largest salivary glands. Wharton duct exits the floor of the mouth near the frenulum of the tongue. The length of Wharton duct is 4 to 5 cm.[15] Autonomic fibers are carried through the facial and lingual nerve to innervate the submandibular gland.

The sublingual glands lie just deep to the mucosa of the floor of the mouth and, unlike the parotid and submandibular glands, lack a single dominant duct. They drain through multiple small ducts, which exit the gland and open along the floor of the mouth. Autonomic innervation of the sublingual gland follows the submandibular gland.

Minor salivary glands are scattered in the oral cavity and oral pharynx. They each have a single duct that secretes into the oral cavity and pharynx. Autonomic innervation primarily comes from the lingual nerve.[15]

The salivary glands are made up of parenchyma and stroma. The parenchyma of the salivary glands is made up of the salivary acinus and associated ducts. Stroma consists of surrounding connective tissue. Salivary acini produce saliva, which is composed of organic and inorganic compounds. Saliva is secreted through a complex ductal system into the mouth and pharynx.[14,15] Serous acini secrete watery saliva that is enzyme rich and contains IgA. Serous saliva aids in digestion, taste, antibacterial properties, and tooth integrity.[15] Mucinous acini produce viscous saliva that contains higher amounts of IgA and other protective enzymes. Mucinous saliva facilitates lubrication, mastication, and swallowing.[15] The parotid gland is composed of primarily serous acini. Both the submandibular and sublingual glands contain serous and mucinous acini. The submandibular gland, however, has more serous than mucinous acini. The sublingual gland is predominately mucinous. Two-thirds of constant salivation is produced by the submandibular gland, and reversed during periods of stimulation when two-thirds of salivation is produced by the parotid gland.[7,15] The basal salivary flow rate in the parotid gland is considerably less than that of the submandibular gland.

A variety of factors are attributed to inflammation of the salivary glands. Viral or bacterial infections are thought to cause salivary gland inflammation.[2,3,16] Some authors have suggested that genetics, immunologic diseases, congenital ductal abnormalities, dehydration, and allergy contribute to the pathology.[3,7,8,17,18] As diagnostic technology has improved, additional predisposing factors have been reported, including salivary stones, mucus plugs, foreign bodies, and stenosis.[1,4,9,19,20]

Viral or bacterial infections may result in sialadenitis from direct inoculation of the ductal epithelium or through ascending oral cavity infections. Retrograde infections can arise from a septic focus in the oral cavity. Alternatively, they may be the result of normal oral flora entering the salivary glands secondary to diminished salivary flow in the dehydrated, toxic, or debilitated patient.[3,7,16] Transient bacteremia with direct ductal inoculation during a systemic illness, such as mumps parotitis, has also been suggested.[16]

It has been difficult to identify one specific cause pertaining to recurrent acute sialadenitis. Histologic specimens of sialadenitis show dilated ducts (sialectases) and stromal lymphocytic infiltration.[6,7] Conventional thought has been that infection is a primary event. The development of sialectases is considered a secondary change predisposing to chronic low-grade inflammation with acute exacerbations.[3,6,7] Other clinicians advocate a sequence of events effecting a structural change, predisposing to recurrent acute inflammation. These authors suggested that decreased salivary flow leads to inflammation and tissue destruction. Tissue destruction exacerbates inflammation and salivary stasis, yielding mucus plugs/debris, stenosis, and postobstructive sialectases.[3,5,18] Microscopic examination has shown that mucus plugs contain desquamated cells.[21] The mucus plugs are secondary to inflammation but are also an obstruction. Other authors proposed that congenital ductal stenosis predisposes to recurrent episodes of inflammation.[3,6,7]

Obstruction by salivary stones or foreign bodies can also result in sialadenitis. These obstructions cause inflammation, salivary stasis, postobstructive dilation, tissue damage, and remodeling that predispose to further inflammatory changes. Several theories describe the formation of a salivary stone. Salivary mucin, bacteria, and desquamated epithelial cells form an early organic nidus. Organic and nonorganic material is deposited around the nidus, which gradually expands.[10,21,22] Another model suggests that infection (inflammation and tissue destruction) changes salivary composition (precipitation of proteins or changes in calcium solubility), which leads to stone formation.[21,22] The retrograde theory for sialolithiasis describes how bacteria, nutrients, or a foreign body from the oral cavity pass into the salivary duct and become the nidus for stone formation.[9,21–23]

The link between genetics, immunologic disease, and allergy and sialadenitis is not completely understood. Early studies excluded a relationship connecting these factors.[6,7,18] Others have supported such an association based on cytologic and pathologic findings of inflammation, vasculitis, tissue destruction, and stenosis.[24,25] IgA deficiency can predispose to infection, and genetic factors influence the overall immune response.[8,17,25]

The general consensus is that sialadenitis is a multifactorial process. Recently, Jabbour and colleagues[1] comprehensively described how multiple factors, independently or in combination, can result in acute, chronic, or recurrent salivary gland inflammation. The appropriately termed "salivary gland inflammatory cycle" is a sequence of events that includes decreased salivary flow, inflammation, ductal dysfunction and metaplasia, and increased mucinous saliva. Each component progresses serially to complete a full circle and return to decreased salivary flow.[1] Predisposing factors of the inflammatory cycle include dehydration, infection, ductal abnormality, and/or immune factors. Additional components that can result from or add to the cycle include the precipitation of proteins with stone formation, and ductal stenosis resulting from chronic inflammation. Both further the inflammatory cycle through obstruction and decreased salivary flow.[1] In the multifactorial cause proposed by Jabbour and colleagues,[1] inflammation is the cause and result of the nonneoplastic inflammatory disease.

Although the inflammatory cycle Is present in parotid and submandibular gland disease, there is a closer association between the parotid gland and an inflammatory or infectious process. Both bacterial and viral infections and idiopathic inflammation occur more commonly in the parotid gland, whereas sialolithiasis occurs most frequently in the submandibular gland.[1,3,16] The parotid gland has a lower rate of secretion and a less mucinous salivary composition than the submandibular gland. Mucinous saliva confers greater antibacterial properties.[3,15] Both increase the parotid glands susceptibility to infection and inflammation. Characteristic inflammatory changes, ductal stenosis, and sialectasis cause recurrent inflammation more commonly in the parotid gland.[1,4,19] The submandibular gland is more likely to form salivary stones. The mucinous saliva is viscous and likely to form a nidus for stone formation (80%–90%).[21,26–29]

CLINICAL PRESENTATION AND DIAGNOSIS

The most common presenting symptoms of acute sialadenitis are swelling, pain, fever, and erythema overlying the affected glands. Symptoms are usually unilateral; in bilateral cases, symptoms are more prominent on one side.[16] Pain is elicited with mastication and/or swallowing. Trismus can be present. The mouth of the duct is erythematous and edematous. Purulence and/or inspissated mucus may be expressed by manual palpation and gentle pressure applied over the salivary gland and duct. In severe cases of infectious sialadenitis, systemic complications can extend regionally into adjacent tissues, or systemically spread to distal sites.[16] Clinical signs vary based on the site of inflammation and an acute or chronic presentation. **Table 1** provides a complete list of sialadenitis etiologies.

Viral parotitis is generally caused by the paramyxovirus. Mumps, historically the most common infectious sialadenitis, has become much less common because of immunization efforts. The effectiveness of the vaccine approaches 90%.[30,31] Clinicians should distinguish mumps from other causes of sialadenitis in the pediatric population, because outbreaks have occurred among highly vaccinated individuals.[30,31] Mumps is a systemic illness that infects the salivary glands without producing purulence. Prodromal symptoms include fever, headache, and malaise, with subsequent gland involvement. Other exocrine glands can be affected, and systemic complications,

Table 1 Causes of sialadenitis			
Viral	**Bacterial**	**Immune**	**Traumatic**
Mumps	*Staphylococcus aureus*	HIV (benign	Penetrating
Epstein-Barr	*Streptococcus viridians*	lymphoepithelial	Blunt
virus	*Haemophilus influenzae*	disease)	Radiation
Parainfluenza	*Peptostreptococcus* spp	Sjögren syndrome	Obstruction/stone
HIV	*Streptococcus pneumoniae*	Juvenile rheumatoid	
	Escherichia coli	arthritis	
	Bacteroides	Ankylosing spondylitis	
		IgA deficiency	
		Ulcerative colitis	
		Rheumatoid arthritis	

such as encephalitis, are not uncommon. Serologic assays are useful in confirming the diagnosis. Other viruses are less commonly associated with salivary gland inflammation (see **Table 1**).

Bacterial sialadenitis most commonly occurs in the parotid gland.[16] It is characterized by acute swelling of the cheek that extends to the angle of the mandible. In the submandibular gland, severe infection may result in floor of mouth edema and respiratory compromise. It is usually distinguished from other inflammatory diseases of the salivary glands by the presence of pus. In the absence of purulence, fever and leukocytosis support the diagnosis. The most common pathogens associated with acute bacterial parotitis are *Staphylococcus aureus* and *Streptococcus* species, and less commonly, anaerobic pathogens (see **Table 1**).[2,16] Any purulence should be sent for aerobic/anaerobic Gram stain and culture. Antistaphylococcal penicillinase-resistant antibiotics should be started while awaiting culture results. Systemic manifestations, such as abscess formation, should be evaluated with imaging.

Chronic sialadenitis is commonly associated with chronic inflammation and obstruction of the salivary glands. Patients frequently present with repeated episodes of acute painful gland swelling, which can be complicated by a superimposed bacterial infection. Often, the symptoms are associated with eating and settle between meals. The main causes for chronic obstructive sialadenitis are salivary stones, mucus plugs, ductal stenosis, and foreign bodies.[9,10,20,32,33]

Pediatric sialolithiasis is relatively uncommon and usually included within the adult literature. It occurs in less than 5% of all cases.[9,20] Similar to adult sialolithiasis, stones are found in the submandibular gland in 80% to 90% of cases, followed by the parotid gland, and rarely the sublingual and minor salivary glands.[10,20,33] Salivary stones in pediatric cases are smaller, occur distally within the duct, and present with shorter symptom duration.[9,22]

There is little literature characterizing ductal stenosis or stricture in obstructive sialadenitis. Stenosis of the duct is more common in the parotid ductal system than in the submandibular gland based on endoscopic findings.[20,21] Obstruction is primarily caused by inflammation in the salivary duct, leading to segments of stricture and dilation. The partial obstruction caused by stenosis is thought to be an important factor in the recurrence and persistence of sialadenitis and the formation of sialoliths.[21] Although the incidence of mucus plugs, foreign bodies, and ductal stenosis was lacking in the past, advancements in diagnostic and therapeutic tools have allowed clinicians to confirm their presence in the development of chronic obstructive sialadenitis.[9,10,20]

Chronic sialadenitis is also connected to immune deficiency and several autoimmune disorders, such as Sjögren syndrome, selective IgA deficiency, HIV, and HLA-B27 syndromes.[17,25,34–39] Diagnostic salivary endoscopy suggests that chronic inflammation and tissue destruction lead to stricture formation and stenosis.[24] Similarly, acute infection may complicate this chronic disease.

Sjögren syndrome is a chronic inflammatory disease of the exocrine glands with many extraglandular manifestations. The salivary glands are the main target. Dry mouth and dry eyes are common signs of Sjögren syndrome. Histopathologic changes include lymphocytic infiltration, sialectases, and tissue destruction. It is rare in children and as a result standardized criteria are lacking. However, acute inflammatory symptoms have been reported as the initial presentation in some cases.[34–36] The presence of salivary gland inflammation has been used to increase the sensitivity of proposed pediatric criteria for Sjögren syndrome.[34]

Reports have also described immune deficiency in association with sialadenitis. Several authors have reported IgA deficiency in patients presenting with recurrent parotitis through serology and immunoflorescence studies.[17,37,38]

Salivary gland involvement in children with HIV is well recognized. Characteristically, one or both glands are firm, nontender, and chronically enlarged. Xerostomia may also be a presenting symptom. Infiltration of CD8-positive lymphocytes, possibly as a result of HIV, Epstein-Barr virus, or an interaction between the two, enlarges the gland.[40] The diagnosis of HIV parotitis is usually clinical with typical findings of HIV.

JRP is a separate clinical entity, and thought to be the most common salivary disease involving children, after mumps. It is characterized by recurrent episodes of inflammation of the parotid gland. Symptoms include jaw swelling, pain, and redness, associated with fever and malaise. Most cases are unilateral; when bilateral cases occur, one side is usually dominant.[4,5] The true incidence of JRP is unknown; most reports are case series. Studies show predominance in males, although the sex distribution is reversed when events continue into adulthood.[3,4,18] The age distribution is biphasic, typically occurring between ages 2 and 6, and again at the start of puberty.[3,4,7,25,41] The natural history is recurrence. However, most authors agree that this is a self-limited disease that resolves sometime after puberty, whereas rare cases extend into adulthood.[3–5]

The diagnosis of JRP is made clinically in patients with a history of recurrence and physical examination findings. Ultrasonographic findings are consistently being used to make the clinical diagnosis.[5] The minimum requirement for diagnosis is two episodes.[4,42] Most patients are only diagnosed after multiple episodes have occurred. Hackett and colleagues[42] reported an average of 4.7 episodes with a range between two and nine events. Typically, symptoms last 4 to 7 days.[25] The interval between attacks varies individually, with episodes occurring every 3 to 4 months to 10 times per year.[3,25] The measure of severity and thus treatment is based on the frequency of disease.

There are case reports that link JRP, immune deficiency, genetics, and allergy.[8,37,38] No causality has been proved; in many early, large series of JRP, these conditions were not found to contribute to this diease.[6,7] Autoimmune disease is not likely. Most consider JRP as self-limiting and autoantibodies are usually absent.[6,7] Instead, clinicians should distinguish JRP from recurrent sialadenitis as a presenting sign of autoimmune disease. A clear cause is unknown, although a multifactorial approach is recognized as the leading hypothesis.[1,5] Each attack may further tissue destruction and function of the gland. Early recognition of JRP and treatment of this pathology are of utmost importance.

DIAGNOSTIC MODALITIES

Certain causes of sialadenitis are easily diagnosed, whereas others require more complex diagnostic procedures. During acute inflammation, suppurative sialadenitis is usually distinguished from other etiologies by the presence of pus at the orifice of the duct. Viral parotitis (mumps) can be confirmed by laboratory studies. Imaging modalities are not commonly used unless local or systemic complications are suspected. Ultrasonography (US) can confirm the presence of an inflamed gland, identify abscess, and guide aspiration. Computed tomography (CT) is the technique of choice when abscess formation or systemic complications are suspected. There is a limitation, however, for all methods of radiologic evaluation when sialolithiasis is the underlying cause. Stones smaller than 2 mm are difficult to detect, although they may cause ductal obstruction.[20]

Sialography has been the gold standard for the evaluation of sialadenitis. After a scout radiograph is taken, radiopaque dye is injected into the ductal system. A second radiograph is taken after a determined time. Sialography can differentiate chronic inflammatory changes from obstructive pathology. In chronic sialadenitis, the normal ductal system is altered, showing sialectases, kinks, and/or strictures. On sialography, sialectases are rounded areas of contrast.[25] The most commonly described appearance of sialectases is an irregular, mulberry-tree like appearance of the ducts.[3] Sialography is contraindicated in the presence of acute inflammation. It is thought to aggravate the inflammation in the already weakened ductal system.[3,16]

US is being used more in the evaluation of salivary glands. US is much easier to perform than sialography, requires much less instrumentation, and is less invasive. It also eliminates the need for radiation exposure. Early reviews suggested that US be used as a primary investigative tool and this has been supported by further research.[3,43,44] US can distinguish glandular from extraglandular lesions, exclude stones, and identify sialectases with sensitivity and accuracy equal to sialography.[25,43,44] Disadvantages to US are the lower limit of salivary stone detection (2 mm) and variable expertise of the US technician.

During periods of acute inflammation, the gland may be enlarged, heterogenous in appearance, and diffusely hypoechoic. There are normally no signs of ductal dilation, calcifications, or calculi. Areas of suppuration are seen as hyperechoic foci, lymph node enlargement, and central necrosis.[44] In chronic sialadenitis, US can identify the presence of salivary stones or strictures, their extent, and effects on the salivary gland. US can detect glandular enlargement and ductal dilation.[43,44] In recurrent parotitis, the gland is characterized by multiple oval hypoechoic areas that correspond to punctate sialectasis on sialography.[43]

CT is often used for surgical planning in cases of sialolithiasis. CT can detect an inflamed gland, and provide information useful in identifying size, number of calculi, and location in the duct or within the salivary gland.[43,45] Magnetic resonance imaging (MRI) and MRI sialaography is useful in cases where CT is contraindicated, but not routinely obtained in cases of sialadenitis. MR sialography has been suggested as an alternative technique for completely evaluating the ductal system and parenchyma accurately.[46] MRI sialography, however, is costly and requires sedation in young patients.

MANAGEMENT

The treatment of sialadenitis is usually conservative and directed toward etiology. Acute infections are treated with appropriate antibiotics. Viral sialadenitis, or mumps, is managed supportively. No antiviral agent is available for treatment of this self-limited disease. Sialadenitis in association with autoimmune disease, immune deficiency, and genetic factors is managed conservatively and according to the underlying systemic condition. Sialolithiasis causing acute symptoms is also managed conservatively. Ultimately, the salivary stone should be removed. Chronic sialadenitis and JRP have a multifactorial cause and management recommendations have not been uniform.[3,5,25] Over the last 20 years, there has been rising interest in the surgical management of sialolithiasis and chronic, or recurrent acute sialadenitis. Many authors have contributed to the advancements of conventional surgical procedures toward nonsurgical and minimally invasive procedures.[12]

The conservative management of acute sialadenitis consists of oral antibiotics, analgesics, adequate hydration, warm massage, and sialogogues. The goal of these conservative measures is to provide symptomatic relief and prevent permanent parenchymal damage. Broad antimicrobial therapy is indicated to cover aerobic and anaerobic pathogens.[2,16] Analgesics are used to provide pain relief. Both have been reported to rapidly decrease swelling and prevent damage to the parenchyma.[3,4,9] Hydration is important because dehydration can exacerbate the inflammatory response.[1,3,16] Warm massage and sialogogues stimulate salivary flow.[3,7] In cases where conservative management fails to resolve acute symptoms, abscess development should be suspected. CT should be obtained for confirmation and preoperative surgical planning. Abscess formation requires incision and drainage.

Acute infection and inflammation is a relative contraindication to surgical intervention. Duct manipulation should not be performed in this setting because of concerns about scarring, bleeding, ductal perforation, and exacerbation of the inflammatory process.[3,16] Thus, medical therapy to decrease swelling, pain, infection, and inflammation should occur before any surgical intervention.

With regard to salivary stones and ductal stenosis, the conventional approach involves blind stone retrieval, blind dilation, intraoral stone resection, and gland excision. Complications include nerve damage, hemorrhage, infection, stenosis, sialocele development, and cosmesis. Advancements to conventional approaches are based on research that demonstrates histologically and functionally normal glands after intervention.[12,33] The goals of treatment have shifted toward gland preservation methods. Larger stones or difficult stenoses may require combined approaches.[12] Other, more current approaches include interventional radiology procedures, lithotripsy, and salivary endoscopy.

Fluoroscopically guided stone retrieval and balloon dilation in the interventional radiology suite has been reported with some success.[47,48] Interventional radiology treatment is limited in the pediatric literature, likely because of the necessary radiation exposure. Lithotripsy has also been successfully used in the pediatric patient.[47,49] It can be used alone or in combination with sialendoscopy.[12,33] During lithotripsy, a compression and expansion shock wave breaks stones into smaller fragments that are easier to flush out spontaneously or with stimulated salivation. The shock waves can be generated externally or internally, by several different sourses.[50] The use of sialendoscopy for obstructive sialadenitis is described later.

Recurrent acute sialadenitis of the submandibular gland in children and JRP are more difficult to manage. Treatment recommendations have ranged from conservative to aggressive and have not been uniformly accepted. This has been, in part, because of its scarcity, uncertain cause, and natural history. Prevention of sialadenitis by using prophylactic antibiotics has been suggested, but there is little evidence to support this practice and it is generally accepted as unsuccessful.[3] Some authors have suggested expectant management because many patients are known to recover spontaneously.[3]

Several techniques have been advocated to control repeated attacks of inflammation. Historically, some authors promoted radiation therapy; it is no longer used because of a lack of supportive evidence and severe complications.[3,18] Traditional surgical management involves gland excision, salivary gland duct ligation, blind duct lavage, and tympanic neurectomy.[3,51] Complications include nerve damage, cosmesis, hemorrhage, infection, sialocele, hematoma, wound infection, salivary fistula.[51] Duct ligation and lavage have variable outcomes.[3] Some studies found that sialography alone resulted in beneficial clinical effects.[3,12] This is likely the result of "flushing" the salivary gland duct and dilation from high-pressure instillation.

Gland preservation is a paradigm shift in the management of sialadenitis and sialolithiasis that encourages the use of sialendoscopy. Nahlieli and colleagues[11] first reported their experiences with rigid sialendoscopy in the early 1990s.[12] Both Nahlieli and Marchal popularized sialendoscopy in adults and advanced this technique using progressively smaller semirigid endoscopes for the treatment of salivary gland diseases.[11,13,52,53] These advancements expanded the diagnostic and therapeutic possibilities in the pediatric population. Analysis has suggested that sialendoscopy is safe, efficacious, and gland preserving.[33] Functional recovery has been documented after salivary endoscopy, which further supported its use.[12,33] Researchers have used this method and other procedures to develop treatment algorithms and improve outcomes.[3,12]

A recent systematic review and meta-analysis by Strychowsky and colleagues[33] reviewed outcomes for sialendoscopy alone and sialendoscopy with combined surgical approaches in adult patients. Success was defined as symptom-free and the absence of residual obstruction. For sialendoscopy alone, 19 studies comprised of 1213 patients were analyzed. The uses of ancillary techniques for intervention (balloon dilation, baskets, forceps) and stone fragmentation (laser, lithotripsy) were included. Success was obtained in 86% of patients. The combined sialendoscopy/surgical group analyzed 11 studies that included 374 patients. The surgical approaches ranged from papillotomy, mucosal incisions, sialolithotomy, or external incision. Success was obtained in 93% of patients. Refractory cases required salivary gland excision in up to 11% of studies for both groups. Complications were minor and temporary.

Through the work of Nahlieli and colleagues, Marchal and colleagues, and that of many others, salivary endoscopy has been validated in pediatrics as a safe and efficacious tool for the diagnosis and treatment of salivary gland disorders.[1,4,9,19,20,41,42,54–58] Shacham and colleagues,[41] Martins-Carvalho and colleagues,[19] and Nahlieli and colleagues[4] report the largest series of interventional pediatric sialendoscopy. After a single procedure, they describe more than 80% to 90% symptom resolution in 70, 38, and 23 patients, respectively. The other referenced studies describe similar success rates.[1,41,42,57,58]

Direct endoscopic visualization can help identify or confirm a specific pathology. Common findings of chronic sialadenitis include a widened Stenson duct; white, avascular appearance of the duct; stenosis; mucus plug/debris; and salivary stones within the duct (Figs. 1–3).[4,19,58] Marchal and Dulguerov[53] reported a 98% success rate at identifying ductal and parenchymal pathology. Although avascularity, debris, and salivary stones are readily visualized, stenosis is commonly diagnosed based on narrowing of the duct under endoscopic control and difficulty of introducing and mobilizing the sialendoscope.[19] Sialendoscopy has been reported to have better sensitivity in diagnosing salivary stones in children than conventional radiology, CT, US, and MRI.[19,22,45,54] These same authors found smaller stones in the pediatric population, finding those missed on radiologic evaluation to be present on endoscopy.

In addition to diagnosis, interventional sialendoscopy has advanced to address various factors causing sialadenitis. Inflammatory changes resulting in tissue damage, strictures, and organic debris can successfully be treated with dilation, lavage, and/or corticosteroid application.[4,24,41,54,55] Dilation of stenosis using the endoscope, lasers, balloon catheters, or high-pressure saline solution has been decribed.[4,19,20,58] Mucus plugs and other debris are flushed with saline irrigation throughout the procedure.

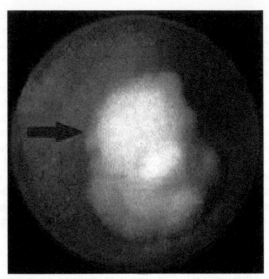

Fig. 1. Mucus plug and debris. Arrow points to mucus plug and debris within the salivary duct.

Corticosteroid application is an accepted practice, although no formal studies have investigated outcomes of the technique.[1,4,5,19,20,33,42,55] Hydrocortisone, triamcinolone, and prednisolone have all been applied. In theory, topical steroid applications prevent scarring and restenosis, and may decrease inflammation in chronic inflammatory sialadenitis, such as JRP.

Pediatric sialendoscopy is also applied successfully to obstructive symptoms resulting from sialolithiasis. Although the efficacy of sialendoscopy alone is well reported, combined procedures may be required, with similar or improved success rates.[19,33,42,45] Retrieval success depends on size and experience. Most authors use additional techniques for stones greater than 3 to 4 mm (parotid and submandibular

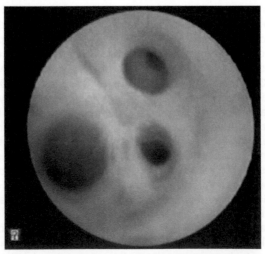

Fig. 2. White avascular appearance of the ductal layer without the natural proliferation of blood vessels.

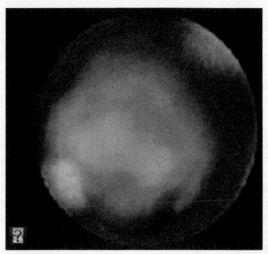

Fig. 3. Salivary stone.

gland, respectively).[26,53] Stone fragmentation can be applied with a microdrill or laser through the sialendoscope's working channel, or lithotripsy before extraction.[19,20,55] Other alternatives to complete sialendoscopic extraction for giant stones (<15 mm), proximal stones, or intraglandular stones include endoscopy combined with intraoral sialolithotomy.[9,19,20,45,59] Lastly, excision of the gland is considered for refractory cases.[42,51]

Postoperative stenting is not a uniform practice.[33] It is considered in cases of significant stenosis or injury. When used, stents are often left in place for 2 to 4 weeks to allow adequate healing time.[33]

As with all surgical procedures, there is a learning curve associated with sialendoscopy. Comfort with equipment and knowledge of surgical anatomy is integral to this technique. Luers and colleagues[60] evaluated sialendoscopic learning with 50 consecutive patients with operative parameters and postoperative performance ratings. They found a significant improvement in outcomes after the first 10 cases and again after the first 30 cases.

Salivary endoscopy is most commonly performed under general anesthesia. However, in cases of inflammatory disease, older children may tolerate an office-based procedure with local anesthesia. Konstantinidis and colleagues[56] reported seven out of eight children who underwent sialendoscopy and dilation after topical anesthetic and intraductal injection. No major complications were reported. More than half of these children were symptom free; two experienced one recurrence and one required repeat sialendoscopy.

Complications of sialendoscopy are uncommon and usually minor, resolving without permanent complication.[1,19,26,33,42,54] Major complications are duct avulsion and immediate postoperative airway compromise. Minor complications include duct wall perforation, nerve paresthesia, postoperative infection, traumatic ranula, and iatrogenic duct stenosis.

Preoperative Planning and Anesthetic Considerations

Perioperative planning for the salivary endoscopy based on the author's preferences is described next. Because the salivary duct is a collapsible tube, constant irrigation improves visualization. The authors use a 1-L bag of saline, intravenous tubing, a 60-mL syringe, and a three-way stopcock. This setup allows an assistant to provide constant irrigant through the irrigation port by filling the syringe from the intravenous bag and changing flow to irrigate through the scope during endoscopy (**Fig. 4**). Cefazolin or clindamycin is given intravenous preoperatively. The oral cavity is cleaned with chlorhexidine rinse. Dexamethasone is also given at a dose of 0.5 mg/kg, up to maximum of 10 mg. Avoidance of glycopyrolate during induction is recommended so that gland palpation and salivary runoff guides identification of the duct papilla.

Multiple-sized semirigid sialendoscopes with fiberoptics are available (Karl Storz, USA; 0.8-, 1.1-, 1.6-mm outer diameter). The smallest sialendoscope only has an irrigation port and no working channel for instruments. Larger sialendoscopes have a working channel that allows passage of guidewires, microdrills, wire baskets, balloon catheters, and laser fibers used to address directed pathology. Both also accommodate grasping and biopsy forceps. The authors have found the 1.6-mm to be quite bulky in the pediatric population and commonly use the 1.1-mm sialendoscope.

Patient Positioning

The patient is positioned on the table with neck extension using a shoulder roll. A bite block or Denhart dental retractor is used to expose the oral cavity. A standard oral endotracheal tube is secured to the opposite side of the mouth. If a large stone is suspected, or for optimal floor of mouth exposure, a nasotracheal tube can be considered. The head of bed is rotated 90 degrees; the surgeon stands on the side of the gland being treated. The video monitor is set up above the patient's head on the opposite side.

Procedural Approach

A plastic cheek retractor can help with oral cavity exposure. The salivary gland duct is visualized next. Gland massage results in salivary runoff, which can guide identification of the duct papilla. Loupe magnification may also assist in duct orifice identification, cannulation, and dilation.

The duct papilla is cannulated and serially dilated with salivary duct probes and/or tapered hollow bore blunt dilators (**Fig. 5**). The papilla is serially dilated until it can accommodate insertion of an endoscope (Karl Storz 4 dilator is the goal to

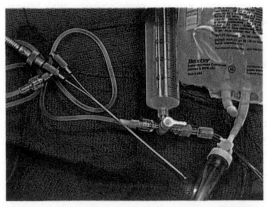

Fig. 4. Three-way stopcock to allow 60-mL syringe for pressure irrigation to aide endoscopic visualization in the duct.

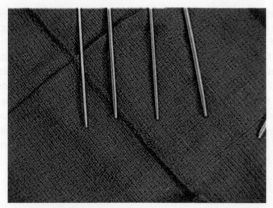

Fig. 5. Tapered hollow bore blunt dilators used for safe and graduated duct dilation with Seldinger technique over a guidewire.

accommodate a 1.1-mm scope). The scope is inserted and advanced under direct visualization with continuous irrigation until secondary and tertiary branches are identified.

Cannulation and dilation, at times, may prove difficult. In the parotid gland, pulling the buccal region anteriorly to straighten Stensen duct can facilitate cannulation and subsequent dilation. The authors find that the submandibular duct is typically more difficult to cannulate because of its relatively less fixed position in the floor of mouth. Persistent difficulty in cannulation of either gland should raise suspicion of duct perforation and/or creation of a false tract. A papillotomy may be performed to facilitate access. Alternatively, sialolithotomy can be performed. An incision is made posterior and lateral to the natural papilla. The duct is then isolated and opened longitudinally. Unfortunately, visualization may suffer because of loss of irrigation and subsequent duct collapse during endoscopy.

Generally, the authors use one or two small probes, and then pass a guidewire through the papilla into the duct. Tapered hollow bore dilators are serially inserted until the largest endoscope can be passed. This form of dilation via the Seldinger technique is atraumatic with less risk of false tract formation or perforation, and may reduce the risk of stenosis (see **Fig. 5**).

Pathology is identified once the sialendoscope is advanced. Salivary stones can be extracted with a wire basket or grasping forceps. Large stones may require fragmentation with microdrills, laser fibers, or lithotripsy before endoscopic extraction. Intraglandular stones may require a combined endoscopic and external approach. Papillotomy is used to retrieve large stones, baskets, or forceps through a narrow duct orifice. Strictures can be dilated with the scope, small balloon catheters, and hydrostatic pressure from the saline irrigant. Likewise, irrigation can clear mucous plugs/debris, fibrinous exudates, and plaques in the duct system. Stenting may be considered in cases of significant stenosis or injury. Corticosteroid may be infused into the duct. The authors prefer triamcinolone, 140 mg, leaving the endoscope in place for 2 minutes to prevent rapid extrusion.

Postoperative Care

Immediate postoperative care requires close observation in the postanesthesia care unit. Patients typically have moderate swelling because of the irrigation. This may result in pharyngeal and floor of mouth swelling that can lead to airway compromise. This is particularly important if the duct was transected and irrigant spills into the interstitial tissues, or if bilateral glands are treated.

Same-day discharge from the postanesthesia care unit is typical. Antibiotics are not routinely prescribed. Pain control is provided as needed. Discomfort usually arises from gland swelling caused by the volume of irrigant. Massage purges the excess fluid and resolves swelling within 1 to 2 days. Sialogogues and adequate hydration maintain salivary flow and assist in flushing the ductal system postoperatively. There are no significant limitations on activity with endoscopy alone. For combined cases with external incisions, standard dressings and postoperative limitations apply.

REFERENCES

1. Jabbour N, Tibesar R, Lander T, et al. Sialendoscopy in children. Int J Pediatr Otorhinolaryngol 2010;74(4):347–50.
2. Brook I, Frazier EH, Thompson DH. Aerobic and anaerobic microbiology of acute suppurative parotitis. Laryngoscope 1991;101(2):170–2.
3. Chitre VV, Premchandra DJ. Recurrent parotitis. Arch Dis Child 1997;77(4): 359–63.
4. Nahlieli O, Shacham R, Shlesinger M, et al. Juvenile recurrent parotitis: a new method of diagnosis and treatment. Pediatrics 2004;114(1):9–12.
5. Katz P, Hartl DM, Guerre A. Treatment of juvenile recurrent parotitis. Otolaryngol Clin North Am 2009;42(6):1087–91 Table of Contents.
6. Konno A, Ito E. A study on the pathogenesis of recurrent parotitis in childhood. Ann Otol Rhinol Laryngol Suppl 1979;88(6 Pt 4 Suppl 63):1–20.
7. Ericson S, Zetterlund B, Ohman J. Recurrent parotitis and sialectasis in childhood. Clinical, radiologic, immunologic, bacteriologic, and histologic study. Ann Otol Rhinol Laryngol 1991;100(7):527–35.
8. Reid E, Douglas F, Crow Y, et al. Autosomal dominant juvenile recurrent parotitis. J Med Genet 1998;35(5):417–9.
9. Nahlieli O, Eliav E, Hasson O, et al. Pediatric sialolithiasis. Oral Surg Oral Med Oral Pathol Oral Radiol Endod 2000;90(6):709–12.
10. Bodner L, Fliss DM. Parotid and submandibular calculi in children. Int J Pediatr Otorhinolaryngol 1995;31(1):35–42.
11. Nahlieli O, Neder A, Baruchin AM. Salivary gland endoscopy: a new technique for diagnosis and treatment of sialolithiasis. J Oral Maxillofac Surg 1994;52(12): 1240–2.
12. Fritsch MH. Sialendoscopy and lithotripsy: literature review. Otolaryngol Clin North Am 2009;42(6):915–26 Table of Contents.
13. Marchal F, Dulguerov P, Lehmann W. Interventional sialendoscopy. N Engl J Med 1999;341(16):1242–3.
14. Carpenter GH. The secretion, components, and properties of saliva. Annu Rev Food Sci Technol 2013;4:267–76.
15. Holsinger FC, Bui DT. Anatomy, function, and evaluation of the salivary glands. In: Myers EN, Ferris RL, editors. Salivary gland disorders. Berlin; Heidelberg (Germany): Springer; 2007. p. 1–16.
16. Brook I. Diagnosis and management of parotitis. Arch Otolaryngol Head Neck Surg 1992;118(5):469–71.
17. Friis B, Karup Pedersen F, Schiodt M, et al. Immunological studies in two children with recurrent parotitis. Acta Paediatr Scand 1983;72(2):265–8.

18. Watkin GT, Hobsley M. Natural history of patients with recurrent parotitis and punctate sialectasis. Br J Surg 1986;73(9):745–8.
19. Martins-Carvalho C, Plouin-Gaudon I, Quenin S, et al. Pediatric sialendoscopy: a 5-year experience at a single institution. Arch Otolaryngol Head Neck Surg 2010;136(1):33–6.
20. Faure F, Querin S, Dulguerov P, et al. Pediatric salivary gland obstructive swelling: sialendoscopic approach. Laryngoscope 2007;117(8):1364–7.
21. Chuangqi Y, Chi Y, Lingyan Z. Sialendoscopic findings in patients with obstructive sialadenitis: long-term experience. Br J Oral Maxillofac Surg 2013;51(4):337–41.
22. Chung MK, Jeong HS, Ko MH, et al. Pediatric sialolithiasis: what is different from adult sialolithiasis? Int J Pediatr Otorhinolaryngol 2007;71(5):787–91.
23. Marchal F, Kurt AM, Dulguerov P, et al. Retrograde theory in sialolithiasis formation. Arch Otolaryngol Head Neck Surg 2001;127(1):66–8.
24. Shacham R, Puterman MB, Ohana N, et al. Endoscopic treatment of salivary glands affected by autoimmune diseases. J Oral Maxillofac Surg 2011;69(2):476–81.
25. Leerdam CM, Martin HC, Isaacs D. Recurrent parotitis of childhood. J Paediatr Child Health 2005;41(12):631–4.
26. Walvekar RR, Razfar A, Carrau RL, et al. Sialendoscopy and associated complications: a preliminary experience. Laryngoscope 2008;118(5):776–9.
27. Cascarini L, McGurk M. Epidemiology of salivary gland infections. Oral Maxillofac Surg Clin North Am 2009;21(3):353–7.
28. Huoh KC, Eisele DW. Etiologic factors in sialolithiasis. Otolaryngol Head Neck Surg 2011;145(6):935–9.
29. Chandak R, Degwekar S, Chandak M, et al. Acute submandibular sialadenitis: a case report. Case Rep Dent 2012;2012:615375.
30. Cohen C, White JM, Savage EJ, et al. Vaccine effectiveness estimates, 2004-2005 mumps outbreak, England. Emerg Infect Dis 2007;13(1):12–7.
31. Centers for Disease Control and Prevention (CDC). Mumps outbreak on a university campus–California, 2011. MMWR Morb Mortal Wkly Rep 2012;61(48):986–9.
32. Koch M, Zenk J, Iro H. Algorithms for treatment of salivary gland obstructions. Otolaryngol Clin North Am 2009;42(6):1173–92 Table of Contents.
33. Strychowsky JE, Sommer DD, Gupta MK, et al. Sialendoscopy for the management of obstructive salivary gland disease: a systematic review and meta-analysis. Arch Otolaryngol Head Neck Surg 2012;138(6):541–7.
34. Houghton K, Malleson P, Cabral D, et al. Primary Sjogren's syndrome in children and adolescents: are proposed diagnostic criteria applicable? J Rheumatol 2005;32(11):2225–32.
35. Baszis K, Toib D, Cooper M, et al. Recurrent parotitis as a presentation of primary pediatric Sjogren syndrome. Pediatrics 2012;129(1):e179–82.
36. Hara T, Nagata M, Mizuno Y, et al. Recurrent parotid swelling in children: clinical features useful for differential diagnosis of Sjogren's syndrome. Acta Paediatr 1992;81(6–7):547–9.
37. Shkalim V, Monselise Y, Mosseri R, et al. Recurrent parotitis in selective IgA deficiency. Pediatr Allergy Immunol 2004;15(3):281–3.
38. Fazekas T, Wiesbauer P, Schroth B, et al. Selective IgA deficiency in children with recurrent parotitis of childhood. Pediatr Infect Dis J 2005;24(5):461–2.
39. Nguyen AM, Francis CL, Larsen CG. Salivary endoscopy in a pediatric patient with HLA-B27 seropositivity and recurrent submandibular sialadenitis. Int J Pediatr Otorhinolaryngol 2013;77(6):1045–7.
40. Pinto A, De Rossi SS. Salivary gland disease in pediatric HIV patients: an update. J Dent Child (Chic) 2004;71(1):33–7.

41. Shacham R, Droma EB, London D, et al. Long-term experience with endoscopic diagnosis and treatment of juvenile recurrent parotitis. J Oral Maxillofac Surg 2009;67(1):162–7.

42. Hackett AM, Baranano CF, Reed M, et al. Sialoendoscopy for the treatment of pediatric salivary gland disorders. Arch Otolaryngol Head Neck Surg 2012; 138(10):912–5.

43. Orlandi MA, Pistorio V, Guerra PA. Ultrasound in sialadenitis. J Ultrasound 2013; 16(1):3–9.

44. Sodhi KS, Bartlett M, Prabhu NK. Role of high resolution ultrasound in parotid lesions in children. Int J Pediatr Otorhinolaryngol 2011;75(11):1353–8.

45. Rahmati R, Gillespie MB, Eisele DW. Is sialendoscopy an effective treatment for obstructive salivary gland disease? Laryngoscope 2013;123(8):1828–9.

46. Gadodia A, Seith A, Sharma R, et al. MRI and MR sialography of juvenile recurrent parotitis. Pediatr Radiol 2010;40(8):1405–10.

47. Ottaviani F, Marchisio P, Arisi E, et al. Extracorporeal shockwave lithotripsy for salivary calculi in pediatric patients. Acta Otolaryngol 2001;121(7):873–6.

48. Drage NA, Brown JE, Escudier MP, et al. Interventional radiology in the removal of salivary calculi. Radiology 2000;214(1):139–42.

49. McJunkin J, Milov S, Jeyakumar A. Lithotripsy for refractory pediatric sialolithiasis. Laryngoscope 2009;119(2):298–9.

50. Capaccio P, Torretta S, Ottavian F, et al. Modern management of obstructive salivary diseases. Acta Otorhinolaryngol Ital 2007;27(4):161–72.

51. Capaccio P, Torretta S, Pignataro L. The role of adenectomy for salivary gland obstructions in the era of sialendoscopy and lithotripsy. Otolaryngol Clin North Am 2009;42(6):1161–71 Table of Contents.

52. Nahlieli O, Baruchin AM. Long-term experience with endoscopic diagnosis and treatment of salivary gland inflammatory diseases. Laryngoscope 2000;110(6): 988–93.

53. Marchal F, Dulguerov P. Sialolithiasis management: the state of the art. Arch Otolaryngol Head Neck Surg 2003;129(9):951–6.

54. Faure F, Froehlich P, Marchal F. Paediatric sialendoscopy. Curr Opin Otolaryngol Head Neck Surg 2008;16(1):60–3.

55. Bruch JM, Setlur J. Pediatric sialendoscopy. Adv Otorhinolaryngol 2012;73:149–52.

56. Konstantinidis I, Chatziavramidis A, Tsakiropoulou E, et al. Pediatric sialendoscopy under local anesthesia: limitations and potentials. Int J Pediatr Otorhinolaryngol 2011;75(2):245–9.

57. Capaccio P, Sigismund PE, Luca N, et al. Modern management of juvenile recurrent parotitis. J Laryngol Otol 2012;126(12):1254–60.

58. Quenin S, Plouin-Gaudon I, Marchal F, et al. Juvenile recurrent parotitis: sialendoscopic approach. Arch Otolaryngol Head Neck Surg 2008;134(7):715–9.

59. Wallace E, Tauzin M, Hagan J, et al. Management of giant sialoliths: review of the literature and preliminary experience with interventional sialendoscopy. Laryngoscope 2010;120(10):1974–8.

60. Luers JC, Damm M, Klussmann JP, et al. The learning curve of sialendoscopy with modular sialendoscopes: a single surgeon's experience. Arch Otolaryngol Head Neck Surg 2010;136(8):762–5.

Comorbid Psychosocial Issues Seen in Pediatric Otolaryngology Clinics

Christen M. Holder, PhD[a], Brooke H. Davis[b], Wendy L. Ward, PhD[a],*

KEYWORDS

- Pediatric psychosocial functioning • Pediatric behavioral problems • Quality of life

KEY POINTS

- Many commonly treated conditions in otolaryngology clinics have serious psychosocial comorbidities, including cognitive, developmental, emotional, social, and behavioral issues.
- Screening for psychosocial and behavioral issues in pediatric otolaryngology patients should be standard of care.
- Screenings can be successfully integrated into busy practices and yield improved clinical outcomes.

INTRODUCTION

The purpose of this article is to review the literature on common disorders seen in pediatric otolaryngology clinics and their related comorbid psychosocial issues and conditions. The article aims to heighten awareness of the cognitive, developmental, behavioral, emotional, and social correlates of these commonly treated conditions. In addition, a screening algorithm is provided for identifying these issues and providing appropriate referrals that are designed to be time efficient to implement in the context of a busy practice.

COMMON DISORDERS SEEN IN PEDIATRIC OTOLARYNGOLOGY CLINICS WITH PSYCHOSOCIAL COMORBIDITIES

- Hearing loss
- Obstructive sleep-disordered breathing (OSDB)
- Cleft lip and palate

The authors have no financial conflicts to disclose.
[a] Department of Pediatrics, Arkansas Children's Hospital, University of Arkansas for Medical Sciences, 1 Children's Way, #512-21, Little Rock, AR 72202, USA; [b] Episcopal Collegiate School, 1701 Cantrell Road, Little Rock, AR 72201, USA
* Corresponding author.
E-mail address: wward@uams.edu

- Psychosocial functioning in the surgery patient
- Attention-deficit/hyperactivity disorder (ADHD)
- Autism spectrum disorder (ASD)

HEARING LOSS

In the United States, hearing loss is the most commonly diagnosed birth defect.[1] Every year, hearing loss occurs in 20,000 newborns. Deaf children are at greater risk for a variety of emotional, behavioral, social, developmental, and cognitive problems. It is important for physicians to know how to recognize these problems.

Deaf children face difficulties in all 3 areas of quality of life: physical functioning, social functioning, and mental health (**Table 1**).[2] More than half of deaf youth have significant impairment in social relationships, and 33.3% have a moderate to severe risk in social functioning.[3] Compared with normal hearing children, deaf children have significantly more depressive symptoms and lower quality of life.[4] Not only is their mental and social health affected, but also their physical health as well. On the positive side, for those who can and do receive cochlear implantation, parents report improvement in social relationships and self-confidence in their child.[5]

Along with a decreased quality of life, deaf youth also suffer from academic, developmental, and behavior impairment. Deaf youth are at greater risk for ADHD, autism, and other developmental and learning disabilities than youth with normal hearing.[3] In fact, about 24% of deaf children have developmental disorders, and 20% of deaf youth are diagnosed with mental retardation.[6] This increase in developmental disorders and cognitive impairments coincides with impairment in school function affecting about 43% of deaf adolescents.[3] Language development and positive social experiences are important to all developing children and often do not proceed smoothly for deaf children. The communication barriers can limit or negatively affect social experience, leading to peer rejection, frustration in social interactions, impulsivity, irritability, and acting out behaviors.[7] Behavioral disorders occur in about 38% of deaf children.[3] Overall, the rates for cognitive, developmental, and behavioral disorders for deaf children are much higher than hearing children, along with related social

Table 1 Psychosocial comorbidities for hearing loss	
Area of Concern	**Specific Deficits**
Cognitive/developmental	IQ deficits Developmental disorders Poor school performance Learning disabilities
Behavioral	Impulsivity Oppositionality
Emotional	Quality-of-life impairment Depressive symptoms Frustration with communication barriers Anger outbursts
Social	Impaired social skill development Impaired quality of friendships
Parent concerns	Lack of knowledge regarding hearing devices Lack of knowledge regarding pros/cons of cochlear implants Lack of knowledge of developmental, emotional, social issues related to hearing loss.

impairments and poor academic functioning. Physicians need to be cognizant of this in order for them to identify and refer appropriately.

The parents' ability to cope with the child's hearing deficits is also important to assess. Parents often do not have adequate information about key aspects of caring for a deaf child, such as alternative forms of communication, developmental concerns, ways to promote social skill development, and ways to promote self-esteem and healthy emotional development. Almost half of parents report that they did not receive the proper education about how to check the function of their child's hearing aids.[8] Another stressful issue for parents is making the decision for cochlear implantation.[5] An important role the physician plays for the family is parent education, so that they may be guided through the diagnosis and treatment process more easily.

Clearly, deaf children are at risk for a diverse range of psychosocial comorbidities including physical, social, psychological, developmental, and behavioral issues. The complex problems of deaf children illustrate the need for preventative interventions aimed at early recognition.[7] Early recognition and intervention are crucial for deaf children because it allows for significantly better developmental outcomes.[9]

OBSTRUCTED SLEEP-DISORDERED BREATHING

OSDB is defined as the obstruction of the upper airway during sleep that negatively affects sleep quality and ventilation and/or oxygenation.[10] OSDB is thought to be caused by "either anatomic narrowing of the upper air way, or increased collapsibility of UAW muscles, or abnormal neural control; usually a combination of all three events."[10(p67)] OSDB affects approximately 10% to 33% of the pediatric population.[11] Predisposing factors include enlarged tonsils and adenoids, obesity, genetic syndromes, craniofacial anomalies, and muscle tone abnormalities.[12–18] Medical complications are numerous: systemic hypertension, impaired cardiac function and structure, cor pulmonale, extraesophageal reflux, impaired somatic growth, failure to thrive, circulating inflammatory mediators, increased insulin resistance, and possible neuronal injury in the hippocampus and frontal cortex.[19–28]

When a patient with OSDB, or obstructive sleep apnea syndrome, a severe form of OSDB,[29] is seen in otolaryngology clinics, it is typically as a consult regarding possible surgical options. Tonsillectomy and adenoidectomy are usually the first line of treatment for children who have significant disease with enlarged tonsils and adenoids and have been shown to help in most of these children.[30] A wide range of additional surgical options are performed when indicated. However, a significant percentage of children continue to have OSDB following surgery[31,32] or are poor candidates for surgery. This population includes mainly obese children,[30] and youth with craniofacial anomalies or neuromuscular difficulties. These children require treatment with a positive airway pressure machine, managed typically by pulmonary or sleep physicians. Psychosocial complications are also numerous and affect behavioral, emotional, and cognitive functioning, including executive functioning deficits, behavior, sustained attention, selective attention, and alertness (**Table 2**).[20,33] In addition, a review of 61 studies of OSDB found increased risk for typical mood being negative, poor emotion regulation, expressive language deficits, visual perceptual difficulties, and impaired working memory.[33] Another multistudy review found reduced attention, hyperactivity, increased aggression, irritability, emotional and peer problems, and somatic complaints. Depression is common.[34] Quality of life is impaired[34] and is similar to children with asthma or rheumatoid arthritis.[33] Improvements in behavior, neurocognition, and quality-of-life scores occur after adenotonsillectomy in patients wherein surgery is appropriate.

Table 2
Psychosocial comorbidities for OSDB

Area of Concern	Specific Deficits
Cognitive/developmental	Poor school performance Inattentiveness Impaired memory Visual perceptual deficits Executive function abnormalities Expressive language deficits
Behavioral	Excessive daytime sleepiness Oppositionality Impulsivity Aggression Hyperactivity
Emotional	Quality-of-life impairment Negative mood Poor emotional regulation Irritability
Social	Impaired relationships with peers
Physical	Nocturnal enuresis Low levels of alertness/sleepiness Somatic complaints

Regardless of treatment options available or whether a successful outcome is achieved, a brief screening of psychosocial comorbidities can be helpful in identifying pediatric patients in need of supportive counseling, behavioral therapy, psychoeducational testing, or other psychosocial services.

CLEFT LIP AND PALATE

Children born with cleft lip and/or palate (CLP) are commonly seen in otolaryngology clinics, because CLPs are the most frequent craniofacial abnormality.[35–37] Cleft lip is diagnosed in 0.3 of 1000 live births; cleft palate is diagnosed in 0.4, and the combination CLP is diagnosed in 0.5 per 1000 births.[36,38] The syndrome is characterized by abnormal development during the gestational period resulting in either failure of the upper lip and nose, or of the roof of the mouth, to fuse properly.[36] The defect can occur as a component of another diagnosed syndrome, or independently (nonsyndromic), and is somewhat more common in Native American and Asian populations.[36,37]

CLP is associated with several inherent developmental and psychosocial difficulties (**Table 3**), including increased rates of depression, attention difficulties, hyperactivity, anxiety disorders, and problems with social interactions.[39–49] Separation anxiety is especially prevalent in children with CLP, as around 24% of these children will be diagnosed with the disorder, compared with only around 4% of the general population.[39,50] These numbers are more than doubled when the children also have cleft-related impairments in speaking and eating.[39] People with cleft lip, cleft palate, or CLP tend to perform worse in language-based cognitive domains and are likely to struggle academically because of learning disabilities, particularly in reading.[36,37,46,51] Some studies have even suggested CLP is associated with decreased brain volumes for the frontal lobes, caudate, putamen, and globus pallidus.[36,46]

Parents of these children also face a great deal of stress for several reasons. Children with CLP often will need care from birth through adulthood, putting a gigantic

Table 3 Psychosocial comorbidities for cleft lip/palate	
Area of Concern	Specific Deficits
Cognitive/developmental	Speech/language concerns Verbal comprehension and memory Learning disabilities (reading) Motor development
Behavioral	Attention/concentration deficits Hyperactivity Attending to directions Inhibiting behavior
Emotional	General anxiety Separation anxiety Depression
Social	Social anxiety Poor social interactions Poor symbolic play
Parent concerns	Financial strain Guilt/shock Feeling they lack good information Less social support May underreport child's psychosocial problems
Physical	Feeding/growth problems Ear infections Dental issues

financial and emotional strain on caregivers.[52–54] They may also experience a great deal of guilt over their child's condition and increased anxiety about their child's well-being and are more likely to underreport their children's psychosocial difficulties because of fear of further stigmatization.[37] Even the decision of whether to pursue further difficult treatments can be a strain on parents.[53,54]

PSYCHOSOCIAL FUNCTIONING IN THE SURGERY PATIENT

Results suggest by 3 or 4 weeks after tonsillectomy or ear tube insertion, psychosocial functioning improves based on both patient and parent report.[55,56] Simply put, when children feel better physically, they feel better emotionally and behave better. In fact, patient quality of life is often positively affected by surgery, as found in children after adenotonsillectomy that had been causing upper airway obstruction.[57]

However, there are several groups of surgical patients with comorbid psychosocial conditions that may benefit from screening and referral (Table 4). First, patients needing tympanostomy tube insertion or having a history of recurrent otitis media are at risk for speech, language, learning, and behavioral problems.[58] Although some of these may improve with tube insertion, others may not. Screening and referral postsurgery can be helpful. Second, patients undergoing tonsillectomy and/or adenoidectomy in the context of obstructive sleep apnea have an increased risk of nocturnal enuresis. After surgery, most patients show improvements in apnea-hypopnea index, quality of life, and behavior.[59] However, not all patients have improvements in nocturnal enuresis after surgery. Research suggests key factors in recidivism include prematurity, obesity, family history of nocturnal enuresis, presence of non-mono-symptomatic nocturnal enuresis, severity of nocturnal enuresis, and arousal difficulties

Table 4
Postsurgery considerations

Area of Concern	Specific Deficits
Cognitive/developmental	Speech/language concerns Poor school performance
Behavioral	Impulsivity Oppositionality
Emotional	Quality-of-life impairment Depressive symptoms Anger outbursts
Physical	Sleep Nocturnal enuresis

during sleep.[60] Also, improvements may not be long-lived after surgery. Improvements in sleep experienced by children after adenotonsillectomy for sleep-disordered breathing were not as great 2.5 years after surgery as they were 6 months after surgery, although still significantly better than baseline levels.[61] Some, but not all, behavioral improvements were maintained.

ADHD

ADHD is one of the most well-known childhood neurodevelopmental disorders. The Diagnostic and Statistical Manual of Mental Disorders, Fifth Edition (DSM-V) estimates approximately 5% of children worldwide have a diagnosis of ADHD, while researchers have estimated that number may be as high as 7% to 9.5%.[50,62–65] When a diagnosis of ADHD is given, 1 of 3 subtypes is identified: combined presentation, predominantly inattention, predominantly hyperactive/impulsive, based on a cluster of symptoms (**Table 5**) that are present before age 12 and can be seen in 2 or more settings (eg, both at home and at school). The term "ADD," or attention deficit disorder, is a misnomer. ADD is an old term that was replaced by ADHD in 1994, with the release of the DSM-IV.[66] Despite its outdated nature, the term ADD continues to be used by many physicians and can cause confusion for families and patients.

Table 5
Symptoms of ADHD

Area of Concern	Specific Deficits
Cognitive/developmental	Poor attention to detail Difficulty staying focused Easily distracted by extraneous stimuli Forgetful of daily activities
Behavioral	Does not seem to listen when spoken to Avoids activities that require sustained attention Poorly organized/loses things frequently Fidgets, squirms, or will not stay in seat Runs and climbs inappropriately Seems to be "driven by a motor"
Social	Difficulty playing quietly Talks excessively Blurts out answers or interrupts others Trouble waiting his/her turn

A diagnosis of ADHD can be associated with several deficits in social, academic, and, later, occupational functioning.[67,68] The course of ADHD is chronic, and although many children with symptoms of ADHD will improve with age, they may never catch up with their peers in terms of controlling inattentiveness or impulsive behaviors.[63,68] As adults, these children are more likely than their peers to be undereducated and underemployed and may be at greater risk for other difficulties, such as conduct problems, depression, and substance abuse.[68] Common treatment components include stimulant and nonstimulant medication, behavioral training for parents and children, and appropriate classroom modifications. An early diagnosis of ADHD allows for earlier interventions, and by being aware of the symptoms, pediatric otolaryngologists can play an integral part in making appropriate referrals.

Pediatric otolaryngologists are likely to see a high prevalence of children with ADHD in their practice. Children who have airway obstruction as a result of adenotonsillar hypertrophy are much more likely to exhibit symptoms of poor attention, hyperactivity, and impulsivity.[69] Studies have also found higher rates of both ADHD and learning disabilities in children who have recurrent otitis media, and that children with these overlapping diagnoses are more likely to struggle with auditory processing and have an increased level of social stress and resulting poorer interpersonal relationships.[67,70,71] Even otolaryngologists working in acute care may see a higher rate of children with ADHD, because of the impulsive nature of the disorder. Perera and colleagues[69] found that among children treated in the emergency room for inserting foreign objects into their nasal/aural cavities, 14.3% had a diagnosis of ADHD, and 25% were repeat offenders. Undergoing adenoidectomy or adenotonsillectomy is associated with an improvement in symptoms of ADHD, indicating the importance of otolaryngology in treatment teams for children with ADHD.

A word of caution is needed in relation to diagnosing ADHD in children who have associated breathing problems disrupting sleep. Up to one-third of children who experience difficulty breathing during sleep will also exhibit symptoms related to ADHD, which can in turn lead to misdiagnosis or overdiagnosis.[69] Recurrent middle ear infections can lead to understandable irritability and impulsivity, another oft-mistaken symptom of ADHD. Similarly, there may be an overdiagnosis of ADHD in children with CLP.[72] Overlapping symptoms, such as poor working memory (especially when language demands are high) and difficulty with expressive language, may be difficult to distinguish from true ADHD.[72] It is important to neither miss a diagnosis of ADHD nor inappropriately medicate a child for a condition they do not have. Although an appropriate referral to a psychiatrist or psychologist is definitely warranted, physicians should communicate clearly in their referral that the child is experiencing sleep difficulties, ear infections, or any other comorbid medical condition.

ASD

Autism represents a diagnosis given to around 1% of the total adult and child population.[50] This figure suggests that around 1 in every 150 children in the United States has a diagnosis of autism.[73] ASD now combines the old diagnoses of autistic disorder, Asperger disorder, and pervasive developmental disorder, not otherwise specified, with the release of the new DSM-V.[50] A child with ASD frequently presents with difficulties managing social communication and social interactions, characterized by problems talking to others, even close family members, and forming relationships.[50,74–76] In addition, there is often an indifference to the lack of relationships as well as patterns of behavior that are restricted and/or repetitive.[50,75,76] These repetitive and restrictive patterns can extend to children's hobbies, interests, and daily activities. The diagnosis is 4 times more prevalent in boys than in girls, and importantly for pediatric physicians, emergence occurs in early childhood.

Other difficulties frequently associated with ASD include hypersensitivity to sensory input (auditory, oral, textural) and difficulty with sensory integration, motor hyperactivity, and coordination, sleep disorders, and aggression to both self and others.[74,77] Although behaviors associated with ASD versus those associated with severe deaf/blindness or intellectual disability (another complicating but related factor) can be hard to distinguish, there is some evidence that those who have an additional ASD diagnosis will have significantly more difficulty with reciprocal social interactions, quality of contact with others, and good use of body language in communication.[76]

Studies have long indicated a higher prevalence of autism in children with hearing issues, with estimates ranging from 1 in 91 to 1 in 110 children.[77–79] Rosenhall and colleagues[80] found that in a group of children and adolescents with ASD, 7.9% had mild to moderate hearing loss and 3.5% were experiencing severe to profound bilateral loss or deafness, a more significant amount than found in the general population. A 2009 to 2010 study conducted by the Galludet Research Institute increased that figure, finding approximately 1 in 59 children who receive special education services for hearing issues at school are also receiving services related to a diagnosis of ASD.[73] On bilateral otoacoustic emission testing, children with ASD were much more likely to have abnormalities in the 1-kHz and 2-kHz bands than controls.[74] Significantly, these are the bands that correspond to voice frequencies and may further increase the difficulty children with autism have communicating with others. Children with ASD are much more likely to have other peripheral and central otologic pathologic abnormality, including abnormalities of the cochlear nerve and auditory pathways, and are about 10 times more likely than the general population to experience hyperacusis, serous otitis media, and related hearing loss.[77,80,81]

Difficulties with hearing loss and lack of language competency have both been found to increase the incidence of behavior problems in children. The presence of both problems in children will further increase risk.[75,77,82] A separate but related issue is the knowledge that children with ASD will face several behavioral issues at home and school, and findings suggest that unfortunately these issues with behavior may mask the presence of hearing loss for families and physicians.[74,80] Adolescents who have both ASD and specific language impairment frequently have poorer functioning in areas of friendship, achieving independence, and obtaining early work experiences than those who have only otolaryngology-related speech issues.[83] Finally, families of children who have not only communication or hearing impairments, but also ASD, face a significantly higher amount of strain as their children will likely need life-long care.[75]

Common courses of treatment for children with ASD include behavioral therapy, speech therapy, sensory integration and desensitization therapies, and pharmacologic treatment of associated symptoms.[74] Hearing loss, especially when undiagnosed, can be a significant hindrance to treatment response in ASD children. Bilateral hearing and the development of appropriate speech skills not only facilitates overall development, but also plays a key role in rehabilitation efforts.[74] Chin and colleagues argue that the otolaryngologists can play an important role in the treatment team for children with ASD. An early diagnosis of both ASD and otorhinolaryngology issues facilitates early treatment, which in turn leads to better outcomes. Although otolaryngologists should not be held responsible for making a diagnosis of ASD, physicians can be aware of warning signs (**Table 6**) and make appropriate referrals to developmental pediatricians or psychologists who specialize in the assessment of ASD. In addition, physicians may be referred clients who already have a diagnosis

Table 6
Warning signs of ASD

Areas of Concern	Specific Deficits
Language	Does not respond to his/her name by 12 mo Does not smile or make other happy expressions by 6 mo Is not engaging in reciprocal gestures or facial expressions by 12 mo
Social	Interacts with caregiver only to get physical needs met (eg, no "cuddling") Does not point to show interest or play pretend by 14–18 mo Avoids eye contact, even with primary caregiver Uninterested in social interaction games (eg, Peek-A-Boo) Does not smile or make other happy expressions by 6 mo
Sensory	Hypersensitivity to sound, smell, touch
Physical	Present to clinic with hearing problems Sleep issues common

of ASD, and an awareness of the symptoms associated with the disorder can ease the treatment process. Physicians should consider changes to their typical examination procedures to facilitate a smoother evaluation process (**Table 7**).

SCREENING ALGORITHM

Given this review of the literature identifies a plethora of comorbid psychosocial conditions and issues commonly seen in pediatric otolaryngology clinics, screening is warranted and should be considered standard of practice. Health care practices are moving more toward integrated interprofessional models of assessment and treatment, which often requires a team approach with several different disciplines working together.[84] Ideally, a pediatric psychologist (a specialty area with training in child and adolescent behavioral medicine) or other behavioral health clinician is a part of this team and can screen/monitor patients for any psychosocial concerns as well as provide support to parents and families. However, some otolaryngology clinics do not yet have an interprofessional team and/or access to a pediatric psychologist, particularly in rural areas or in smaller practices. Therefore, a brief screening algorithm is offered here (**Fig. 1**). This algorithm provides guidance in screening methods and a decision-tree for making referrals. The algorithm includes screening questions for physicians, nurses, or other health care professionals to ask patients and/or caregivers to identify a variety

Table 7
Changes to examination procedures to accommodate children with ASD

Category of Change	Specific Recommendation
Environment	Place patients in a low-stimulus interview room (low lights, less noise) Encourage parents to bring the child's favorite toy to the examination Limit the number of people in the room during examination
Physician behavior	Speak softly and in soothing tones around the child Allow child to engage in soothing activities (rocking, spinning, electronic toys, and so on) Use the parents as a consult on how best to interact with the child Avoid surprise by providing verbal warnings and moving slowly before undertaking any medical examination or procedures

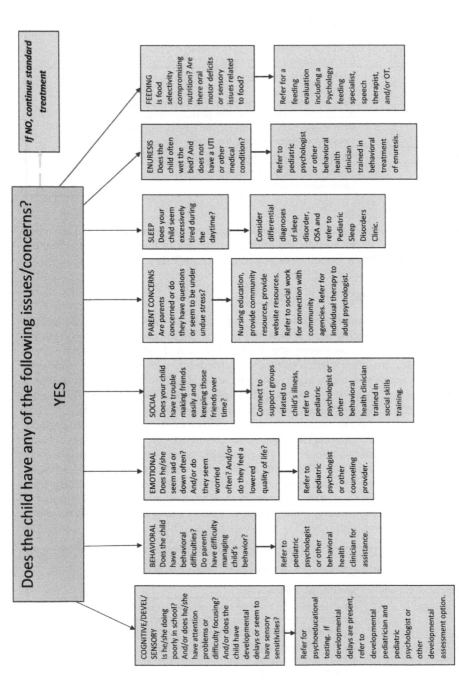

Fig. 1. Screening for psychosocial issues in pediatric otolaryngology clinics. (*Adapted from* Durkin K, Conti-Ramsden G, Simkin Z. Functional outcomes of adolescents with a history of specific language impairment (SLI) with and without autistic symptomatology. J Autism Dev Disord 2012;42:123–38; and Bodenner K, Jambhekar J, Com G, et al. Assessment and treatment obstructive sleep-disordered breathing in children. Clin Pediatr (Phila) 2014;53(6):544–8.[85])

of psychosocial conditions or issues with the intent of referral for a more thorough assessment from a pediatric psychologist or other behavioral health professional.

Individual treatment teams may use oral or written questions when screening. Given the absence of research regarding which method provides more accurate information, whichever modality seems pragmatically easiest and available in the clinical setting should be used. In many settings, the authors suspect an interview format is preferred due to clinic process and patient flow in the care area. Health care providers are strongly encouraged to develop a supportive, open, trusting interaction with positive initial interactions and less sensitive questions before asking those contained in this article, eliciting greater truthfulness and allowing for accurate screening. It is expected that health care professionals use clinical judgment when referring patients for further assessment and intervention, particularly in determining whether the behavior occurs at a frequency and intensity that is significantly problematic for the patient and/or interferes with progress in medical treatment.

Health care professionals should not only be aware of the psychosocial conditions and issues outlined here and screen for them at the initial visit but also re-screen on an approximately annual basis as symptoms can change. Furthermore, health care professionals should actively engage in building strong collaborations with local referral options who will receive their patients, to facilitate communication regarding referrals and seek accurate and timely feedback about the results of those evaluations and related recommendations. In the absence of having a pediatric psychologist in your local area, physicians may seek referral options from the American Psychological Association, Division 54, pediatric psychology's online membership directory and/ or e-mail the listserv manager to post a request on the listserv (http://www.apadivisions.org/division-54/membership/directory/index.aspx) or from state psychological associations.

SUMMARY

In summary, many patients seen in otolaryngology clinics have a wide range of comorbid psychosocial conditions or issues including cognitive, developmental, academic, behavioral, social, physical, and emotional functioning. This article reviewed the relevant literature and presented a screening algorithm for use within a busy clinic environment to positively affect accurate identification and referral.

REFERENCES

1. Ross D, Holstrum WJ, Gaffney M, et al. Hearing screening and diagnostic evaluation of children with unilateral and mild bilateral hearing loss. Trends Amplif 2008;12(1):27–34.
2. Huttunen K. Parents' views on the quality of life of their children 2-3 years after cochlear implantation. Int J Pediatr Otorhinolaryngol 2009;73:1789–94.
3. Landsberger SA, Diaz DR, Spring NZ, et al. Psychiatric diagnoses and psychosocial needs of outpatient deaf children and adolescents. Child Psychiatry Hum Dev 2014;45(1):42–51.
4. Theunissen S. Depression in hearing-impaired children. Int J Pediatr Otorhinolaryngol 2011;75:1313–7.
5. Incesulu A. Children with cochlear implants: parental perspective. Otol Neurotol 2003;24:605–11.
6. Van Gent T. Characteristics of children and adolescents in the Dutch national in- and outpatient mental health service for deaf and hard of hearing youth over a period of 15 years. Res Dev Disabil 2012;33:1333–42.

7. Leigh I. Correlates of psychosocial adjustment in deaf adolescents with and without cochlear implants: a preliminary investigation. J Deaf Stud Deaf Educ 2009;14:244–59.

8. Muñoz K. Parent hearing aid experiences in the United States. J Am Acad Audiol 2013;24:5–16.

9. Holt R, Svirsky M. An exploratory look at pediatric cochlear implantation: is earliest always best? Ear Hear 2008;29:492–511.

10. Jambhekar SK, Com G, Ward-Bengnoche W. Obstructive sleep disordered breathing in children: assessment and treatment at arkansas children's hospital. J Ark Med Soc 2010;107(4):65–8.

11. Faruqui F, Khubchandani J, Price JH, et al. Sleep disorders in children: a national assessment of primary care pediatrician practices and perceptions. Pediatrics 2011;10(1542):540. http://dx.doi.org/10.1542/peds.2011-0344.

12. Brietzke SE, Kezirian E, Thaler ER, et al. Novel sleep apnea surgical treatments. Otolaryngol Head Neck Surg 2012;147(2):34. http://dx.doi.org/10.1177/0194599812449008a87.

13. Marcus CL, Carole L. Sleep-disordered breathing in children. Am J Respir Crit Care Med 2001;164(1):16–30.

14. Marcus CL. Obstructive sleep apnea syndrome: differences between children and adults. Sleep 2000;23(Suppl 4):S140–1.

15. Marcus CL, Carole L. Sleep-disordered breathing in children. Curr Opin Pediatr 2000;12(3):208–12.

16. Katz N, Tamar E, Pillar G. Functional aspects and upper airway control during wakefulness and sleep. In: Kheirandish-Gozal L, Gozal D, editors. Sleep disordered breathing in children: a comprehensive clinical guide to evaluation and treatment. New York; London: Springer; Heidelberg Dordrecht; Humana Press; 2012. p. 13–27. http://dx.doi.org/10.1007/978-1-60761-725-9.

17. Maalej S, et al. Predictive factors of obstructive sleep apnea syndrome. Tunis Med 2010;88(2):92–6.

18. O'Gorman S, Horlocker T, Huddleston J, et al. Does self-tirating CPAP therapy improve postoperative outcome in patients at risk for obstructive sleep apnea syndrome? A random controlled clinical trial. Chest 2013;144(1):72–8. http://dx.doi.org/10.1378/chest.1119434.

19. Chhangani BS, Melgar T, Patel D. Pediatric obstructive sleep apnea. Indian J Pediatr 2009;77(1):81–5. http://dx.doi.org/10.1007/s12098-009-0266-z.

20. Beebe DW, Gozal D. Obstructive sleep apnea and the prefrontal cortex: towards a comprehensive model linking nocturnal upper airway obstruction to daytime cognitive and behavioral deficits. J Sleep Res 2002;11(1):1–16. http://dx.doi.org/10.1046/j.1365-2869.2002.00289.x.

21. Halbower AC, Deganokar M, Parker P, et al. Childhood obstructive sleep apnea associates with neuropsychological deficits and neuronal brain injury. PLoS Med 2006;3(8):e301. http://dx.doi.org/10.1371/journal.pmed.0030301.

22. Marcus CL, Chapman D, Ward SD, et al. Clinical practice guideline: diagnosis and management of childhood obstructive sleep apnea syndrome. Pediatrics 2002;109(4):704–12. http://dx.doi.org/10.1542/peds.109.4.704.

23. Amin R, Carroll JL, Jeffries JL, et al. Twenty-four-hour ambulatory blood pressure in children with sleep-disordered breathing. Am J Respir Crit Care Med 2004; 169(8):950–6.

24. Amin RS, Kimball TR, Bean JA, et al. Left ventricular hypertrophy and abnormal ventricular geometry in children and adolescents with obstructive sleep apnea.

Am J Respir Crit Care Med 2002;165(10):1395–9. http://dx.doi.org/10.1164/rccm.2105118.

25. Gozal D, Kheirandish-Gozal L. Neurocognitive and behavioral morbidity in children with sleep disorders. Curr Opin Pulm Med 2007;13(6):505–9. http://dx.doi.org/10.1097/MCP.0b013e3282ef6880.

26. Flint J, Kothare SV, Zihlif M, et al. Association between inadequate sleep and insulin resistance in obese children. J Pediatr 2007;150(4):364–9. http://dx.doi.org/10.1016/j.jpeds.2006.08.063.

27. Gozal D, Serpero LD, Capdevila OS, et al. Systemic inflammation in non-obese children with obstructive sleep apnea. Sleep Med 2008;9(3):254–9. http://dx.doi.org/10.1016/j.sleep.2007.04.013.

28. Zanation AM, Senior BA. The relationship between extraesophageal reflux (EER) and obstructive sleep apnea (OSA). Sleep Med Rev 2005;9(6):453–8. http://dx.doi.org/10.1016/j.smrv.2005.05.003.

29. Marcus CL, Brooks LJ, American Academy of Pediatrics, et al. Diagnosis and management of childhood obstructive sleep apnea syndrome. Pediatrics 2012;130(3):714–55. http://dx.doi.org/10.1542/peds.2012-1672.

30. Mitchell RB, Kelly J. Outcome of adenotonsillectomy for obstructive sleep apnea in obese and normal-weight children. Otolaryngol Head Neck Surg 2007;137(1):43–8.

31. Guilleminault C, Huang YS, Glamann C, et al. Adenotonsillectomy and obstructive sleep apnea in children: a prospective survey. Otolaryngol Head Neck Surg 2007;136(2):169–75.

32. Mitchell RB. Adenotonsillectomy for obstructive sleep apnea in children: outcome evaluated by pre- and postoperative polysomnography. Laryngoscope 2007;117(10):1844–54.

33. Beebe DW. Neurobehavioral morbidity associated with disordered breathing during sleep in children: a comprehensive review. Sleep 2006;29(9):1115–34.

34. Crabtree V, Varni JW, Gozal D. Health-related quality of life and depressive symptoms in children with suspected sleep-disordered breathing. Sleep 2004;27:1131–8.

35. Sagheri D, Ravens-Sieberer U, Braumann B, et al. An evaluation of Health-Related Quality of Life in a group of 4-7 year-old children with cleft lip and palate. J Orofac Orthop 2009;70:274–84. http://dx.doi.org/10.1007/s00056-009-9906-1.

36. Roberts RM, Mathias JL, Wheaton P. Cognitive functioning in children and adults with nonsyndromal cleft lip and/or palate: a meta-analysis. J Pediatr Psychol 2012;37:786–97. http://dx.doi.org/10.1093/jpepsy/jss052.

37. Zeytinoglu S, Davey MP. It's a privilege to smile: impact of cleft lip palate on families. Fam Syst Health 2012;30:265–77. http://dx.doi.org/10.1037/a0028961.

38. Genisca AE, Frias JL, Broussard CS, et al. Orofacial clefts in the national birth defects prevention study, 1997-2004. Am J Med Genet 2009;149:1149–58.

39. Tyler MC, Wehby GL, Robbins JM, et al. Separation anxiety in children ages 4 through 9 with oral clefts. Cleft Palate Craniofac J 2013;50:520–7. http://dx.doi.org/10.1597/11-239.

40. Tobiasen JM, Hiebert JM. Clefting and psychosocial adjustment. Influence of facial aesthetics. Clin Plast Surg 1993;20:623–31.

41. Hunt O, Burden D, Hepper P, et al. Self-reports of psychosocial functioning among children and young adults with cleft lip and palate. Cleft Palate Craniofac J 2006;43:598–605.

42. Hunt O, Burden D, Hepper P, et al. Parent reports of the psychosocial functioning of children with cleft lip and palate. Cleft Palate Craniofac J 2007;44:304–11.

43. Snyder H, Pope A. Psychosocial adjustment in children and adolescents with a craniofacial anomaly: diagnosis-specific patterns. Cleft Palate Craniofac J 2010; 47:264–72. http://dx.doi.org/10.1597/08-227.1.
44. Wehby GL, Tyler MC, Lindgren S, et al. Oral clefts and behavioral health of young children. Oral Dis 2012;18:74–84.
45. Lingyi P, Zucheng W. Behavior problems in children with cleft lip and/or palate. Chin Ment Health J 2001;15(6):381–3.
46. Richman LC, McCoy TE, Conrad AL, et al. Neuropsychological, behavioral, and academic sequelae of cleft: early developmental, school age, and adolescent/ young adult outcomes. Cleft Palate Craniofac J 2012;49:387–96. http://dx.doi.org/10.1597/10-237.
47. Demir T, Karacetin G, Baghaki S, et al. Psychiatric assessment of children with nonsyndromic cleft lip and palate. Gen Hosp Psychiatry 2011;33:594–603. http://dx.doi.org/10.1016/j.genhosppsych.2011.06.006.
48. Sousa AD, Devare S, Ghanshani J. Psychological issues in cleft lip and cleft palate. J Indian Assoc Pediatr Surg 2009;14(2):55–8. http://dx.doi.org/10.4103/0971-9261.55152.
49. Murray L, Arteche A, Bingley C, et al. The effect of cleft lip on socio-emotional functioning in school-aged children. J Child Psychol Psychiatry 2010;51(1): 94–103. http://dx.doi.org/10.1111/j.1469-7610.2009.02186.x.
50. American Psychiatric Association. Diagnostic and statistical manual of mental disorders. 5th edition. Washington, DC: American Psychiatric Association; 2013.
51. Conrad AL, Richman L, Nopoulos P, et al. Neuropsychological functioning in children with non-syndromic cleft of the lip and/or palate. Child Neuropsychol 2009;15:471–84. http://dx.doi.org/10.1080/09297040802691120.
52. Colburn N, Cherry R. Community-based team approach to the management of children with cleft palate. Child Health Care 1985;13(3):122–8.
53. Nelson PA, Kirk SA, Caress AL, et al. Parents' emotional and social experiences of caring for a child through cleft treatment. Qual Health Res 2012;22:346–59. http://dx.doi.org/10.1177/1049732311421178.
54. Nelson P, Glenny AM, Kirk S, et al. Parents experiences of caring for a child with a cleft lip and/or palate: a review of the literature. Child Care Health Dev 2011; 38(1):6–20. http://dx.doi.org/10.1111/j.1365-2214.2011.01244.x.
55. Howard K, Lo E, Sheppard S, et al. Behavior and quality of life measures after anesthesia for tonsillectomy or ear tube insertion in children. Paediatr Anaesth 2010;20(10):013–23.
56. Kim DY, Rah YC, Kim DW, et al. Impact of tonsillectomy on pediatric psychological status. Int J Pediatr Otorhinolaryngol 2008;72(9):1359–63.
57. Flanary VA. Long-term effect of adenotonsillectomy on quality of life in pediatric patients. Laryngoscope 2003;113(10):1639–44.
58. Rosenfeld RM, Schwartz SR, Pynnonen MA, et al. Clinical practice guideline: tympanostomy tunes in children. Otolaryngol Head Neck Surg 2013;149(Suppl 1):S1–35.
59. Mitchell RB, Boss EF. Pediatric obstructive sleep apnea in obese and normal-weight children: impact of adenotonsillectomy on quality of life and behavior. Dev Neuropsychol 2009;34(5):650–61.
60. Kovacevic L, Jurewica M, Dabaja A, et al. Enuretic children with obstructive sleep apnea syndrome: should they see otolaryngology first? J Pediatr Urol 2013;9(2):145–50.
61. Wei JL, Bond J, Mayo MS, et al. Improved behavior and sleep after adenotonsillectomy in children with sleep-disordered breathing: long-term follow-up. Arch Otolaryngol Head Neck Surg 2009;135(7):642–6.

62. Willcutt E. The prevalence of DSM-IV attention-deficit/hyperactivity disorder: a meta-analytic review. Neurotherapeutics 2012;9:490–9. http://dx.doi.org/10. 1007/s13311-012-0135-8.

63. Barkley RA. Fact sheet: attention deficit hyperactivity disorder topics. Available at: http://www.russellbarkley.org/factsheets/adhd-facts.pdf. Accessed October 25, 2013.

64. Garfield CF, Dorsey ER, Zhu S, et al. Trends in attention deficit hyperactivity disorder ambulatory diagnosis and medical treatment in the United States, 2000-2010. Acad Pediatr 2012;12(2):110–6. http://dx.doi.org/10.1016/j.acap.2012. 01.003.

65. Perera H, Fernando SM, Yasawardena AD, et al. Prevalence of attention deficit hyperactivity disorder in children presenting with self-inserted nasal and aural foreign bodies. Int J Pediatr Otorhinolaryngol 2009;73:1362–4. http://dx.doi. org/10.1016/j.ijporl.2009.06.011.

66. American Psychiatric Association. Diagnostic and statistical manual of mental disorders. 4th edition. Washington, DC: American Psychiatric Association; 1994.

67. Padolsky I. The neuropsychological and neurobehavioral consequences of ADHD comorbid with LD and otitis media. J Dev Phys Disabil 2008;20:11–20. http://dx.doi.org/10.1007/s10882-007-9075-3.

68. Barkley R. Attention-deficit hyperactivity disorder: a handbook for diagnosis and treatment. 3rd edition. New York: Guilford Press; 2005.

69. Ayral M, Baylan MY, Kinis V, et al. Evaluation of hyperactivity, attention deficit, and impulsivity before and after adenoidectomy/adenotonsillectomy surgery. J Craniofac Surg 2013;24(3):731–4. http://dx.doi.org/10.1097/SCS. 0b013e31828011ea.

70. Adesman A, Altshuler LA, Lipkin PH, et al. Otitis media in children with learning disabilities and children with attention deficit disorder with hyperactivity. Pediatrics 1990;35(3):442–6.

71. Winskel H. The effects of an early history of otitis media on children's language and literacy skill development. Br J Educ Psychol 2006;76(4):727–44. http://dx. doi.org/10.1348/000709905X68312.

72. Richman LC, Ryan S, Wilgenbusch T, et al. Overdiagnosis and medication for attention-deficit hyperactivity disorder in children with cleft: diagnostic examination and follow-up. Cleft Palate Craniofac J 2004;41(4):351–4.

73. Szymanski C, Brice P, Lam K, et al. Deaf children with autism spectrum disorders. J Autism Dev Disord 2012;42:2027–37. http://dx.doi.org/10.1007/ s10803-012-1452-9.

74. Rafal Z. Conductive hearing loss in children with autism. Eur J Pediatr 2013;172: 1007–10. http://dx.doi.org/10.1007/s00431-013-1980-0.

75. Vernon M, Rhodes A. Deafness and autism spectrum disorders. Am Ann Deaf 2009;154(1):5–14.

76. Hoevenaars-van den Boom M, Antonissen A, Knoors H, et al. Differentiating characteristics of deafblindness and autism in people with congenital deafblindness and profound intellectual disability. J Intellect Disabil Res 2009;53(6): 548–58. http://dx.doi.org/10.1111/j.1365-2788.2009.01175.x.

77. Chin RY, Moran T, Fenton JE. The otological manifestations associated with autistic spectrum disorders. Int J Pediatr Otorhinolaryngol 2013;77:629–34. http://dx.doi.org/10.1016/j.ijporl.2013.02.006.

78. Kogan MD, Blumberg S, Schieve L, et al. Prevalence of parent-reported diagnosis of autism spectrum disorder among children in the US, 2007. Pediatrics 2009;124(4):1–8.

79. Centers for Disease Control and Prevention. Prevalence of autism spectrum disorder—autism and developmental disability monitoring network, 14 sites. United States, 2002. MMWR Morb Mortal Wkly Rep 2007;56:12–24.

80. Rosenhall U, Nordin V, Sandstrom M, et al. Autism and hearing loss. J Autism Dev Disord 1999;29(5):349–57.

81. Sun W, Deng A, Jayaram A, et al. Noise exposure enhances auditory cortex responses related to hyperacusis behavior. Brain Res 2012;1485:108–16. http://dx.doi.org/10.1016/j.brainres.2012.02.008.

82. Stevenson J, McCann D, Watkin P, et al. The relationship between language development and behaviour problems in children with hearing loss. J Child Psychol Psychiatry 2010;51(1):77–83.

83. Durkin K, Conti-Ramsden G, Simkin Z. Functional outcomes of adolescent with a history of Specific Language Impairment with and without autistic symptomatology. J Autism Dev Disord 2012;42:123–38. http://dx.doi.org/10.1007/s10803-011-1224-y.

84. Ward W, Cadieux A, Dreyer M, et al. Consensus-based recommendations regarding screening for a variety of behavioral health issues in stage III weight management programs, in press. Available at: www.childrenshospitals.net/obesity.

85. Bodenner K, Jambhekar J, Com G, et al. Assessment and treatment of obstructive sleep disordered breathing in children. Clinical Pediatrics 2014;53(6): 544–8.

Pediatric Stridor

Jonathan B. Ida, MD, MA*, Dana Mara Thompson, MD, MS

KEYWORDS

- Pediatric stridor • Upper airway obstruction • Airway endoscopy • Laryngoscopy
- Bronchoscopy

KEY POINTS

- Stridor is a symptom of upper airway obstruction, and can not only be heard but also visualized.
- Complete and efficient evaluation and diagnosis of the stridorous child is critical for safe and timely management and intervention.
- A wealth of ancillary diagnostic studies are available for airway evaluation, which can tailor further intervention, but operative endoscopy remains the mainstay of diagnosis and intervention.
- A thorough understanding of airway anatomy and associated obstructive lesions equips the surgeon for intervention with decreased risk of further injury.
- Creation of simulation scenarios and a multidisciplinary approach to the child with stridor may improve the physician and the team approach and subsequently the outcome.

INTRODUCTION

Stridor is a symptom and not a diagnosis (**Table 1**). It is defined by a partial obstruction of the airway caused by abnormal apposition of 2 tissue surfaces in close proximity, with resultant turbulent airflow. This condition produces a high-pitched sound known as stridor. The degree of obstruction can range from minimal to life threatening, and stridor may be inconsequential or a sign of impending airway collapse. Those untrained in the evaluation and management of a stridorous child are uncomfortable with the symptom and fearful of the potential implications. In some circumstances, without adequate airway protection or intervention, respiratory collapse may ensue, particularly in young children.

The evaluation and airway management of infants and children with stridor continues to evolve, with technological advancements and improved understanding of

Disclosures: The authors have no conflicts of interest or disclosures to report.
Pediatric Otolaryngology – Head and Neck Surgery, Ann & Robert H. Lurie Children's Hospital of Chicago, Northwestern University Feinberg School of Medicine, 225 East Chicago Avenue, Chicago, IL 60611, USA
* Corresponding author. Division of Pediatric Otolaryngology, Ann & Robert H. Lurie Children's Hospital of Chicago, 225 East Chicago Avenue, Box 25, Chicago, IL 60611.
E-mail address: jida@luriechildrens.org

Otolaryngol Clin N Am 47 (2014) 795–819
http://dx.doi.org/10.1016/j.otc.2014.06.005
0030-6665/14/$ – see front matter © 2014 Elsevier Inc. All rights reserved.

oto.theclinics.com

Abbreviations	
BVCP	Bilateral vocal cord paralysis
CT	Computed tomography
DISE	Drug-induced sleep endoscopy
ED	Emergency department
EoE	Eosinophilic esophagitis
GERD	Gastroesophageal reflux disease
HIB	*Haemophilus influenzae* B
HPV	Human papillomavirus
LPR	Laryngopharyngeal reflux
MRI	Magnetic resonance imaging
OSA	Obstructive sleep apnea
RRP	Recurrent respiratory papillomatosis
SGH	Subglottic hemangioma
SGS	Subglottic stenosis
UVCP	Unilateral vocal cord paralysis

the impact of inflammatory triggers and trauma in the causation of airway obstruction and stridor.[1,2] Preventive measures have been used to curtail pediatric stridor. The widespread use of *Haemophilus influenzae* B (HIB) vaccine has essentially eliminated HIB-induced epiglottitis. The incidence of stridor caused by acquired subglottic stenosis (SGS) in neonates has declined dramatically over several decades because of improved airway management of the intubated infant; however, those surviving may have multiple medical comorbidities that influence evaluation, management, and outcome. The advancements in technology for optical visualization of the airway and expanded surgical armamentarium have allowed surgeons to push the limits of endoscopic surgery for airway management in children with stridor.[3,4] Serendipitous discovery of the application of propranolol for management of airway hemangiomas has revolutionized treatment.[5,6] Adoption of slide tracheoplasty for complete tracheal rings has greatly reduced the morbidity and mortality traditionally associated with these lesions.[7,8] This article reviews the pathophysiology of stridor, and discusses key concepts and advances in diagnosis and management of common causes of stridor.

ANATOMY AND PATHOPHYSIOLOGY OF STRIDOR
Physics of Stridor

The phenomenon of stridor is mediated by 2 basic principles of physics: Poiseuille's law and the Bernoulli principle. Poiseuille's law of fluid dynamics describes the relationships among the variables involved in the rate of laminar flow of a fluid through a tube. This equation can be directly extrapolated to airflow through a tube:

$$Q = \Delta P \pi r^4 / 8 \eta L$$

The outstanding relationship in this equation is the proportion of flow rate (Q) to the radius of the tube to the fourth power, resulting in an exponential effect on flow rate related to any change in radius. When applied to the 4-mm diameter of a neonatal airway, 1 mm of edema reduces the cross-sectional area leading to a 75% reduction in airflow. Because of decreased cross-sectional area, airflow velocity increases and induces the effect of the Bernoulli principle. This principle states that as the velocity of airflow increases, the pressure exerted by airflow decreases. The application of the

Table 1
Diagnosis and management of common airway lesions

Level of Obstruction	Cause	Diagnostic Studies	Management/Treatment Options
Pharynx	Vallecular cyst	Laryngoscopy, CT	Surgical excision
	Glossoptosis	Laryngoscopy, sleep-state endoscopy, polysomnogram	CPAP, posterior glossectomy, suture tongue base advancement, tracheotomy if severe
Supraglottis	Laryngomalacia	Laryngoscopy, feeding evaluation	Acid suppression treatment Supraglottoplasty if severe
	Laryngocele	Laryngoscopy, CT	Surgical excision
	Epiglottitis	Flexible laryngoscopy	Steroids, antibiotics Secure airway if indicated
Glottis	Bilateral vocal fold paralysis	Fiber optic laryngoscopy CT Chest if indicated MRI head if indicated	Tracheotomy, Cordotomy/cordectomy laryngotracheoplasty
	Glottic web	Laryngoscopy, genetic testing	Open or endoscopic web lysis with keel
	Recurrent respiratory papilloma	Flexible laryngoscopy, operative endoscopy, biopsy	Endoscopic excision, cidofovir
Subglottis	Inflammatory croup	Laryngoscopy, airway films	Corticosteroids, nebulized saline
	Reflux or EoE related	Gastroenterology consult pH/impedance probe Empiric suppression therapy	Acid suppression treatment
	Subglottic stenosis	Airway films, airway endoscopy	Endoscopic or open airway expansion surgery (LTR/CTR)
	Hemangioma	Airway endoscopy	Propranolol, corticosteroids, open excision, laser excision
Trachea	Primary tracheomalacia	Airway fluoroscopy, airway endoscopy	Observation, and medical management of inflammation Tracheotomy if severe
	Secondary tracheomalacia from extrinsic compression	Airway fluoroscopy, airway endoscopy, CTA chest, 3D reconstruction MRI	Surgical management of vascular ring
	Complete tracheal rings	CTA chest, 3D reconstruction, airway endoscopy, cardiac w/u	Slide tracheoplasty
	Airway foreign body	Airway films and chest radiographs	Airway endoscopy with removal

Abbreviations: CPAP, continuous positive airway pressure; CT, computed tomography; EoE, eosinophilic esophagitis; CTA, CT angiography; MRI, magnetic resonance imaging; 3D, three-dimensional.

Bernoulli principle in a narrowed pediatric airway predicts that increased airflow velocity exerts negative pressure on the walls of the lumen, precipitating airway collapse (**Fig. 1**). It is the resultant alteration of laminar flow and turbulence of the airflow that creates a vibratory resonant effect on tissues that are closely approximated, which then creates the sound described as stridor. Stridor can be heard during inspiration, expiration, or both phases of respiration. The phase of respiration in which stridor is heard usually correlates with a specific anatomic site and whether or not the site of obstruction is fixed or dynamic, as described later.

Anatomy of Stridor

Stridor can originate from a narrowing at any level of the airway. There are occasions when there are multiple levels of the airway involved.[9,10] The site of obstruction and the nature of its structural support combined with increased airflow and the patient's respiratory effort influence the observed characteristics of stridor (**Fig. 2**).

Supraglottis and pharynx

Stridor related to supraglottic disease or narrowing is typically inspiratory. The supraglottis in an infant is funnel shaped, and although large in diameter relative to other parts of the larynx it contains multiple moving parts connected by soft tissue attachments. This anatomy results in a high level of structural mobility, which is an inherent requirement of the supraglottic functions of respiration, deglutition, and airway protection. In the infant, supraglottic stridor is the result of collapse of these mobile structures into the airway on inspiration. Because of the funnel shape of the supraglottis, expiration tends to separate the supraglottic structures, relieving the obstruction temporarily. The most common cause of infantile supraglottic stridor is laryngomalacia. In this condition a structurally small, tubular supraglottis and redundant supraarytenoid tissue narrow the airway, resulting in pathologically increased airflow rate, and collapse based on the principles of airflow previously described (**Fig. 3**). With supraglottic growth and neuromuscular maturation the child is less prone to symptoms of stridor caused by collapse. As children age, supraglottic conditions causing stridor tend to be less dynamic and more likely inflammatory, infectious, or acquired from complications of surgery or intubation. Only a fixed obstruction, such as severe supraglottic stenosis, could cause an expiratory component of stridor at this site.

Dynamic pharyngeal collapse presents with noisy breathing called stertor (snoring) and must be differentiated from stridor. Stertor can be heard on inspiration, expiration, or both and is caused by the reverberation of soft structures from the level of the

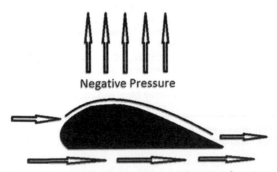

Negative Pressure

Fig. 1. The Bernoulli principle. Increased airspeed over the top of a wing results in decreased pressure above the wing. The resulting vacuum results in lift.

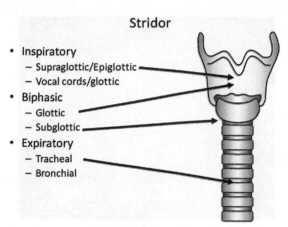

Fig. 2. Level of obstruction correlates with phase of stridor.

nasopharynx and pharynx. Stertor can occur in conjunction with stridor. Recognition and differentiation of this overlap are critical for appropriate treatment of upper airway obstruction. Stertor and stridor concurrently occur when there is extrinsic compression of the larynx or supraglottis by the tongue base as exemplified by a vallecular cyst (**Fig. 4**) or glossoptosis. Stertor and stridor are also heard when adenotonsillar hypertrophy and laryngomalacia coexist.[11]

Glottis

Stridor related to glottic disease or narrowing can be inspiratory or biphasic. The glottis includes the arytenoid cartilages and adductor and abductor muscles of the larynx. Because of the supporting muscular and cartilaginous structures, the glottis is more limited in its capacity for expansion or collapse. Stridor at this site is usually from a fixed, rather than a dynamic, obstruction. The degree of obstruction and phase of respiration in which the subsequent turbulent airflow is heard depends on how much of the diameter of the airway at this level is compromised. For example, a unilateral vocal fold paralysis (UVCD) may present with inspiratory stridor caused by

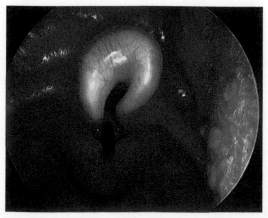

Fig. 3. Laryngomalacia. Note the tubular epiglottis and crowding of supraglottic structures.

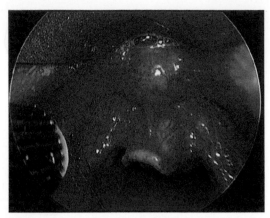

Fig. 4. Vallecular cyst. Note the proximity to the epiglottis.

partial obstruction, particularly in the neonate or in the setting of another airway lesion, and a bilateral paralysis or glottic stenosis presents with biphasic stridor caused by rapid airflow occurring in both directions without relief from the obstruction.

Subglottis
Stridor related to subglottic disease or narrowing is typically heard during both phases of respiration (ie, biphasic). The subglottis, the most inferior aspect of the larynx, comprises the cricoid cartilage, the only complete cartilage ring of the airway and the smallest portion of the infant larynx. The rigid and fixed nature of the cricoid cartilage and its noncompliant diameter, combined with sensitive respiratory mucosa in this region, make it uniquely prone to complications of inflammation or trauma.[12] Stridor emanating from this site generally results from clinically significant airway obstruction that is difficult to manage (**Figs. 5** and **6**).

Trachea
Stridor related to tracheal conditions or narrowing is typically expiratory but can be biphasic with fixed obstructive lesions. The trachea is divided into intrathoracic and extrathoracic components. Respiratory effort modulates intrathoracic pressures

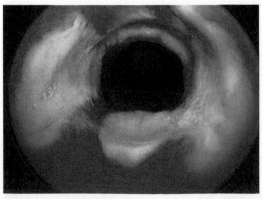

Fig. 5. Acute subglottic injury from intubation, with denuded mucosa and exposed cartilage.

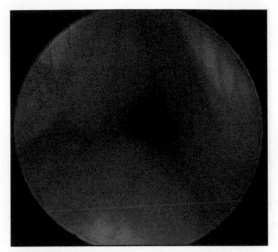

Fig. 6. Grade 3 subglottic stenosis caused by neonatal intubation.

leading to dynamic changes in the diameter of the airway and subsequent turbulent airflow. The intrathoracic trachea is more susceptible to such pressure gradient changes, and more likely to collapse with triggers of increased pressure such as the act of coughing. The intrathoracic trachea expands during inspiration, when intrathoracic pressure is negative, and collapses with the positive intrathoracic pressure of expiration.[13] The physics of this pressure gradient change explain why the trachea is the primary site of the airway implicated in pure expiratory stridor. As seen in **Fig. 7**, congenital tracheomalacia is a classic example of expiratory stridor caused by dynamic collapse of the airway. Structures in close proximity but extrinsic to the airway, such as a vascular ring (**Fig. 8**), can also cause tracheal compression and expiratory stridor.[14,15] Similar to a fixed subglottic lesion, a fixed tracheal obstruction, as exemplified by complete tracheal rings (**Fig. 9**), produce biphasic stridor.

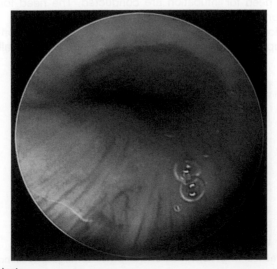

Fig. 7. Tracheomalacia.

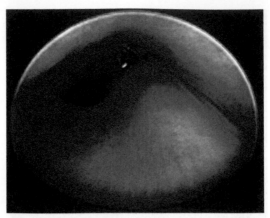

Fig. 8. Vascular compression of the trachea.

A list of common or notable causes of pediatric stridor is shown in **Box 1**.

EVALUATION OF THE STRIDOROUS PATIENT
History

The evaluation of a stridorous patient requires an initial observation of the patient's respiratory pattern, assessment of the severity of airway obstruction, and determination of the potential need for urgent or emergent airway intervention. The phase of respiration in which stridor occurs can help the clinician determine the level at which the obstruction is located. Patients who present with acute onset of stridor are most likely to have infection, inflammation, or foreign object aspiration as the cause. The initial point of evaluation is most often the emergency department (ED), where the goal of the ED physician is to assess risk for impending respiratory collapse. In this setting, vital signs, respiratory rate and effort, and oxygenation are assessed. Airway and chest radiographs are performed. A rapid evaluation for impending airway collapse and the need for intubation are conducted. The need for otolaryngology and anesthesia consultations for airway control is determined.

The otolaryngologist can provide additional diagnostic information using fiberoptic nasopharyngoscopy and laryngoscopy in the cooperative and clinically stable patient.

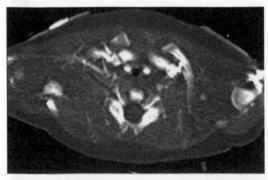

Fig. 9. Complete tracheal rings identified on computed tomography scan. Note the narrow trachea at this level.

Box 1
Causes of pediatric stridor by anatomic subsite

Pharynx/hypopharynx
- Glossoptosis
- Laryngopharyngeal reflux
- Vascular malformation
- Vallecular cyst

Supraglottis
- Laryngomalacia
- Laryngocele
- Stenosis
- Vascular malformation
- Neck mass

Glottis
- Vocal cord paralysis (bilateral>unilateral)
- Intubation injury
- Laryngeal cleft
- Glottic web
- Stenosis
- Laryngeal trauma/fracture

Subglottis
- Croup
- Intubation granulation/edema
- Acquired stenosis
- Hemangioma
- Cysts
- Congenital cricoid malformation
- Foreign body

Tracheobronchus
- Tracheobronchomalacia
- Foreign body
- Complete tracheal rings
- Vascular compression
- Stenosis
- Bacterial tracheitis
- Neck/chest mass

The otolaryngologist has the expertise to assess the need for diagnostic or therapeutic intervention in the operating room or for establishing a surgical airway. Some institutions have created a critical airway assessment team with supporting bronchoscopic equipment in the ED to facilitate management in cases of critical airway obstruction.[16]

With the advancement of simulation as an educational tool, institutions are encouraged to develop simulation programs for the assessment of acute stridor requiring urgent intervention.[17]

Most children present with chronic or gradual onset stridor in which the airway is restricted but stable and allows the physician to conduct a methodical evaluation. A carefully taken history helps to narrow the differential diagnosis and direct the diagnostic evaluation. Chronology of the event is important, because many causes can be predicted by symptom onset. For example, stridor associated with laryngomalacia is generally present within the first 2 weeks of life,[18] whereas stridor associated with subglottic hemangiomas (SGH) begins around 2 months of life and is likely to be progressive.[19] Other causes have a latency between lesion occurrence and onset of symptoms. For example, bilateral vocal cord paralysis (BVCP) may take several months to become symptomatic,[20] whereas congenital SGS may only become clinically significant in early childhood as recurrent croup.[21] Accompanying complaints or symptom triggers can guide the diagnosis and management of stridor. Hoarseness could signify a glottic mass (papilloma) or neurologic cause affecting the vagal nerve and vocal fold function. Feeding difficulty could indicate acid reflux or an anatomic anomaly such as a laryngeal cleft or tracheoesophageal fistula.

A query of the past medical history can also provide diagnostic clues to stridor. Stridor in the context of an intubation history is characteristic of acquired laryngotracheal stenosis. A history of neck, chest, or neurologic trauma or surgical procedures may indicate obstruction from a vocal cord weakness. Because children with chronic stridor are often misdiagnosed with other conditions such as asthma, a lack of response to typical therapies may indicate a structural cause in the tracheobronchial tree.

In patients with episodic stridor, an attempt should be made to identify the potential triggers and evaluate the severity of the paroxysms, to identify patients at risk for critical airway compromise and emergent respiratory events. Such patients require a diagnostic evaluation in an inpatient setting with appropriate monitoring during the evaluation (**Box 2**).[22]

Physical Examination

Observation of the respiratory phase of stridor helps determine the level of obstruction, but combining this assessment with other characteristics of the noise such as volume, pitch, and respiratory effort quickly helps identify patients at risk for impending respiratory failure or in need of noninvasive airway support. Retractions of the suprasternal and intercostal region are reliable signs of increased respiratory effort. Mental status changes signify advancing hypoxia or hypercarbia with the impending need for intervention. Pulse oximetry is included in the physical examination and is a rapid test that can provide prognostic data in children with stridor, such as in laryngomalacia.[23]

A complete head and neck examination helps locate the stridor source. For example, a micrognathic child with stridor may have posterior displacement of the tongue and glossoptosis, leading to collapse of the supraglottis. Cutaneous hemangiomas, particularly those in a segmental beard distribution, may indicate subglottic disease (**Figs. 10** and **11**).[24] Lymphatic malformations or other facial, neck, or chest masses may cause extrinsic compression of the airway. Visual examination of the chest wall and auscultation complete the noninvasive portion of the physical examination. The presence of a pectus excavatum suggests significant upper airway obstruction and is often an indication for surgical intervention of the inciting upper airway lesion.[23] Identification of the stigmata of a specific syndrome can aid in the diagnosis, because many well-known syndromes are linked to congenital airway anomalies, such

---

Box 2
Stridor history

Timing

- Initiation of symptoms
- Duration of symptoms/episodes
- Episodic versus continuous
- Worsening, steady, or improving

Severity

- Retractions
- Cyanosis
- Fatigue/mental status change
- Weight loss or failure to thrive
- Associated feeding difficulties

Character

- Pitch high versus low
- Phase
- Vibratory
- Positional

Associated symptoms/influence

- Feeding or sleep related
- Strenuous activity
- Spitting up/reflux
- Weight loss
- Dysphagia/aspiration
- Fevers
- Neck mass
- Lymphadenopathy

Medical history

- Intubation history
- Prior surgeries
- Neurologic conditions
- Syndromes/genetics

---

as Down syndrome with congenital SGS,[25] VATER/VACTRL with TEF and tracheomalacia, Pallister-Hall with laryngeal cleft, or CHARGE syndrome with cranial nerve palsies (**Box 3**).[26]

Awake fiberoptic nasopharyngoscopy and laryngoscopy is an indispensable part of the physical examination of the stridorous child. It provides dynamic, real-time visualization of the pharynx, hypopharynx, supraglottis, and vocal cords, thereby providing a safe and simple way of diagnosing common, stridor-inducing lesions such as laryngomalacia, vocal cord paralysis, and laryngopharyngeal reflux (LPR). In some cases the

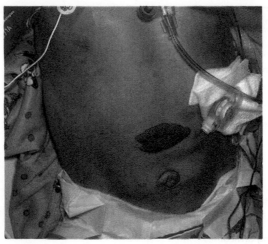

Fig. 10. Cutaneous hemangioma associated with the subglottic hemangioma in **Fig. 11.**

subglottic region is visualized enough to screen for SGS. Awake flexible tracheoscopy in infants with stridor has been shown to be safe when used by experienced practitioners.[27]

Diagnostic Radiography

Colleagues in radiology, cardiology, gastroenterology, and pulmonology can have a role in the evaluation of the child with stridor by providing and interpreting additional procedures or tests. In many tertiary medical centers this evaluation is done in the context of a multidisciplinary aerodigestive team, as discussed later.

Airway radiographs can quickly, safely, and inexpensively identify airway lesions as indicated by various radiographic signs. A classic example is the steeple sign on plain neck film seen in children with croup or SGS as the cause of stridor (**Fig. 12**). Other examples of obstructive lesions that can be screened for on plain films include epiglottitis, subglottic cysts (**Fig. 13**), SGH, tracheal stenosis, and complete tracheal rings. These lesions are generally confirmed by endoscopy (**Fig. 14**). Stridor from

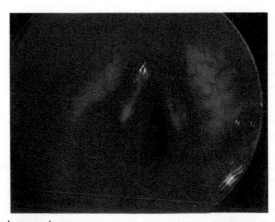

Fig. 11. Subglottic hemangioma.

| Box 3 |
| Syndromes and conditions commonly associated with obstructive airway lesions |
| Down syndrome |
| Pierre Robin sequence |
| Chiari malformation |
| Pallister-Hall syndrome |
| DiGeorge syndrome |
| CHARGE association |
| Facial hemangioma |
| Cerebral palsy |
| Mucopolysaccharidoses |
| Noonan syndrome |
| Beckwith-Wiedemann syndrome |
| Goldenhar syndrome |
| Cornelia de Lange syndrome |
| Crouzon syndrome |
| Treacher-Collins syndrome |
| Opitz syndrome |
| Klippel-Feil syndrome |
| Congenital high airway obstruction syndrome |

aerodigestive tract foreign bodies is best screened by radiographs with the understanding that some common foreign bodies are radiolucent, such as food debris or plastic.[28] Airway fluoroscopy can be used in certain cases for identification of dynamic airway lesions such as tracheomalacia.[29]

Computed tomography (CT) with three-dimensional reconstruction can assist the practitioner in evaluating airway lesions and planning surgical intervention.[30] CT

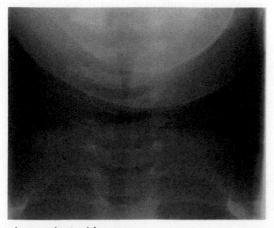

Fig. 12. Steeple sign in a patient with croup.

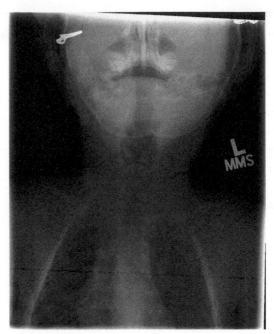

Fig. 13. Subglottic cysts on plain neck film.

and/or magnetic resonance imaging (MRI) are used to evaluate neck or chest masses and aberrant vasculature, such as vascular rings or innominate artery compression. The child with congenital heart disease and stridor should alert the clinician to vascular compression or complete tracheal rings. As cardiologists have become more facile with the technology, echocardiography has become a more widely used screening test to identify intrathoracic aberrant vasculature that may cause tracheal compression and stridor without exposing the child to radiation.[31]

Multidisciplinary Assessment

In most tertiary care centers the evaluation of a child with stridor is done in a multidisciplinary fashion, whereby gastroenterology and pulmonology participate with the

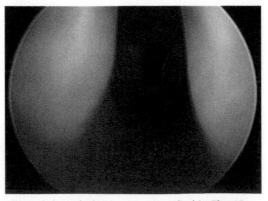

Fig. 14. Endoscopic view of the subglottic cysts identified in **Fig. 13**.

otolaryngologist in a collaborative experience. With this approach, diagnostic testing by each discipline can be performed under the same anesthetic when necessary.

Gastroenterology

There is a well-established association between gastroesophageal reflux disease (GERD), LPR, and impact on inflammatory and obstructive disorders of the airway.[1] The presence of GERD and LPR affect the outcome of airway intervention and can lead to recurrence and failure of even carefully executed procedures. Similar to acid reflux disease, eosinophilic esophagitis (EoE) can be a trigger of airway inflammation and obstruction, with similar untoward effects on airway healing.[2] The inclusion of pediatric gastroenterology is therefore critically important in the evaluation of the child who presents with symptomatic airway obstruction that is recurrent or chronic. The gastroenterologist contributes diagnostic testing for GERD and EoE and helps elucidate their relationship to stridor and airway disorder. Conditions affected by LPR/GERD include laryngomalacia, SGS, and recurrent croup.[32] Specific quantification of acid reflux via impedance probe testing can delineate the severity of reflux and determine whether extraesophageal reflux is present. The presence of significant acid reflux in the setting of stridor mandates multidisciplinary action and aggressive treatment. Visualization of the esophagus by esophagoscopy with histopathologic evaluation of biopsies provides complementary information about pathologic esophagitis. Eosinophils can confirm the diagnosis of GERD, but the presence of more than 15 eosinophils per high-powered field helps differentiate GERD from EoE.[33]

Pulmonology

Pulmonary health is among the most important factors in outcome when treating chronic airway lesions. Poor pulmonary capacity and lung disease are critical factors contributing to the need for repeated airway intervention, intubation, and emergence of airway lesions that cause stridor. The pulmonologist participates in the evaluation of the child with stridor by providing assistance with diagnosis and management of lower airway disorder, physiologic tests of airflow, and flexible bronchoscopy. In age-appropriate patients, pulmonary function testing can identify obstructive lesions through characteristic flow-volume loops. For example, tracheomalacia displays a droop in the forced expiratory portion of the flow-volume loop, caused by obstruction during increased intrathoracic pressure. Flexible bronchoscopy is an important tool for the evaluation of dynamic tracheal lesions, like tracheomalacia, and evaluation of the lower tracheobronchial tree. Flexible bronchoscopy also provides the opportunity for directed lower airway lavage for cytology and identification of lipid-laden macrophages or pepsin, which signal the presence of aspiration of food matter and refluxate, respectively.[34,35] Cultures and bronchial brushings can also be valuable.

Among refractory or complex causes of stridor, a multidisciplinary aerodigestive approach between the otolaryngologist, pulmonologist, and gastroenterologist provides patients with airway disorders with a level of care that is greater than the sum of the individual providers' care. This platform allows all 3 services to participate and deliberate, by which patients may be seamlessly treated by multiple services, especially during endoscopic evaluation and treatment.

Operative Endoscopy

Definitive diagnosis of a stridor-inducing airway lesion is often impossible without endoscopic visualization. Although parts of the airway can or must be visualized in the clinic with the patient awake, other lesions require anesthetics and specialized equipment to completely visualize and completely evaluate the airway beyond the larynx. This type of evaluation is done with age-appropriate laryngoscopes and bronchoscopes, an operating room team, and pediatric anesthesiology adept in collaborative airway management.[36] Excellent communication with the anesthesia provider is critical for safe endoscopy and to allow the surgeon sufficient time to acquire information and provide intervention if indicated. A mutually agreed approach before induction is essential. The anesthetist's ability to keep the child spontaneously breathing without an endotracheal tube in the airway allows optimal examination and diagnosis of potential causes of stridor. The introduction of drug-induced sleep endoscopy (DISE) allows the determination of levels of stridor and obstruction that may occur during sleep.[37] DISE maneuvers, such as a jaw thrust and other manipulations, can localize the obstruction to the supraglottis, hypopharynx, or tongue base.[38] Under a deeper plane of anesthesia, evaluation of the entire upper airway is conducted to evaluate not just for the primary lesion resulting in obstruction, but to determine whether secondary lesions are present and how they might influence management or the expected success of interventions.[9,10] For example, it has been shown that unilateral vocal cord immobility is a major risk factor for airway reconstruction failure.[39]

With advances in endoscopic management such as balloon dilation and endoscopic laryngeal cleft repair[3,4] the surgeon should always be prepared for surgical intervention if indicated. This type of laryngotracheal manipulation can lead to intermittent laryngospasm with unintentional airway obstruction or intentional temporary obstruction as encountered during balloon dilation of the airway. These potential scenarios and their management should be discussed and mutually agreed upon by the surgeon and anesthesiologist before initiation of the procedure.

The technique of suspension laryngoscopy allows precision in diagnosis and expanded capability for endoscopic intervention. The larynx is exposed and suspended in a fixed position, which affords the surgeon 2-handed manipulation of the airway, and integration of an operating microscope for optimal visualization. Suspension allows the surgeon to perform an advanced diagnostic evaluation such as arytenoid palpation for mobility to rule out vocal fold fixation, inspect the interarytenoid region for a cleft, and size the airway with serial endotracheal tubes to determine the presence or absence of SGS according the Myer-Cotton scale.[40] Suspension also allows intervention such as steroid injection for hemangioma or stenosis, balloon dilation, or the application of laser technology for the management of vascular anomalies or stenosis. The use of an operating microscope in conjunction with suspension is an important surgical skill for better visualization and precise 2-handed instrumentation during endoscopic intervention. For those lesions that cannot be managed endoscopically, operative endoscopy provides an opportunity to garner information necessary to provide further medical and surgical intervention for a more extensive lesion, such as a grade 3 SGS.

COMMON AND ILLUSTRATIVE CAUSES OF STRIDOR

As a symptom resulting from multiple potential causes, the epidemiology of stridor is not well delineated. The most common cause of stridor in the neonate is laryngomalacia. Chronic stridor originates more frequently from a congenital airway abnormality.[23,41] The most common cause of noncongenital stridor that occurs in older infants and young toddlers is viral laryngotracheobronchitis, otherwise known as croup.[42] In general, congenital abnormalities of the larynx and trachea, infectious causes, and traumatic injury predominate in pediatric stridor, whereas tumors (eg, papillomas or hemangiomas) are rare by comparison.[19,43,44]

Laryngomalacia

Congenital laryngomalacia is the most common cause of neonatal stridor, and is typified by inspiratory stridor that is aggravated by feeding, sleep, irritability, and supine position. Diagnosis relies primarily on awake flexible endoscopy, in which the findings of a congenitally small, tubular epiglottis and prominent supra-arytenoid tissues are seen. There are multiple causal theories to explain the typical findings, with an abnormal sensorimotor integration of neuromuscular tone being predominant.[45]

Most infants with laryngomalacia (60%) have inconsequential stridor and outgrow the symptoms by 12 to 24 months of age. Up to 88% have feeding difficulty and benefit from acid suppression treatment or surgery.[46] About 20% have airway obstruction or dysphagia that warrants surgical intervention.[23,45] This spectrum of disease presentation is associated with the presence or absence of medical comorbidities such as GERD, underlying neurologic disorder, congenital heart disease, or genetic anomaly or syndromes. The presence of a secondary or synchronous airway lesion (58%)[10] can exacerbate symptoms because of the additive airflow limitations. Indications for surgical intervention include apnea, recurrent cyanotic events, failure to thrive, hypoxia, and pulmonary hypertension. Because of airway obstruction, many patients have feeding difficulty caused by poor coordination of the suck-swallow breath sequence. Feeding difficulty can lead to failure to thrive and even aspiration. Supraglottoplasty has been shown to open the airway in more than 80% of patients with severe laryngomalacia, to improve swallowing, and to decrease aspiration risk in carefully selected patients who otherwise would not be at risk for aspiration.[46–48]

Cervicomedullary compression of the brainstem, such as a spinal anomaly or Chiari malformation, can cause the clinical symptoms and physical examination findings of severe laryngomalacia. Neurosurgical correction of the compression may result in reversal of laryngomalacia symptoms and examination findings without need for supraglottoplasty.[49] Identification of these patients requires a high index of suspicion.

Persistent or occult laryngomalacia has been identified in a group of otherwise healthy pediatric patients with obstructive sleep apnea (OSA) refractory to adenotonsillectomy. This form of laryngomalacia may present only during sleep. In the authors' experience the use of DISE improves the ability to diagnose patients with this form of OSA. Supraglottoplasty seems to be effective for patients with this form of laryngomalacia, and as DISE becomes more widely used in children in the future more frequent reports about this entity are expected.[37,50]

Vocal Cord Paralysis

UVCP is far more common than BVCP, and does not generally cause stridor, except in neonates or in the presence of another airway lesion. UVCP is most commonly iatrogenic, particularly in neonates undergoing thoracic procedures.[51] These patients have a weak, hoarse cry, and often have dysphagia and aspiration caused by glottic insufficiency. Arytenoid fixation can present identically to or concomitantly with vocal cord paralysis and should be differentiated on endoscopy.

BVCP presents with stridor and obstruction, and requires intervention for airway improvement and protection. BVCP can be congenital or acquired, generally requiring tracheostomy as a temporary measure while awaiting recovery of neurologic function, followed by definitive intervention if there is no recovery. Congenital BVCP can be caused by a Chiari malformation, an intracranial neurologic abnormality, a hereditary disease, or may be idiopathic. Diagnosis is generally made with awake fiberoptic nasopharyngoscopy. Additional testing includes cytomegalovirus titers, MRI of the head, genetic evaluation, and neurosurgical evaluation. An acquired BVCP without a surgical history strongly suggests a neurologic lesion and imaging is mandated.

Surgical management can range from tracheotomy to open and endoscopic surgical procedures and choice is individualized around patient factors, comorbidities and risk for aspiration, and the patient's risk tolerance for alteration in voice. Tracheotomy bypasses the obstructed airway but may not be a good long-term solution. Surgical management of BVCP is intended to open the posterior glottic airway by distraction of the vocal cords, which risks future aspiration or a detrimental effect on the voice.[52]

Open laryngotracheoplasty using a posterior cartilage graft to augment the posterior glottis, with or without arytenoid lateralization, is an acceptable and successful option for children, as is open vocal cord lateralization, with 60% to 70% surgery-specific decannulation rates.[53] Endoscopic management options include CO_2 laser arytenoidectomy and vocal fold posterior cordectomy. An innovative minimally invasive alternative in carefully selected patients includes endoscopic partial arytenoidectomy with suture lateralization of the vocal cord. A successful innovative option in experienced hands is the endoscopic posterior cricoid split with costal cartilage graft placement.[54]

Croup

Croup is the most common cause of acute stridor in young children and toddlers, and is commonly caused by a viral infection of the larynx and upper trachea. Stridor in the presence of a barking cough and upper respiratory infection are the pathognomonic signs. A radiographic steeple sign confirms the diagnosis and precludes the need for laryngoscopy in most patients. Treatment includes supportive oxygenation, humidification, and intravenous corticosteroids.[42]

Recurrent croup can be a sign of an underlying anatomic airway problem, such as subglottic cysts, hemangiomas, or congenital stenosis, which predispose to recurrent or recalcitrant stridor with a smaller airway diameter. In addition, recurrent croup has been reported as a sequela of chronic airway inflammation from gastrointestinal sources, EoE in particular.[21] Recurrent croup, particularly when it is becoming more severe and more frequent with age, should be further investigated with airway endoscopy.[55] A subtle structural grade 1 SGS may be discovered and inflammatory triggers may then lead to symptoms. The list of inflammatory triggers is long and they may be difficult to precisely identify, diagnose, or control. Most children become less symptomatic over time as the airway grows, and parents should be provided assurance and encouraged to seek symptomatic relief if a serious structural abnormality is not identified. Certain patients may be good candidates to receive steroid prescriptions for symptomatic control and prevention of hospitalization, but the frequency of steroid usage should be monitored and limited.

Subglottic Stenosis

SGS can be congenital or acquired, both of which have unique presentations. Congenital SGS can present insidiously and not immediately after birth. As the breathing requirements of the infant or young child increase, worsening exertional dyspnea is caused by the congenitally narrowed airway.

Acquired SGS is a result of intubation injury. These patients tend to present in the hospital setting after extubation. Length of time to develop a SGS in a child is unknown but presentation is often 3 to 6 weeks after extubation. Respiratory syncytial virus bronchiolitis has been shown to be a risk factor for intubation injury.[56] The symptom spectrum of SGS includes oxygen desaturation, stridor, and increased work of breathing with use of accessory muscles of respiration. Medical management with inhaled racemic epinephrine and systemic steroids may provide symptomatic relief. Escalating noninvasive airway management includes positive pressure ventilation with or without heliox. SGS is a common reason for otolaryngologic consultation from intensive care units, and endoscopy is required for diagnosis. Balloon dilation of the airway is performed in the acute setting for immediate relief and to prevent a long-term airway stenosis. Early dilation may improve outcomes because the stenosis is often immature and thin, and repeat dilations may be necessary.

If the airway cannot be restored with endoscopic techniques, tracheostomy or open airway reconstruction may be necessary. The airway can be expanded using laryngotracheal reconstruction techniques, or cricotracheal resection. Choice of operation depends on location of the stenosis and degree of obstruction. The details are beyond the scope of this article. Although successful surgical correction of airway stenosis is a realistic goal for an experienced surgeon, the evolution and future of airway reconstruction remain the development of innovative techniques for voice preservation while achieving airway patency.[57,58]

Subglottic Hemangioma

SGH is a rare vascular tumor of the larynx, which presents after 4 to 6 weeks of life and undergoes 3 to 6 months of rapid proliferation, after which a slow involution phase follows, with complete resolution in most patients by 5 to 7 years of age. Patients present with stridor that worsens with crying because of vascular engorgement, and edema from increased air flow turbulence across the subglottic mucosa. Symptoms improve with steroids, resulting in an erroneous diagnosis of croup. Subglottic lesions are associated with cutaneous lesions, particularly facial lesions in the beard distribution.[24] Airway films may be diagnostic, showing an asymmetric, smooth swelling of the subglottis (**Fig. 15**). Diagnosis generally requires endoscopy, which shows a smooth, round, compressible mass, most commonly in the left posterior portion of the subglottis,[19] but it may be circumferential.

Treatment modalities for SGH have evolved over the past 30 years and most are now managed with propranolol alone or in combination with other modalities. The

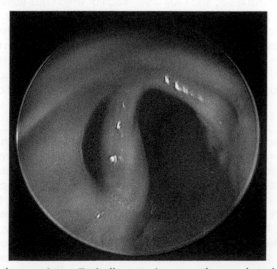

Fig. 15. Subglottic hemangioma. Typically posterior, smooth, round, and compressible.

choice and extent of intervention depend on the size of the lesion and severity of associated symptoms. For large and symptomatic lesions tracheotomy to bypass the lesion until resolution was the standard of care with which all other modalities were compared. The historical role for systemic steroids has been for lesions that are minimally symptomatic, or to mitigate the growth rate. However, the need for prolonged therapy with significant side effects limits use of systemic steroids for treatment of SGH at this time. Steroids are now mostly used as an adjunct to propranolol.

The serendipitous discovery of the effect of propranolol on hemangiomas, reported in 2008,[6] has revolutionized therapy for SGH and it is now considered first-line treatment.[2] Although it is generally well tolerated, the potentially concerning side effects of propranolol include hypoglycemia, hypotension, bradycardia, bronchospasm, dizziness, and depressed mood/fatigue. A rare and more severe side effect is arrhythmia such as heart block. Because of these risks, patients are generally treated in conjunction with cardiology, or with a preliminary cardiology consultation. Treatment is initiated at 1 mg/kg of propranolol 3 times a day, then advanced to 2 mg/kg, and is continued for 6 to 12 months. Most institutions monitor patients for adverse reactions (as discussed earlier) at the onset of therapy.[59] Treatment regimens continue to be developed and modified, and more data about the outcomes of its use are reported prolifically, appearing in the medical and general literature.[60–62]

Recurrent Respiratory Papillomatosis

Although fundamentally rare, recurrent respiratory papillomatosis (RRP) is the most common benign neoplasm of the larynx in children. Caused by human papillomavirus (HPV) infection and highly variable in behavior, these warty growths tend to affect areas of mucosal transition, but can extend throughout the airway. Hoarseness and airway obstruction are the typical signs of RRP, but this is variable depending on the size and specific laryngeal location of the lesions. Lesions may be lifelong, may respond quickly to excision, or may be recurrent into late childhood or adolescence and then resolve. The mainstay of therapy is judicious excision to maintain airway patency and phonatory ability, while minimizing voice damage from repeated excision. Multiple modalities for endoscopic excision exist, including cold microdebrider, potassium titanyl phosphate laser, and CO_2 laser, each of which has advantages. The primary chronic outcome measure of repeated excision is voice quality, and current and future research is oriented toward identifying optimal treatment strategies.[63] Adjuvant therapies include cidofovir and avastin, which have shown success in reducing the frequency of excision and severity of recurrence, respectively.[64,65] There is hope among the otolaryngology community that HPV vaccination, which has become widespread in recent years, could be a bellwether for the future of RRP prevention.

Tracheomalacia

The structural integrity of tracheal rings relies on a specific shape, in which the cartilage of the ring is round and accounts for two-thirds to three-quarters of the circumference of the trachea. Rings that are abnormally shaped or that have abnormal proportions of cartilage to soft tissue are significantly more prone to collapse. Tracheomalacia is most commonly congenital, but can also be acquired through external compression from vasculature or a mass. Most tracheomalacia does not require surgical intervention, but severe tracheomalacia, particularly in infancy, can require tracheostomy for airway patency. Because the airway obstruction is worse on expiration, many patients with tracheomalacia have significant expiratory stridor, and have difficulty clearing secretions when coughing.[66] In general, patients with

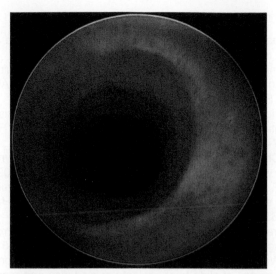

Fig. 16. Complete tracheal rings in an infant. Note the completely round and narrow rings.

isolated tracheomalacia only require supportive measures. The inclusion of a pulmonologist in their care is critical for optimum management.

Complete Tracheal Rings

Complete tracheal rings are a congenital abnormality, in which the posterior trachealis muscle of the trachea does not develop, resulting in fused, circular tracheal cartilages that are significantly smaller than the expected size of the trachea (**Fig. 16**). These patients present with significant airway obstruction and biphasic stridor, or with difficulty at intubation for another procedure. This abnormality frequently occurs concomitantly with congenital cardiovascular defects, particularly pulmonary artery slings,[67] can vary from a single complete ring to a segment that is the length of the trachea, and can include bronchial cartilage rings. Over the decades many procedures were used for treatment, with limited success and high mortality. Within the last 15 years, a previously known procedure, the slide tracheoplasty, has been applied to this airway deformity with great success, and has greatly improved disease-specific survival.[8,15] It has been suggested anecdotally that about 80% of patients with tracheal rings require surgical intervention in infancy, 10% require it later in childhood because of worsening exertional dyspnea, and about 10% never need intervention.[68]

SUMMARY

Pediatric stridor must be recognized as a symptom of upper airway obstruction, and as such it can be a minor transient sign with little clinical significance or it can herald impending airway collapse or respiratory failure. Proper evaluation of the stridorous patient requires an understanding of aerodigestive anatomy and physiology, diagnostic modalities, and potential interventions and complications. There are many ancillary studies that may or may not assist in the diagnosis and management of a stridorous patient, and it is important to use these in an efficient manner, focusing the diagnostic approach through a stepwise evaluation. Many interventions for airway obstruction require a high level of care from the physicians and hospital, and complications may be catastrophic. Complete evaluation of a stridorous patient is often best performed with a multidisciplinary approach.

REFERENCES

1. Hartl TT, Chadha NK. A systematic review of laryngomalacia and acid reflux. Otolaryngol Head Neck Surg 2012;147:619–26.
2. Hill CA, Ramakrishna J, Fracchia MS, et al. Prevalence of eosinophilic esophagitis in children with refractory aerodigestive symptoms. JAMA Otolaryngol Head Neck Surg 2013;139:903–6.
3. Lang M, Brietzke SE. A systematic review and meta-analysis of endoscopic balloon dilation of pediatric subglottic stenosis. Otolaryngol Head Neck Surg 2014;150:174–9.
4. Rahbar R, Chen JL, Rosen RL, et al. Endoscopic repair of laryngeal cleft type I and type II: when and why? Laryngoscope 2009;119:1797–802.
5. Denoyelle F, Garabedian EN. Propranolol may become first-line treatment in obstructive subglottic infantile hemangiomas. Otolaryngol Head Neck Surg 2010;142:463–4.
6. Leaute-Labreze C, Dumas de la Roque E, Hubiche T, et al. Propranolol for severe hemangiomas of infancy. N Engl J Med 2008;358:2649–51.
7. Grillo HC, Wright CD, Vlahakes GJ, et al. Management of congenital tracheal stenosis by means of slide tracheoplasty or resection and reconstruction, with long-term follow-up of growth after slide tracheoplasty. J Thorac Cardiovasc Surg 2002;123:145–52.
8. Rutter MJ, Cotton RT, Azizkhan RG, et al. Slide tracheoplasty for the management of complete tracheal rings. J Pediatr Surg 2003;38:928–34.
9. Rutter MJ, Link DT, Liu JH, et al. Laryngotracheal reconstruction and the hidden airway lesion. Laryngoscope 2000;110:1871–4.
10. Schroeder JW Jr, Bhandarkar ND, Holinger LD. Synchronous airway lesions and outcomes in infants with severe laryngomalacia requiring supraglottoplasty. Arch Otolaryngol Head Neck Surg 2009;135:647–51.
11. Durvasula VS, LB, Bower CM, et al. Adenoidectomy and tonsillectomy are common in patients undergoing supraglottoplasty. American Academy of Otolaryngology Annual Meeting. Vancouver (Canada), 2013.
12. Colton House J, Noordzij JP, Murgia B, et al. Laryngeal injury from prolonged intubation: a prospective analysis of contributing factors. Laryngoscope 2011; 121:596–600.
13. Boogaard R, Huijsmans SH, Pijnenburg MW, et al. Tracheomalacia and bronchomalacia in children: incidence and patient characteristics. Chest 2005; 128:3391–7.
14. McLaren CA, Elliott MJ, Roebuck DJ. Vascular compression of the airway in children. Paediatr Respir Rev 2008;9:85–94.
15. Russell HM, Backer CL. Pediatric thoracic problems: patent ductus arteriosus, vascular rings, congenital tracheal stenosis, and pectus deformities. Surg Clin North Am 2010;90:1091–113.
16. Johnson K, Geis G, Oehler J, et al. Simulation to implement a novel system of care for pediatric critical airway obstruction. Arch Otolaryngol Head Neck Surg 2012;138:907–11.
17. Amin MR, Friedmann DR. Simulation-based training in advanced airway skills in an otolaryngology residency program. Laryngoscope 2013;123:629–34.
18. Landry AM, Thompson DM. Laryngomalacia: disease presentation, spectrum, and management. Int J Pediatr 2012;2012:753526.
19. Rahbar R, Nicollas R, Roger G, et al. The biology and management of subglottic hemangioma: past, present, future. Laryngoscope 2004;114:1880–91.

20. Chen EY, Inglis AF Jr. Bilateral vocal cord paralysis in children. Otolaryngol Clin North Am 2008;41:889–901, viii.
21. Cooper T, Kuruvilla G, Persad R, et al. Atypical croup: association with airway lesions, atopy, and esophagitis. Otolaryngol Head Neck Surg 2012;147: 209–14.
22. Altman KW, Wetmore RF, Marsh RR. Congenital airway abnormalities in patients requiring hospitalization. Arch Otolaryngol Head Neck Surg 1999;125:525–8.
23. Thompson DM. Laryngomalacia: factors that influence disease severity and outcomes of management. Curr Opin Otolaryngol Head Neck Surg 2010;18:564–70.
24. Orlow SJ, Isakoff MS, Blei F. Increased risk of symptomatic hemangiomas of the airway in association with cutaneous hemangiomas in a "beard" distribution. J Pediatr 1997;131:643–6.
25. Shott SR. Down syndrome: analysis of airway size and a guide for appropriate intubation. Laryngoscope 2000;110:585–92.
26. Verloes A. Updated diagnostic criteria for CHARGE syndrome: a proposal. Am J Med Genet A 2005;133A:306–8.
27. Hartzell LD, Richter GT, Glade RS, et al. Accuracy and safety of tracheoscopy for infants in a tertiary care clinic. Arch Otolaryngol Head Neck Surg 2010; 136:66–9.
28. Bloom DC, Christenson TE, Manning SC, et al. Plastic laryngeal foreign bodies in children: a diagnostic challenge. Int J Pediatr Otorhinolaryngol 2005;69:657–62.
29. Berg E, Naseri I, Sobol SE. The role of airway fluoroscopy in the evaluation of children with stridor. Arch Otolaryngol Head Neck Surg 2008;134:415–8.
30. Dillman JR, Attili AK, Agarwal PP, et al. Common and uncommon vascular rings and slings: a multi-modality review. Pediatr Radiol 2011;41:1440–54 [quiz: 1489–90].
31. Li S, Luo G, Norwitz ER, et al. Prenatal diagnosis of congenital vascular rings and slings: sonographic features and perinatal outcome in 81 consecutive cases. Prenat Diagn 2011;31:334–46.
32. Venkatesan NN, Pine HS, Underbrink M. Laryngopharyngeal reflux disease in children. Pediatr Clin North Am 2013;60:865–78.
33. Liacouras CA, Furuta GT, Hirano I, et al. Eosinophilic esophagitis: updated consensus recommendations for children and adults. J Allergy Clin Immunol 2011;128:3–20.e6 [quiz: 21–2].
34. Gopalareddy V, He Z, Soundar S, et al. Assessment of the prevalence of micro-aspiration by gastric pepsin in the airway of ventilated children. Acta Paediatr 2008;97:55–60.
35. Kieran SM, Katz E, Rosen R, et al. The lipid laden macrophage index as a marker of aspiration in patients with type I and II laryngeal clefts. Int J Pediatr Otorhinolaryngol 2010;74:743–6.
36. Collins CE. Anesthesia for pediatric airway surgery: recommendations and review from a pediatric referral center. Anesthesiol Clin 2010;28:505–17.
37. Vroegop AV, Vanderveken OM, Boudewyns AN, et al. Drug-induced sleep endoscopy in sleep-disordered breathing: report on 1,249 cases. Laryngoscope 2014;124:797–802.
38. Reber A, Paganoni R, Frei FJ. Effect of common airway manoeuvres on upper airway dimensions and clinical signs in anaesthetized, spontaneously breathing children. Br J Anaesth 2001;86:217–22.
39. White DR, Cotton RT, Bean JA, et al. Pediatric cricotracheal resection: surgical outcomes and risk factor analysis. Arch Otolaryngol Head Neck Surg 2005;131: 896–9.

40. Myer CM 3rd, O'Connor DM, Cotton RT. Proposed grading system for subglottic stenosis based on endotracheal tube sizes. Ann Otol Rhinol Laryngol 1994;103: 319–23.
41. Zoumalan R, Maddalozzo J, Holinger LD. Etiology of stridor in infants. Ann Otol Rhinol Laryngol 2007;116:329–34.
42. Zoorob R, Sidani M, Murray J. Croup: an overview. Am Fam Physician 2011;83: 1067–73.
43. Derkay CS, Wiatrak B. Recurrent respiratory papillomatosis: a review. Laryngoscope 2008;118:1236–47.
44. Larson DA, Derkay CS. Epidemiology of recurrent respiratory papillomatosis. APMIS 2010;118:450–4.
45. Thompson DM. Abnormal sensorimotor integrative function of the larynx in congenital laryngomalacia: a new theory of etiology. Laryngoscope 2007;117:1–33.
46. Richter GT, Wootten CT, Rutter MJ, et al. Impact of supraglottoplasty on aspiration in severe laryngomalacia. Ann Otol Rhinol Laryngol 2009;118:259–66.
47. Durvasula VS, Lawson BR, Bower CM, et al. Supraglottoplasty in premature infants with laryngomalacia: does gestation age at birth influence outcomes? Otolaryngol Head Neck Surg 2014;150:292–9.
48. Lee KS, Chen BN, Yang CC, et al. CO_2 laser supraglottoplasty for severe laryngomalacia: a study of symptomatic improvement. Int J Pediatr Otorhinolaryngol 2007;71:889–95.
49. Petersson RS, Wetjen NM, Thompson DM. Neurologic variant laryngomalacia associated with Chiari malformation and cervicomedullary compression: case reports. Ann Otol Rhinol Laryngol 2011;120:99–103.
50. Chan DK, Truong MT, Koltai PJ. Supraglottoplasty for occult laryngomalacia to improve obstructive sleep apnea syndrome. Arch Otolaryngol Head Neck Surg 2012;138:50–4.
51. Clement WA, El-Hakim H, Phillipos EZ, et al. Unilateral vocal cord paralysis following patent ductus arteriosus ligation in extremely low-birth-weight infants. Arch Otolaryngol Head Neck Surg 2008;134:28–33.
52. Harnisch W, Brosch S, Schmidt M, et al. Breathing and voice quality after surgical treatment for bilateral vocal cord paralysis. Arch Otolaryngol Head Neck Surg 2008;134:278–84.
53. Hartnick CJ, Brigger MT, Willging JP, et al. Surgery for pediatric vocal cord paralysis: a retrospective review. Ann Otol Rhinol Laryngol 2003;112:1–6.
54. Inglis AF Jr, Perkins JA, Manning SC, et al. Endoscopic posterior cricoid split and rib grafting in 10 children. Laryngoscope 2003;113:2004–9.
55. Jabbour N, Parker NP, Finkelstein M, et al. Incidence of operative endoscopy findings in recurrent croup. Otolaryngol Head Neck Surg 2011;144:596–601.
56. Jorgensen J, Wei JL, Sykes KJ, et al. Incidence of and risk factors for airway complications following endotracheal intubation for bronchiolitis. Otolaryngol Head Neck Surg 2007;137:394–9.
57. Krival K, Kelchner LN, Weinrich B, et al. Vibratory source, vocal quality and fundamental frequency following pediatric laryngotracheal reconstruction. Int J Pediatr Otorhinolaryngol 2007;71:1261–9.
58. Tirado Y, Chadha NK, Allegro J, et al. Quality of life and voice outcomes after thyroid ala graft laryngotracheal reconstruction in young children. Otolaryngol Head Neck Surg 2011;144:770–7.
59. Parikh SR, Darrow DH, Grimmer JF, et al. Propranolol use for infantile hemangiomas: American Society of Pediatric Otolaryngology Vascular Anomalies Task Force practice patterns. JAMA Otolaryngol Head Neck Surg 2013;139:153–6.

60. Bajaj Y, Kapoor K, Ifeacho S, et al. Great Ormond Street Hospital treatment guidelines for use of propranolol in infantile isolated subglottic haemangioma. J Laryngol Otol 2013;127:295–8.
61. Buckmiller LM, Munson PD, Dyamenahalli U, et al. Propranolol for infantile hemangiomas: early experience at a tertiary vascular anomalies center. Laryngoscope 2010;120:676–81.
62. Drolet BA, Frommelt PC, Chamlin SL, et al. Initiation and use of propranolol for infantile hemangioma: report of a consensus conference. Pediatrics 2013;131: 128–40.
63. van Nieuwenhuizen AJ, Rinkel RN, de Bree R, et al. Patient reported voice outcome in recurrent respiratory papillomatosis. Laryngoscope 2010;120: 188–92.
64. Tanna N, Sidell D, Joshi AS, et al. Adult intralesional cidofovir therapy for laryngeal papilloma: a 10-year perspective. Arch Otolaryngol Head Neck Surg 2008; 134:497–500.
65. Zeitels SM, Barbu AM, Landau-Zemer T, et al. Local injection of bevacizumab (Avastin) and angiolytic KTP laser treatment of recurrent respiratory papillomatosis of the vocal folds: a prospective study. Ann Otol Rhinol Laryngol 2011;120: 627–34.
66. Carden KA, Boiselle PM, Waltz DA, et al. Tracheomalacia and tracheobronchomalacia in children and adults: an in-depth review. Chest 2005;127:984–1005.
67. Yu JM, Liao CP, Ge S, et al. The prevalence and clinical impact of pulmonary artery sling on school-aged children: a large-scale screening study. Pediatr Pulmonol 2008;43:656–61.
68. de Alarcon A, Rutter MJ. Revision pediatric laryngotracheal reconstruction. Otolaryngol Clin North Am 2008;41:959–80, x.

Diagnosis and Management of Patients with Clefts

A Comprehensive and Interdisciplinary Approach

Larry D. Hartzell, MD[a],*, Lauren A. Kilpatrick, MD[b]

KEYWORDS

- Cleft • Diagnosis • Management • Team • Interdisciplinary • Surgery • Follow-up

KEY POINTS

- Proper care of a patient born with a cleft lip and/or cleft palate (CL ± P) requires a team-based approach.
- Close monitoring by members of an accredited cleft team is essential throughout the patient's development.
- Speech and ear problems are common issues that require early evaluation and treatment.

INTRODUCTION

CL ± P is one of the most common birth defects. Patients with CL ± P are frequently encountered in general pediatric clinics but even more commonly in an otolaryngology practice. Problems with ear disease, hearing, infections, breathing, sleep disturbance, and feeding and speech disorders are often encountered with clefts. These patients often require multiple surgeries and many need therapy during their development.

Early and accurate diagnosis of a patient's cleft is critical for proper management. The primary care provider (PCP) and cleft surgeon must be aware of the potential issues that may arise with CL ± P and be familiar with the process for appropriate management, referral, and follow-up. Referral to a cleft team accredited by the American Cleft Palate-Craniofacial Association should be made either prenatally or soon after a child's birth.

Once referred to a cleft team's care, a coordinated evaluation must be completed to properly identify the need for surgical and medical management as well as possible

Disclosure: There are no financial disclosures for these authors.
^a Arkansas Children's Hospital, Department of Otolaryngology Head and Neck Surgery, University of Arkansas for Medical Sciences, 1 Children's Way, Slot 836, Little Rock, AR 72202, USA;
^b Department of Pediatric Otolaryngology, University of North Carolina School of Medicine, Chapel Hill, NC, USA
* Corresponding author.
E-mail address: LDHartzell@uams.edu

Otolaryngol Clin N Am 47 (2014) 821–852
http://dx.doi.org/10.1016/j.otc.2014.06.010
0030-6665/14/$ – see front matter © 2014 Elsevier Inc. All rights reserved.

oto.theclinics.com

therapy. This requires a fully functioning interdisciplinary cleft team that can provide comprehensive and cohesive care.

The object of this article is to provide a general understanding of clefts and describe an overview of the specific care each patient with CL ± P may receive. The embryology, epidemiology, classification, descriptive evaluations, surgical and medical interventions, and follow-up care are described.

EMBRYOLOGY

In the fourth week of embryogenesis, the developing median frontonasal prominence and paired maxillary prominences and mandibular prominences emerge around the primitive oral cavity.[1,2] At the end of the fourth week of embryonic development, the inferior frontonasal prominence divides into medial nasal prominences and lateral nasal prominences. The nasal alae are formed by elevation of the lateral nasal prominences. The upper lip and primary palate complete formation at the end of the sixth week of embryogenesis by fusion of the bilateral maxillary prominences with the 2 medial nasal prominences.[1,2]

The secondary palate has a distinct embryologic origin from the lip and primary palate. Bilateral palatal shelves of the maxillary processes begin a vertical growth phase in the sixth week of embryonic development and transition to horizontal growth in the seventh week. The palatal shelves then fuse in the midline and fuse to the primary palate anteriorly as well as the nasal septum. Ossification of the anterior aspect of the secondary palate occurs in the eighth week, differentiating the hard palate from the more posterior soft palate. Palatal development is complete by the 10th week of embryogenesis.[1,2]

Failure of fusion during embryonic development of the face results in orofacial clefting. Clefts can be divided into CL ± P and isolated CP due to their distinct developmental patterns.[1,2] Teratogen exposure and timing of insult are critical factors in labiopalatal clefting.[3,4]

EPIDEMIOLOGY

The overall incidence of orofacial clefts is estimated at 1 in 700 live births.[5,6] Prevalence varies by race and ethnicity, with high rates of oral clefts in Asian populations (0.79 to 3.74 per 1000 individuals), intermediate rates in white populations (0.91 to 2.69 per 1000 individuals), and low rates in African populations (0.18 to 1.67 per 1000 individuals).[7,8] CL ± P more often affects male infants, whereas CP occurs more frequently in female infants.

Syndromic cleft malformations represent a minority of cases, accounting for 10% to 37% of patients with CL ± P and 40% to 50% of patients with CP.[9–13] Gorlin and colleagues[14] indicate more than 400 syndromes that may be implicated in orofacial clefting. Van der Woude syndrome is the most common syndrome associated with CL ± P, accounting for approximately 2% of all cases (**Fig. 1**).[14,15] It is heralded by lower lip pits and is inherited in an autosomal dominant pattern with incomplete penetrance. CHARGE syndrome and Down syndrome represent additional recognizable malformations in the cleft lip population.

Stickler syndrome is the most commonly associated syndrome in patients with isolated CP, accounting for 5% of patients in some studies.[13] This syndrome demonstrates an autosomal dominant pattern of inheritance and is due to collagen defects. Affected individuals are at risk for SNHL and ophthalmologic involvement, including myopia, retinal detachment, cataracts, and glaucoma (**Fig. 2**).[9,13] 22q11.2 Deletion syndrome, historically referred to as velocardiofacial syndrome or DiGeorge

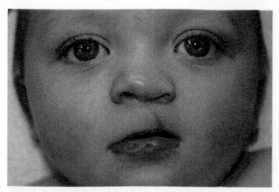

Fig. 1. Patient with Van der Woude syndrome, including cleft lip and lip pits.

syndrome, is the second most common syndrome observed in patients with CP; phenotypic expression may include conotruncal cardiac defects, velopharyngeal insufficiency, and characteristic facies (flattened malar eminences and square nasal root, among other features [**Fig. 3**]).[16] Pierre Robin sequence (PRS) is not a syndromic entity but occurs frequently in patients with CP and is commonly associated with multiple orofacial clefting syndromes. A classic triad of micrognathia, glossoptosis, and U-shaped CP occurs sequentially, resulting in postnatal airway obstruction and/or feeding difficulty. Isolated, or nonsyndromic, PRS is estimated to account for 17% to 63% of cases.[17–19] A referral to a geneticist or additional subspecialists (ie, ophthalmology) is warranted for many patients with clefts.

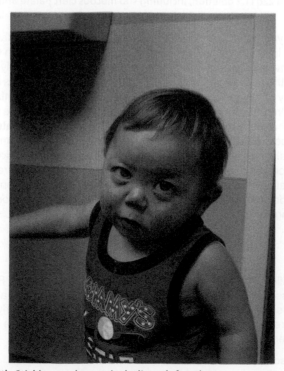

Fig. 2. Patient with Stickler syndrome, including cleft palate.

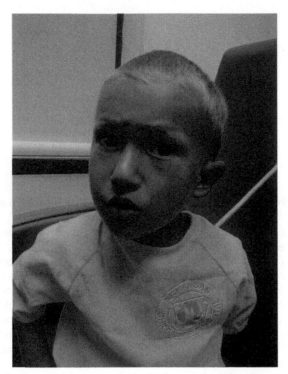

Fig. 3. Patient with 22q11.2 deletion, including sub mucous cleft palate and velopharyngeal insufficiency.

Cases of nonsyndromic CL ± P or CP are largely due to multiple factors, including complex genetic interactions and exogenous factors. The risk of both CL ± P or CP in first-degree relatives (ie, parent, offspring, or sibling) is approximately 3% to 4% and thus higher than the general population.[20–22] Maternal use of retinoids and anticonvulsants, specifically phenytoin, greatly increases the risk of having an infant with an orofacial cleft.[23,24] Pregestational diabetes in mothers also increases the risk of orofacial clefts, among other congenital malformations, and seems to correlate with glycemic control.[25] Folic acid deficiency has been implicated in the development of orofacial clefts with several case-control studies reporting a positive effect of folic acid supplementation on decreasing risk of orofacial clefting.[26–28] A multicenter randomized clinical trial investigating folic acid supplementation and oral cleft prevention is currently ongoing.[29] An additional exogenous risk factor for development of orofacial clefts is maternal smoking, which increases risk by 1.3 or 1.2 times for CL ± P or isolated CP, respectively.[30]

CLASSIFICATION

Numerous classification schemes exist to describe orofacial clefting. Rare facial clefts are typically classified using the Tessier system, with clefts located along axes identified by numbers, which are assigned relative to the midline.[31] Early classifications for oral clefts were based on observed morphology.[32–35] Of these, the Veau classification divided patients into 4 subgroups[33]:

1. Clefts of the soft palate
2. Clefts of the soft and hard palate, posterior to the incisive foramen

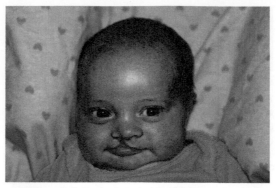

Fig. 4. Unilateral incomplete cleft lip and CP before repair.

3. Complete unilateral cleft lip and CP
4. Complete bilateral cleft lip and CP

Cefts may more simply be described in terms of anatomy and embryologic origin. Clefts of the lip or palate can be similarly subcategorized into (**Figs. 4–11**)

- Unilateral versus bilateral
- Complete versus incomplete

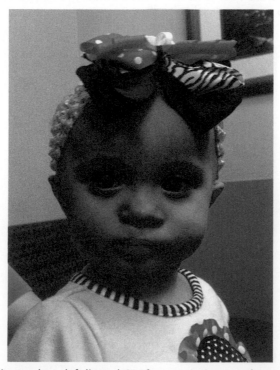

Fig. 5. Unilateral incomplete cleft lip and CP after repair. Same patient as in **Fig. 4**.

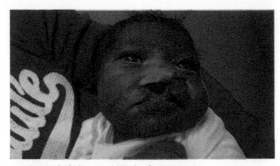

Fig. 6. Unilateral complete cleft lip and CP before repair.

A complete cleft lip describes a cleft of the lip and alveolus extending into the floor of the nose. A Simonart band can be seen in complete cleft lips and is a soft tissue band connecting the disrupted lip segments. An incomplete cleft lip has an intact nasal sill and may or may not involve a cleft alveolus. Incomplete cleft lips can be further divided as mini-microform, microform, or minor-form, depending on the height of the defect from the normal Cupid bow peak.[36]

A complete CP involves both the primary (anterior to the incisive foramen) and secondary (posterior to the incisive foramen) palate. An incomplete CP involves the secondary palate only but may be of the hard and soft palate, soft palate only, or a submucous CP. A submucous CP describes a dehiscence of the central palatal musculature with intact palatal mucosa; patients may exhibit a bifid uvula, zona pellucida (bluish discoloration due to absent muscle centrally), and a hard palate notch due to absence of the posterior nasal spine.[16]

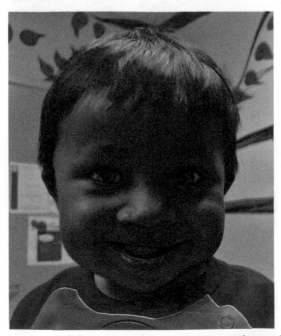

Fig. 7. Unilateral complete cleft lip and CP after repair. Same patient as in **Fig. 6**.

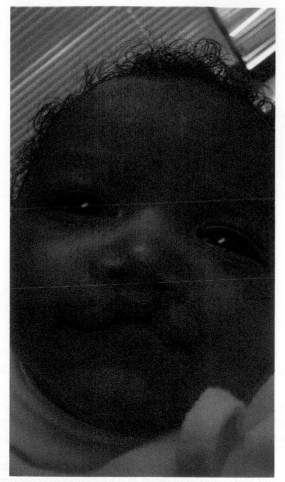

Fig. 8. Bilateral incomplete cleft lip and CP before repair.

INITIAL EVALUATION

Patients born with a CL ± P may present at different ages, ranging from intrauterine to adulthood. The needs at these different stages can be different, requiring a comprehensive evaluation tailored to the individual. It is important that a fully functioning and accredited cleft team becomes involved from the beginning. The composition of each team may be different but the aim is the same: to provide complete interdisciplinary care. Each team has a coordinator whose major role is to determine the most appropriate timing and place for patient evaluation and to arrange for the appropriate subspecialty assessments (**Fig. 12**).

Prenatal Evaluation

Although a significant number of infants are born with CL ± P to parents who were unaware of the child's condition, a growing number of women (10% of cases[37]) discover during routine fetal ultrasound that their child has a cleft. A vast majority of infants who are diagnosed with a cleft prenatally have a cleft lip because it is much more difficult to

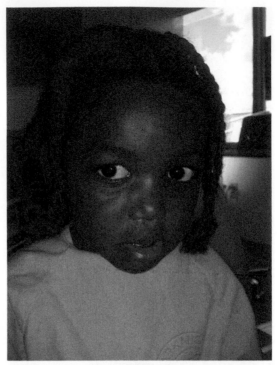

Fig. 9. Bilateral incomplete cleft lip and CP after repair. Same patient as in **Fig. 8**.

diagnose a CP accurately with ultrasound.[38–40] Other anomalies may be identified by ultrasound at this time because there is an elevated incidence of additional congenital anomalies and genetic abnormalities (10%–25% of cases depending on the type and degree of cleft).[40–42]

Receiving the news of a fetal birth defect in a developing child may be a shock to the pregnant mother and family and may result in a multitude of emotions and additional questions. Soon after diagnosis, a referral to the cleft team for a prenatal visit can prove beneficial for the mother as well as her family and friends.[39,43] The majority of this visit includes counseling and education. The goal should be to provide

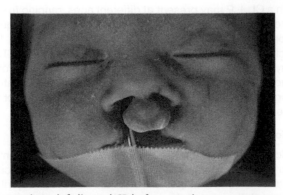

Fig. 10. Bilateral complete cleft lip and CP before repair.

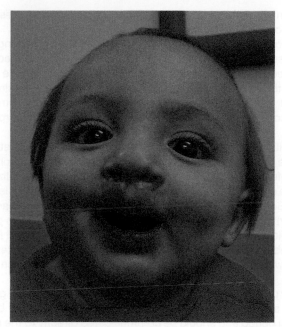

Fig. 11. Bilateral complete cleft lip and CP after repair. Same patient as in **Fig. 10**.

reassurance to the family of the type and quality of care the child receives and what they can expect from an evaluation and treatment plan once their infant is born.[44]

Nutritionist
It is helpful to include a nutritionist familiar with CL ± P (ideally the nutritionist associated with the cleft team) as part of this prenatal visit. A discussion of the feeding

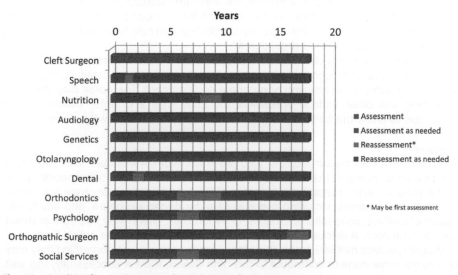

Fig. 12. Timeline for evaluation of patients with CL ± P.

challenges the infant may face tempered by an encouraging description of the different feeding options is helpful.

The topic of breastfeeding may be discussed if that is something the mother is interested in pursuing. Most infants with CP struggle with breastfeeding (as well as standard bottle feeding) due to an inability to achieve an appropriate sucking mechanism.[45] The mother may attempt breastfeeding at first, if she desires, but feeding and weight must be monitored closely to assure adequacy of nutrition and avoid negative health consequences.[46] The use of a feeding plate is controversial and not widely used.[47]

Most infants with CP cannot successfully breastfeed or even use standard bottles. In this setting, the mother and support team are encouraged to explore other feeding options. It is helpful to discuss and demonstrate the different specialized nipples and bottles, which the child may use during this prenatal visit (ie, Pigeon Cleft Palate Nipple and Cleft Palate Bottle, Haberman Special Needs Feeder, and/or Mead Johnson Cleft Lip/Palate Nurser). Providing them with some of these items can also prove beneficial especially if a child is delivered in an area with limited resources and little experience with CL $\pm$ P. Hubbard and colleagues[48] found hospital admission rates for feeding issues in patients with clefts are reduced by approximately 50% when prenatal counseling is given.

As an indicator of proper nutrition, a weight gain of at least 15 to 30 g per day should be expected. To monitor this closely, weekly weight checks should be performed in the early neonatal period and should be communicated directly to the cleft team nutritionist. Rarely, alternative feeding options may be required, such as extended nasogastric tube feeding (NGT) or gastrostomy tube (GT) placement.

Nursing

In addition to visiting with a nutritionist and surgeon, a mother's visit with a nurse who is a member of the cleft team is helpful while still pregnant. Providing reassurance to the family about the quality and type of care the child will receive is paramount. A discussion in conjunction with the surgeon regarding the timeline of evaluations and surgeries may take place at this time to help prepare the family for what may lie ahead. When possible, pictures of children before and after surgical management can be shown. Photographs may provide an excellent form of comfort because they see what their child may look like immediately at birth and also how he or she will transform through the various indicated procedures.

The overall goal of the cleft team should be discussed during this prenatal visit: to provide individualized coordinated care to allow the child to successfully engage in society and achieve healthy and appropriate development. The nurse may consider describing the other various specialists the child may encounter during clinical follow-ups to show the family the comprehensive care their child will receive.

Surgeon

A prenatal visit with the surgeon can also prove exceedingly valuable. This visit helps plant the initial seeds of trust and confidence that will prove essential especially early in the child's health management. During this visit, the physician may ask about maternal health status, including prenatal care, teratogen exposure, and any family history of clefting, congenital anomalies, or syndromes, which may help further direct the neonatal care. A discussion about cleft etiology can take place at this time.

Many expectant mothers feel guilt as they wonder if there was something they may or may not have done to contribute to this birth defect. If done successfully, this visit can help the mother and family remove some of these negative feelings and instead develop the positive sentiments that typically come with the arrival of a new child. The opportunity to ask questions should be offered multiple times throughout the visit and, when possible, information about resources available to the family and contact information for the team should be provided.

Overall, the goal of the prenatal visit should be to answer questions and provide information and materials that allow the mother and her close associates to prepare physically and emotionally for an infant's arrival. Women are encouraged to deliver in whatever setting their obstetrician feels is most appropriate and to make contact with the cleft team soon after the child is born.

Infant Evaluation

For any infant born with a cleft, a thorough examination is essential. As discussed previously, associated anomalies are common in patients born with clefts. A thorough head and neck examination (including airway) as well as heart and extremity evaluations can discover most of the common related findings in CL ± P. Depending on the type and degree of cleft, other specialists (such as audiology, speech, nutrition, genetics, and surgery) should be consulted to provide further evaluation and care for such infants (see **Fig. 12**).

Primary care

It is critical that each patient born with CL ± P establish a close relationship with the managing PCP. Regular follow-ups, especially early in a child's development, are beneficial to the emotional and physical needs of patients and their families.[49] Accurate communication between the PCP and the cleft team members is essential.

Cleft team evaluation

Once a child is stabilized, a consultation to the cleft team, including the infant's managing cleft surgeon and nurse, should be initiated. This referral provides the infant with prompt access to the appropriate members of the cleft team whose services the child may require and establishes a mechanism for close follow-up (see **Fig. 12**).

If a prenatal consultation was not performed, the information described previously should be shared at this time. This discussion includes information about clefts; descriptions of surgical interventions, including a timeline of procedures and evaluations; specific issues the patient may encounter (eg, feeding, hearing, speech, and dental), and information about the cleft team composition and timing of evaluations. Whether the initial visit takes place while still in the hospital or in an outpatient setting, this visit is the first opportunity for the nurse and/or managing surgeon to evaluate a patient and determine the degree and type of clefting. A thorough examination and history take place at this time to evaluate the cleft and identify any associated anomalies.[50]

Specific attention should be directed at this time toward the common problems encountered in CL ± P, including feeding, hearing, and breathing. Depending on findings, appropriate referrals should be generated and evaluations performed. In many cases, multispecialty evaluations can be accomplished during the same visit (inpatient or outpatient), which expedites patient care and provides convenience to the patient and family.

Breathing is one of the first things evaluated when an infant is born, and neonates with CL ± P are at higher risk for airway compromise. This is particularly true in the context of associated anomalies and if syndromic. PRS is the main source of upper airway obstruction in CL ± P although other causes need to be ruled out (**Fig. 13**).[51] If a patient is in respiratory distress, indicated interventions may be pursued (discussed later).

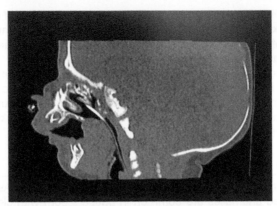

Fig. 13. CT scan of patient with PRS showing micrognathia and glossoptosis into CP.

Speech pathology

An evaluation by a speech and language pathologist (SLP) familiar with clefts is often beneficial in neonates with CL ± P. Early assessment and proper Intervention allow for determination of oral and pharyngeal function. Most infants with CP, as well as some with cleft lip alone, have difficulty with standard feeding approaches and SLP intervention can help them successfully feed and grow.[52]

The degree of clefting as well as the presence of an associated syndrome has been shown closely associated with the severity of feeding problems. Feedings often take longer in CL ± P and frequent burping and breaks are typically required because infants often swallow large amounts of air.

The SLP can greatly support patients with learning appropriate techniques for feeding as well as determining the most effective feeding method (breastfeeding, standard bottle feeding vs specialized nipples/bottles, and so forth).[52–55] The use of a palatal obturator or feeding plate is controversial although widely used in some institutions and regions of the world.[56,57] This option is rarely considered, however, at the authors' institution due to limited proved benefit in this setting combined with increased time and monetary cost.

Initially, a neonate with CL ± P may have difficulty despite using specialized nipples/bottles and having close SLP assistance. In these cases, NGT may be required. Rates of NGT placement have been found close to 30% in neonates with CP.[58] Oral feeding efforts should continue while NGT is in place and successful oral feeding is frequently accomplished. Some infants may eventually require GT placement.[59] Even if GT surgery is performed, regular speech therapy and close follow-up examinations by the cleft team are important to avoid or at least minimize oral aversion and eventually achieve successful oral feeding.

Nutrition

As discussed previously, feeding and nutrition difficulties are frequently present in CLP.[60] Close weight monitoring (initially weekly) is important in neonates. Increasing formula calories or adding calories to expressed breast milk, changing formula type, and so forth may all be required. Occasionally, an infant may present with failure to thrive and require admission to the hospital.[61,62] A team nutritionist can serve a pivotal role in making these decisions. A coordinated effort between SLP, nutritionist, nurse, and managing physician nearly always achieves successful feeding, nutrition and growth.

Audiology
Universal newborn hearing screening (NBHS) is mandated in a majority of states in the United States, such that more than 95% of newborn infants are screened for hearing loss.[63] Infants born with a cleft (in particular, CP) are at a higher risk of failing their NBHS; pass rates for these patients are only 72% in some studies compared with greater than 97% in patients without clefts.[64–66] In many cases, the cause of the failed hearing screen is middle ear effusion, which is present almost universally in patients with CPs.[67,68] Rates of congenital sensorineural hearing loss (SNHL) have been found as high as 5% in cleft populations.[69] Rates of conductive hearing loss (CHL) and mixed hearing loss are also much higher in CLP.[64,70]

The NBHS includes otoacoustic and/or automated auditory brainstem response testing, preferably before an infant is discharged home from the hospital. If a child refers (does not pass) the screening test, an appropriate and timely referral should be made to obtain repeat hearing screening and possibly further evaluation, testing, and possible intervention as indicated. A prompt evaluation becomes especially important in CL ± P. Identification of hearing loss should take place by 3 months of age and intervention should transpire by 6 months of age for confirmed hearing loss (see **Fig. 12**).[71]

Genetics
Many institutions consult genetics once a cleft is diagnosed. This consultation can prove helpful in identifying associated anomalies and may allow for classification into a specific syndrome. More than 400 syndromes have been found associated with CL ± P although most cleft cases are multifactorial.[50,72] A thorough history and examination with investigation into teratogen exposure and maternal factors (such as smoking, diabetes, prenatal vitamins, and so forth) may elucidate the cleft etiology and allow for meaningful genetic counseling; genetic testing is also an increasingly used tool. This evaluation can serve a critical role in helping the family adjust to the news that their child was born with a cleft. A discussion about recurrence risks and prevention can also be enlightening to the family and assist with future pregnancy planning.[73] The authors make efforts to have all cleft patients evaluated by genetics within the first 6 months of life (see **Fig. 12**).

Social work
Patients born with CL ± P may have multiple medical issues, as described previously, which require extensive work-ups, treatments, procedures, and frequent hospital visits. The financial, intellectual, and emotional issues can be challenging for many families. It is important to recruit the assistance of a social worker when indicated to provide the family with information and resources.[74]

CHILDHOOD/ADOLESCENT NEW PATIENT EVALUATION

Because the modern day population is dynamic and mobile, patients frequently present as a new patients to cleft teams after already having received treatments. The cleft team coordinator and director must possess a thorough understanding of the major medical and psychosocial issues that patients with CL ± P may encounter. This knowledge allows for a timely and effective approach to the evaluation of such patients (see **Fig. 12**). Newly established PCPs should also be aware of the various issues their patients may encounter to ensure quality and individualized care for their steward.

Airway and Breathing
The airway of any patient with CL ± P needs to be carefully considered and monitored. A compromised airway can result in poor weight gain, low school performance,

dysfunctional behaviors, and overall health detriment. Patients with CP are in an elevated risk category for airway anomalies, especially if there is an associated syndrome.[75] Although maxillary and mandibular hypoplasias are frequently the source of obstruction, other anomalies can be present and require a systematic and comprehensive evaluation.

The incidence of obstructive sleep apnea (OSA) or sleep disturbed breathing is also elevated in CL ± P compared with the general population and should be screened for during any evaluation, especially in patients with an identified syndrome.[76] In many cases, sleep-related problems can be corrected but require an appropriate workup, including a referral to an otolaryngologist and cleft surgeon.[77] A formal sleep study is often recommended. If adenotonsillectomy is indicated to provide relief for OSA or for other reasons, such as chronic tonsillitis, a partial (ie, superior) adenoidectomy should be performed to lessen the risk of postoperative hypernasality in this at-risk group.[78,79]

Otology and Audiology

As discussed previously, hearing loss of various types is common in patients with clefts. Eustachian tube dysfunction may persist longer in CL ± P and has been found to often persist into adolescence and adulthood.[70,80] As such, frequent audiometric and otologic evaluations, especially during the early developmental years, are important (see **Fig. 12**). Any new patient to a cleft team should receive an audiogram and otologic examination followed by indicated intervention.

In patients with tympanostomy tubes, evaluations should take place at least yearly. Tube otorrhea is common and routine treatments should be pursued. The development of atelectasis of the tympanic membrane, tympanic membrane perforations, cholesteatoma, and other otologic diseases have been found more common in CL ± P and need to be closely monitored throughout a child's growth. Even in adolescence and adulthood, the incidence of otologic disease is high.[70,81] Regular otologic and audiometric follow-up throughout development by an otolaryngologist and audiologist is important in many patients with CL ± P.[82]

Speech

Speech and language are critical aspects for successful communication in society. Children born with CL ± P have an elevated risk of speech delay or disorder.[83–85] It is important to evaluate speech for each patient with CL ± P in a timely fashion.[86] A majority of speech disorders in CL ± P are related to either articulation disorder or velopharyngeal dysfunction (VPD), although other disorders are also commonly identified.[87] Providing early intervention and therapy can prove beneficial in this population and should be pursued.[88] Speech assessment starting at or before 18 months of age is recommended with reassessment every 6 to 12 months as indicated (see **Fig. 12**).[89]

Dental/Orthodontics

Close attention needs to be paid to dental hygiene and care in patients with CL ± P.[90] The ability of the patient to access appropriate dental care may, however, prove challenging.[91] The complexity of care required may also be difficult for a general dentist to manage.[92,93] A vast majority of patients with CL ± P, however, are able to receive routine dental care.[94] The type of assessments and treatments vary depending on a patient's age. Orthodontic care is required in most patients with CL ± P. The involvement of a craniofacial-trained orthodontist as a key member of the cleft team is essential.[95] Most patients should begin routine dental care at approximately 2 years old and receive an evaluation by an orthodontist by 6 or 7 years of age (see **Fig. 12**).

Cleft Surgery

A surgeon's involvement with a new patient who has already been managed by a different cleft team depends on the specific diagnosis and treatments already received. The outcomes of previous interventions as well as the age and maturity of the patient are heavily considered. The surgical procedures and techniques offered and performed during this period are described in detail later. Surgeries, such as lip revision, palatal fistula repair, speech surgery, and alveolar bone grafting, among others, may be considered at this time.

Neuropsychology

Less than average IQ scores have been identified in several children with CL ± P. As such, many struggle with schoolwork and are frequently found to have learning disabilities.[96] It is important to assess each patient for evidence of cognitive and/or behavioral deficits that might benefit from further evaluation and treatment. This is typically evaluated once formal schooling has begun (see **Fig. 12**).

Social Work

Social adjustment has been found significantly affected in many children with clefts.[96] There are also many challenges a patient's family may be facing and access to social work should always be considered and offered.[97,98] Children with CL ± P who are of school age are at particular risk of low self-esteem, negative peer relationships, and social isolation.[99–101]

Nutrition

As described previously, the nutritional status of patients with CL ± P needs to be followed closely. Dietary habits should be inquired about as well as nutritional supplementation in these growing individuals. A nutritionist can also serve a critical role in preparation for procedures, such as palatoplasty and alveolar bone grafting, where dietary restrictions are frequently used (see **Fig. 12**).

EARLY INTERVENTIONS
Airway and Breathing

If a patient with CL ± P has associated PRS, difficulty with breathing and/or feeding may be present, and conservative measures should be attempted first.[102] These measures are successful in managing approximately 70% of cases.[103] Prone or side positioning is successful in alleviating the obstruction in at least half of all patients with PRS.[104,105] If a patient continues to struggle, a nasopharyngeal airway can be placed to bypass the obstruction and allow for appropriate ventilation.[106,107]

With continued respiratory difficulty and/or dysphagia, flexible laryngoscopy should be performed to confirm the suspicion of glossoptosis and rule out associated airway anomalies, which are present in greater than 20% of cases.[51] Depending on the results of the endoscopic evaluation, surgery may be indicated.

Multiple surgical techniques are available to address the issues related to micrognathia in PRS. Surgery is a topic of much controversy and debate, however.[104,108–112] Tongue-lip adhesion,[113–117] mandibular distraction osteogenesis,[118–121] and tracheotomy each have specific indications, benefits, and complications. The decision-making and surgical techniques for management of airway compromise in PRS are, however, beyond the scope of this article.

If a patient with PRS is having significant respiratory distress, intubation may be required. This intervention can be challenging and experienced personnel should be involved. Fortunately, with proper training and instrumentation, intubation can be safely performed in nearly all cases without resulting in emergent tracheotomy or death.[122] Additional reasons, other than PRS, can exist for respiratory distress in patients with CL ± P and should be thoroughly explored using standard protocols.

Feeding

Early intervention for dysphagia or feeding disorders was described previously. A team approach to this problem is most effective, which may include a PCP or neonatologist, SLP, nutritionist, and cleft surgeon. The cause of dysphagia should be thoroughly explored and different options for management considered. Some patients may require prolonged nasogastric feeding whereas others may require GT placement (discussed previously).

Ears

As discussed previously, the incidence of failed hearing screens is high in the cleft population. A study by Chen and colleagues[64] discovered that 28% of infants with CP failed their hearing screen. The failed hearing screen is frequently attributable to the presence of fluid, which is almost universally found in patients with CP. Chen also found, however, that 43% of infants with failed hearing screens who go on to have pressure equalization tube (PET) placement had persistent hearing loss in follow-up evaluations. The main associated findings that predicted hearing loss after tubes in this study were isolated CP, female gender, and a syndromic diagnosis.

If hearing loss is discovered, a thorough examination is required to evaluate a patient's anatomy and determine pathology. A sedated audiometric brainstem response (ABR) test may be indicated at this point to determine the degree and type of hearing loss. In the presence of fluid, however, the ABR frequently shows a more severe hearing loss. In this setting, most otolaryngologists recommend PET placement, which can be accomplished during the same anesthetic as the sedated ABR. This approach is supported in a recent consensus statement by the American Academy of Otolaryngology Head and Neck Surgery.[123]

Historically, early and frequent PET placement was recommended due to research in the 1960s by Paradise[124] showing the universality of middle ear effusions in CP. Rates of chronic otitis media with effusion in greater than 90% of ears are consistently reported.[70] The reasoning for treating middle ear effusions is to assist with language, communication, and psychosocial development as well as prevention of hearing loss and ear disease.[125–127] Paradise showed improved hearing, higher IQ, and better language skills in children who underwent PET placement and had close follow-up.[124] Tympanostomy tube placement was found to improve hearing results in CL ± P and is recommended.[128,129] The authors follow this philosophy at their institution with a majority of CL ± P patients receiving PET either early at 3 months due to hearing loss in the presence of effusion or at the time of palatoplasty if effusion has been present for greater than 3 months (usually at 9 to 12 months of age).[81]

Some recent literature has looked, however, at the possible consequences of PET placement and questioned the developmental, otologic, and audiologic benefits of treating middle ear effusions in CL ± P.[130,131] A study by Phua and colleagues[132] retrospectively compared 2 groups of patients with CP who underwent routine PET placement compared with a selective group. They found no difference in persistent CHL between the 2 groups; however, there was an increased incidence of otologic complications in the routine tympanostomy group and they recommend a more selective approach to PET placement. The speech and language benefits of PET placement for persistent effusion have also been questioned when looking at long-term outcomes; however, these findings were in noncleft populations.[133–136]

Presurgical Orthopedics

Depending on the type and degree of cleft lip, presurgical orthopedics may be considered and provide benefit. Different options, such as lip taping,[137] nasoalveolar molding (NAM),[138–140] and lip adhesions,[141–143] can assist with narrowing the cleft width and improving the affiliated soft tissue, aligning the alveolar margins and improving nostril formation and position (**Fig. 14**). The decision to used any one of these techniques is frequently based on subjective evaluations, surgeon preference and training, family compliance, and resource availability. The use of these different methods to improve surgical preparation and postoperative outcomes is controversial with variable supportive data and is discussed further later.[144,145]

SURGICAL MANAGEMENT

A timeline for the following interventions is shown in **Fig. 15**.

Lip Adhesion

Ideal candidates for lip adhesion are patients with wide complete unilateral cleft lip or bilateral cleft lips who cannot be managed in a presurgical orthopedic program (ie, lip taping or NAM) (**Fig. 16**). The goal of lip adhesion is to improve symmetry and minimize cleft width. Surgery is performed under general anesthesia at approximately 1 month of age. Key points for definitive cleft lip repair are marked to ensure these critical tissues are not violated during lip adhesion. I-shaped bookend flaps of the mucosa are elevated on the adjacent lip segments and extend into the gingivobuccal sulcus and nasal vestibule as necessary to obtain adequate mobilization and decreased tension during closure. Mucosal closure is performed first followed by a horizontal mattress suture through the orbicularis oris muscle bilaterally using large-gauge permanent suture. The cutaneous portion is also closed with absorbable suture. Silicone nostril retainers can be used to shape the ala and lengthen the columella after this procedure (**Fig. 17**). A tongue suture is placed for any postoperative airway obstruction, and the infant is admitted for overnight observation. Syringe feedings and soft arm restraints are used for approximately 10 to 14 days postoperatively. Complications are uncommon with dehiscence rates occurring in fewer than 5% of cases.[146]

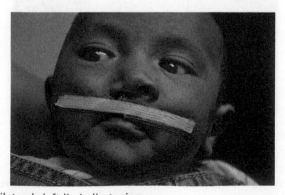

Fig. 14. Wide unilateral cleft lip in lip taping.

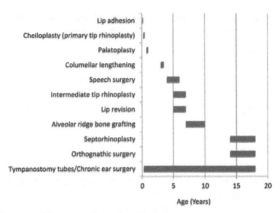

Fig. 15. Timing of surgical interventions for CL ± P.

Cheiloplasty (with or Without Primary Rhinoplasty)

Definitive lip repair occurs at approximately 3 months of age to ensure adequate weight/growth and hemoglobin level, decrease risk of postanesthetic apnea, and minimize nasal airway compromise. Numerous techniques are described for unilateral cleft lip repair. In North America, the most commonly used technique is the rotation advancement, initially popularized by Millard.[147,148] Adaptations of the rotation-advancement technique by Mohler[149] or Noordhoff[150] are also frequently used. The triangular flap technique is less commonly used.[151,152] Recent studies indicate that a majority of surgeons use the same technique for complete and incomplete cleft lip repair.[148] Similarly, multiple techniques exist for repair of the bilateral cleft lip.[153–156] The authors' institution uses the Millard technique for both unilateral and bilateral complete cleft lip repairs (discussed later) (see **Figs. 4–11**).

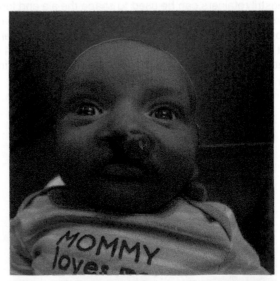

Fig. 16. Bilateral complete cleft lip and CP before lip adhesion. Note the rotated and asymmetric premaxilla.

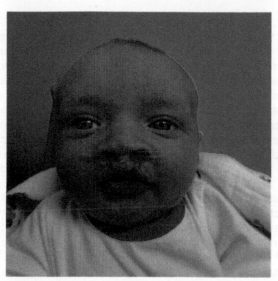

Fig. 17. Bilateral complete cleft lip and CP after lip adhesion with nostril retainers in place. Same patient as in **Fig. 16**. Note the improved symmetry of the lip.

Similar to lip adhesion, cheiloplasty is performed under general anesthesia. Critical points are marked at the high and low points of Cupid bow, columellar base, alar bases, and corresponding high point of Cupid bow on the cleft side. Measurements are confirmed using calipers. Dissection proceeds so as to rotate the noncleft side inferiorly and advance the cleft side medially. A C flap is created from the medial aspect of the noncleft side to recreate the nasal sill and may be used to lengthen the columella. Mucosa from the cleft edge (the M flap) is used to cover the premaxilla, and the orbicularis oris is reapproximated to create a competent oral sphincter and lengthen the lip. Subcutaneous, cutaneous, and mucosal sutures are then used for closure.[147] If warranted, due to alar and nasal tip distortion, a primary tip rhinoplasty can be performed in conjunction with lip repair. Subcutaneous dissection over the medial and lateral crura on the cleft side of the nose is performed and the cartilage and alar base are repositioned medially. Mattress sutures are typically used to prevent alar hooding after rhinoplasty.

Similarly, repair of the bilateral cleft lip begins with marking the critical points. Bilateral fork flaps are created from the lateral aspects of the prolabium, which are used during a later surgery to lengthen the columella. A small E flap is created from the vermilion of the prolabium to lengthen the central lip and join lateral vermilion-mucosal flaps to create the median tubercle of the lip. After mucosal coverage of the premaxilla and labial mucosal closure, the orbicularis oris is advanced bilaterally and closed in the midline as the prolabium contains no muscle. The alar bases are repositioned medially to create the nasal sill in appropriate contour. Multilayer closure is again used to complete the repair.[153]

Postoperative care is similar to lip adhesion surgery with the exception of suture removal in the operating room 7 days postoperatively. Silicone nostril retainers may again be used at the time of repair and/or after suture removal.

Complications may involve dehiscence or hypertrophic scarring. Scar massage, including the use of silicone scar gel, usually begins at 1 month postoperatively. Persistent erythema or thickened scar may be managed with laser or steroid injection, respectively.

Palatoplasty

Repair of the CP usually occurs at age 9 to 12 months to allow for sufficient growth and appropriate oropharyngeal airway. Speech outcomes are improved if palate repair is performed before 12 months of age.[157] Several techniques are also described for palatoplasty and choice of technique is often dependent on the type of cleft involved. In the United States, a majority of surgeons perform 1-stage CP repair. A 2-stage procedure, with delayed hard palate closure, has been well described and its supporters propose maxillary growth is most impaired by hard palate closure before age 1 year.[158] The most common surgical techniques for palatoplasty in the United States include a Bardach style (2 flaps) with or without intravelar veloplasty, V-to-Y advancement, and Furlow palatoplasty (double-opposing Z-plasty).[159–162]

For unilateral and bilateral complete CP, the authors prefer the 2-flap or 3-flap palatoplasty, respectively, with intravelar veloplasty. Bilateral mucoperiosteal flaps are elevated with preservation of the greater palatine vascular pedicle. Sharp dissection is performed to posteriorly reposition the palatal musculature. The hamulus of the maxilla may be fractured if necessary for mobilization of the flaps. Vomer flaps are also elevated to aid in closure of the nasal layer. A multilayer closure with absorbable suture is then performed. This procedure is often combined with bilateral myringotomy and tube placement.

For incomplete CP extending anteriorly into the hard palate, the technique is modified into a V-to-Y closure pattern. Incomplete cleft of the soft palate only is typically repaired using the Furlow technique. Posteriorly based muscle-and-mucosa flaps and anteriorly based mucosa-only flaps of both the nasal and oral layers are incised, elevated, and then transposed to lengthen the palate and realign the palatal musculature.[160]

After palatoplasty, patients are admitted for observation with a temporary tongue stitch in place in the event of airway obstruction. Postoperative antibiotics are used for 1 week. Patients remain on a liquid diet only via free-flowing sippy cup or standard cup and use soft arm restraints (no-no's) for 3 weeks.

Possible complications after palatoplasty include airway compromise, hemorrhage, infection, palatal fistula, and VPD. Risk of airway obstruction may be decreased by shorter length of procedure and frequent release of the tongue retractor intraoperatively. Steroids are not routinely used for palatoplasty at our institution. Fistula rates vary widely in the literature but have been reported to be as high as 45%. Moreover, a fistula recurs in one-half of patients after fistula repair.[163] A majority of surgeons report fistula rates of less than 10%, with more than half of surgeons reporting rates less than 5%.[161] Several studies indicate higher fistula rates are associated with the Furlow technique especially for wide clefts.[164] VPD results from incomplete closure of the soft palate (velum) with the lateral and posterior pharyngeal walls during oral pressure consonant production. The Furlow technique has been shown to improve speech outcomes in most studies.[165]

Columellar Lengthening

For patients with bilateral cleft lip, columellar lengthening may be necessary to increase nasal projection (**Figs. 18** and **19**). This outpatient surgery takes place at approximately 3 years of age. The bilateral fork flaps preserved during the primary lip repair can be elevated and advanced to lengthen the columella.[166] NAM and primary nasal correction are additional techniques that have reduced the overall need for columellar lengthening.[167]

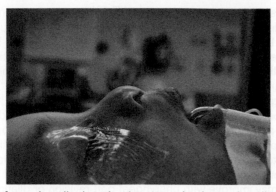

Fig. 18. Patient before columellar lengthening. Note the short columella with limited nasal projection.

Secondary Speech Surgery

Although a wide range of rates of VPD has been reported, an estimated 20% of patients who undergo palatoplasty have VPD.[168] Assessment by an SLP familiar with clefts begins at age 15 to 18 months and continues at regular intervals to monitor for signs of VPD among other speech disorders. Nasopharyngoscopy or fluoroscopy for patients showing signs of VPD provides evidence of the closure pattern of the velopharyngeal port and aid in surgical planning if necessary. Surgical intervention typically occurs no earlier than age 4 to 5 years due to the level of maturity needed for adequate speech testing.

Intervention options for VPD include prostheses, posterior pharyngeal wall augmentation, palatal lengthening, and pharyngeal reconstruction procedures (ie, pharyngeal flap and sphincter pharyngoplasty). Injection pharyngoplasty with or without nasal endoscopic assistance may be attempted for small central gaps.[169,170] Double-opposing Z-plasty, especially after previous palatoplasty using straight-line closure technique, can reorient the levator musculature and increase palatal length.[171] A superiorly based pharyngeal flap is performed in patients with adequate lateral pharyngeal wall movement and sagittal or circular velopharyngeal closure patterns. A musculomucosal flap incised inferiorly and laterally from the posterior pharyngeal wall and is elevated and sutured into a submucosal pocket of the soft palate. This

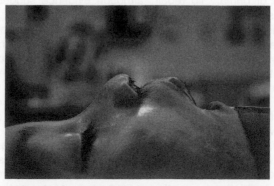

Fig. 19. Patient immediately after columellar lengthening. Same patient as in **Fig. 18**. Note the improvement in length and nasal projection.

surgery is successful in 63% to 98% of cases.[172–174] Sphincter pharyngoplasty is typically recommended for patients with coronal velopharyngeal closure patterns and limited to absent lateral pharyngeal wall motion. Bilateral superiorly based musculomucosal flaps are rotated medially and inset to augment the posterior pharyngeal wall and assist with velopharyngeal closure.[175] Success rates after sphincter pharyngoplasty are similar to pharyngeal flap.[176]

Patients undergoing sphincter pharyngoplasty or pharyngeal flap surgery are typically admitted postoperatively for observation. Complications include residual VPD, flap dehiscence, and OSA. Nearly all patients report snoring and/or apneic pauses in the immediate postoperative period after VPD surgery, with resolution for a majority of cases within 1 to 2 weeks. OSA may occur after both pharyngeal flap and sphincter pharyngoplasty but is more commonly associated with pharyngeal flap.[177] OSA on polysomnogram may improve with pharyngeal port revision or dilation, although flap takedown or continuous positive airway pressure may be necessary if OSA is deemed severe and revision attempts fail.

Lip Revision and/or Intermediate Tip Rhinoplasty

Secondary surgery on the lip or nasal tip of a patient with a cleft lip may be considered at approximately ages 5 to 7 years or thereafter. A diamond excision may be performed for a vermilion mismatch; a white roll triangular flap can be used for an under-rotated high point and vermilion mismatch; and a V-to-Y mucosal advancement can correct a whistle lip deformity. A complete lip takedown incorporating any of the aforementioned techniques may be necessary for extensive scarring along the entire lip and/or severe under-rotation, especially if there is evidence of muscular dehiscence. An intermediate tip rhinoplasty can also be performed at this age to provide nasal tip symmetry, improve nasal vestibular banding, and improve alar hooding. A full description of these and other revision techniques is beyond the scope of this article.

Alveolar Ridge Bone Grafting

For patients with a cleft alveolus, ideal timing of bone grafting occurs prior to eruption of the secondary dentition and specifically prior to eruption of the cuspid.[178,179] Presurgical orthodontic preparation is often necessary for proper alignment of the alveolar arches and to establish a cleft width suitable for grafting. Postsurgical orthodontics is typically delayed for several months to facilitate graft maturation. Gingivoperiosteoplasty is another technique to address the alveolus and is performed at some institutions at the time of primary lip repair, although evidence suggests it may have detrimental effects on maxillary growth.[180,181]

Alveolar bone graft surgery involves elevation of gingival, labial, and palatal tissues to expose the alveolar bone and create separate oral and nasal layers. Fresh autogenous bone is considered by most surgeons to be the ideal donor material and typically is harvested from the iliac crest. Substitute materials, such as bone morphogenic proteins and cadaveric bone, are used by some surgeons and may be valuable tools in revision cases or for large donor requirements. The nasal layer is closed, followed by placement of the donor graft material and subsequent closure of the labial and palatal mucosa over the graft.

Postoperatively, patients are admitted for observation. A strict liquid diet is maintained for at least 2 to 3 weeks after surgery. Nutritional counseling is requested prior to surgery for adequate planning with respect to caloric and protein intake and vitamin supplementation. Antibiotics are continued for 2 weeks postoperatively. With an iliac donor site, the authors recommend light physical activity for 6 weeks to avoid fracture.

Complications include dehiscence, recurrent fistula, infection, and graft failure. Revision surgery to augment the maxilla may be necessary in approximately 20% of patients and is higher in patients with bilateral cleft alveolus.[182]

Septorhinoplasty

Significant septal deviation and nasal asymmetry, specifically in patients with a unilateral cleft lip, can be addressed between the ages of 14 and 18 years, when the face has largely completed its growth. An external rhinoplasty approach via a transverse columellar and marginal incisions is used to expose the cartilaginous framework. A septoplasty is typically required in unilateral clefts due to significant deviation and functional obstruction. Cartilage repositioning and occasionally grafting may be necessary to create a symmetric nasal tip.

Orthognathic Surgery

Patients who undergo surgical correction for cleft lip and CP in infancy commonly develop maxillary hypoplasia. Approximately 25% to 30% require orthognathic surgery to establish proper dental occlusion. Facial growth may be restricted by scar tissue formation from surgical procedures or by an intrinsic mechanism related to the CP.[183,184] Perioperative orthodontic treatment is paramount, and extensive treatment planning between orthodontist and surgeon is necessary.

FOLLOW-UP CARE

Interdisciplinary teams have become the standard of care for the evaluation and management of patients with orofacial clefts. The American Cleft Palate-Craniofacial Association (ACPA) established guidelines for team development in the United States and strives for family-centered, coordinated care efforts for families and patients with CL ± P.[185]

Specialties commonly represented on the team include the primary surgeon (otolaryngology, oral maxillofacial surgery, or plastic surgery), speech pathology, audiology, dentistry, orthodontics, otolaryngology, pediatrics, genetics, nutrition, social work, and psychology. Additional subspecialists (neurosurgery, ophthalmology, craniofacial surgery, and so forth) serve an important role in complex patients as well. Each team should have a designated coordinator as a patient advocate and team facilitator. Regular coordinated meetings, including patient evaluations by team members, should occur to optimize patient care. **Fig. 12** shows the recommended timing for evaluation by team specialists. In most cases, evaluations take place yearly throughout a patient's development.

SUMMARY

The care of a patient with CL ± P is a lifelong process extending from the prenatal period into adulthood. A comprehensive, systematic evaluation by a cleft team throughout development is critical. With close follow-up, adequate education, and proper management, patients with CL ± P can thrive and achieve a high level of functioning in society in a majority of cases. Collaboration and utilization of resources assist patients and managing cleft teams in reaching this goal.

SUMMARY OF KEY POINTS

- A multidisciplinary team approach is required for comprehensive care of the patient with orofacial clefting.

- Patients with CL ± P may exhibit respiratory issues, feeding difficulty, chronic ear disease, hearing loss, learning disability, speech disorder, and/or dental and orthodontic abnormalities requiring intervention from infancy to adulthood.
- Early intervention and timely referral to a multidisciplinary team for patients with CL ± P are essential to improve patient outcomes and provide family support.

REFERENCES

1. Sperber G, editor. Formation of the primary and secondary palate. New York: Oxford University Press; 2002. p. 5–13.
2. Sperber GH, Sperber SM, editors. Embryology of orofacial clefting. New York: McGraw-Hill; 2009. p. 3–20.
3. Shi M, Christensen K, Weinberg CR, et al. Orofacial cleft risk is increased with maternal smoking and specific detoxification-gene variants. Am J Hum Genet 2007;80:76–90.
4. Yamade T, Mishima K, Fujiwara K, et al. Cleft lip and palate in mice treated with 2,3,7,8-tetrachlorodibenzo-p-dioxin: a morphological in vivo study. Congenit Anom (Kyoto) 2006;46:21–5.
5. Mossey P, Castillia E. Global registry and database on craniofacial anomalies. Geneva (Switzerland): World Health Organization; 2003.
6. Mossey PA, Little J, Munger RG, et al. Cleft lip and palate. Lancet 2009;374: 1773–85.
7. Wantia N, Rettinger G. The current understanding of cleft lip malformations. Facial Plast Surg 2002;18:147–53.
8. Vanderas A. Incidence of cleft lip, cleft palate, and cleft lip and palate among races: a review. Cleft Palate J 1987;24:216–25.
9. Shprintzen RJ, Siegel-Sadewitz VL, Amato J, et al. Anomalies associated with cleft lip, cleft palate, or both. Am J Med Genet 1985;20:585–95.
10. Jones M. Etiology of facial clefts: prospective evaluation of 428 patients. Cleft Palate J 1988;25:16–20.
11. Croen LA, Shaw GM, Wasserman CR, et al. Racial and ethnic variations in the prevalence of orofacial clefts in California, 1983–1992. Am J Med Genet 1998; 79:42–7.
12. Stoll C Alembik Y, Dott B, et al. Cleft Palate Craniofac J.
13. Jones MC, Jones KL, editors. Syndromes of orofacial clefting. New York: McGraw-Hill; 2009. p. 107–27.
14. Gorlin RJ, Cohen MM Jr, Hennekam RCM, editors. Orofacial clefting syndromes. New York: Oxford University Press; 2001.
15. Velez A, Alamillos FJ, Dean A, et al. Congenital lower lip pits (Van der Woude syndrome). J Am Acad Dermatol 1995;32:520–1.
16. Strong EB, Buckmiller LM. Management of the cleft palate. Facial Plast Surg Clin North Am 2001;9:15–25.
17. Shprintzen R. The implications of the diagnosis of Robin sequence. Cleft Palate Craniofac J 1992;29:205–9.
18. Holder-Espinasse M, Abadie V, Cormier-Daire V, et al. Pierre robin sequence: a series of 117 consecutive cases. J Pediatr 2001;139:588–90.
19. van den Elzen AP, Semmekrot BA, Bongers EM, et al. Diagnosis and treatment of the Pierre Robin sequence: results of a retrospective clinical study and review of the literature. Eur J Pediatr 2001;160:47–53.
20. Mitchell L, editor. Epidemiology of cleft lip and palate. New York: McGraw-Hill; 2009. p. 35–42.

21. Mitchell LE, Christensen K. Analysis of the recurrence patterns for nonsyndromic cleft lip with or without cleft palate in the families of 3,073 Danish probands. Am J Med Genet 1996;61:371–6.
22. Christensen K, Mitchell LE. Familial recurrence-pattern analysis of nonsyndromic isolated cleft palate–a Danish registry study. Am J Hum Genet 1996; 58:182–90.
23. Lammer EJ, Chen DT, Hoar RM, et al. Retinoic acid embryopathy. N Engl J Med 1985;313:837–41.
24. Abrishamchian AR, Khoury MJ, Calle EE. The contribution of maternal epilepsy and its treatment to the etiology of oral clefts: a population based case-control study. Genet Epidemiol 1994;11:343–51.
25. McLeod L, Ray JG. Prevention and detection of diabetic embryopathy. Community Genet 2002;5:33–9.
26. Botto LD, Olney RS, Erickson JD. Vitamin supplements and the risk for congenital anomalies other than neural tube defects. Am J Med Genet C Semin Med Genet 2004;125C:12–21.
27. Shaw GM, Lammer EJ, Wasserman CR, et al. Risks of orofacial clefts in children born to women using multivitamins containing folic acid periconceptionally. Lancet 1995;346:393–6.
28. van Rooij IA, Ocké MC, Straatman H, et al. Periconceptional folate intake by supplement and food reduces the risk of nonsyndromic cleft lip with or without cleft palate. Prev Med 2004;39:689–94.
29. Wehby GL, Goco N, Moretti-Ferreira D, et al. Oral cleft prevention program (OCPP). BMC Pediatr 2012;12:84.
30. Little J, Cardy A, Munger RG. Tobacco smoking and oral clefts: a meta-analysis. Bull World Health Organ 2004;82:213–8.
31. Tessier P. Anatomical classification facial, cranio-facial, and latero-facial clefts. J Maxillofac Surg 1976;4:69.
32. Davis JS, Ritchie HP. Classification of congenital clefts of the lip and palate. J Am Med Assoc 1922;79:1323.
33. Veau V, editor. Division palatine. Paris: Masson; 1931. p. 554–63.
34. Fogh-Andersen P, editor. Epidemiology and etiology of clefts. Baltimore (MD): Williams and Wilkins; 1971.
35. Kernahan D. The striped Y–a symbolic classification for cleft lips and palates. Plast Reconstr Surg 1971;47:469.
36. Yuzuriha S, Mulliken JB. Minor-form, microform, and mini-microform cleft lip: anatomical features, operative techniques, and revisions. Plast Reconstr Surg 2008;15:90–8.
37. Hegge FN, Franklin RW, Watson PT, et al. Fetal malformations commonly detectable on obstetric ultrasound. J Reprod Med 1990;35:391–8.
38. Hegge FN, Prescott GH, Watson PT. Fetal facial abnormalities identified during obstetric sonography. J Ultrasound Med 1986;5:679–84.
39. Matthews MS, Cohen M, Viglione M, et al. Prenatal counseling for cleft lip and palate. Plast Reconstr Surg 1998;101:1–5.
40. Gillham JC, Anand S, Bullen PJ. Antenatal detection of cleft lip with or without cleft palate: incidence of associated chromosomal and structural anomalies. Ultrasound Obstet Gynecol 2009;34:410–5.
41. Saltzman DH, Benacerraf BR, Frigoletto FD. Diagnosis and management of fetal facial clefts. Am J Obstet Gynecol 1986;155:377–9.
42. Meizner I, Katz M, Bar-Ziv J, et al. Prenatal sonographic detection of fetal facial malformations. Isr J Med Sci 1987;23:881–5.

43. O'Hanlon K, Camic PM, Shearer J. Factors associated with parental adaptation to having a child with a cleft lip and/or palate: the impact of parental diagnosis. Cleft Palate Craniofac J 2012;49:718–29.
44. Mulliken JB, Benacerraf BR. Prenatal diagnosis of cleft lip: what the sonologist needs to tell the surgeon. J Ultrasound Med 2001;20:1159–64.
45. da Silva Dalben G, Costa B, Gomide MR, et al. Breast-feeding and sugar intake in babies with cleft lip and palate. Cleft Palate Craniofac J 2003;40:84–7.
46. Livingstone VH, Willis CE, Abdel-Wareth LO, et al. Neonatal hypernatremic dehydration associated with breast-feeding malnutrition: a retrospective survey. CMAJ 2000;162:647–52.
47. Turner L, Jacobsen C, Humenczuk M, et al. The effects of lactation education and a prosthetic obturator appliance on feeding efficiency in infants with cleft lip and palate. Cleft Palate Craniofac J 2001;38:519–24.
48. Hubbard BA, Baker CL, Muzaffar AR. Prenatal counseling's effect on rates of neonatal intensive care admission for feeding problems cleft lip/palate infants. Mo Med 2012;109:153–6.
49. Yetter JF 3rd. Cleft lip and cleft palate. Am Fam Physician 1992;46:1211–21.
50. Brito LA, Meira JG, Kobayashi GS, et al. Genetics and management of the patient with orofacial cleft. Plast Surg Int 2012;2012:782821.
51. Cruz MJ, Kerschner JE, Beste DJ, et al. Pierre Robin sequences: secondary respiratory difficulties and intrinsic feeding abnormalities. Laryngoscope 1999;109:1632–6.
52. Miller CK. Feeding issues and interventions in infants and children with clefts and craniofacial syndromes. Semin Speech Lang 2011;32:115–26.
53. Bessell A, Hooper L, Shaw WC, et al. Feeding interventions for growth and development in infants with cleft lip, cleft palate or cleft lip and palate. Cochrane Database Syst Rev 2011;(2):CD003315.
54. Reid J. A review of feeding interventions for infants with cleft palate. Cleft Palate Craniofac J 2004;41:268–78.
55. Glenny AM, Hooper L, Shaw WC, et al. Feeding interventions for growth and development in infants with cleft lip, cleft palate or cleft lip and palate. Cochrane Database Syst Rev 2004;(3):CD003315.
56. Chandna P, Adlakha VK, Singh N. Feeding obturator appliance for an infant with cleft lip and palate. J Indian Soc Pedod Prev Dent 2011;29:71–3.
57. Jones JE, Henderson L, Avery DR. Use of a feeding obturator for infants with severe cleft lip and palate. Spec Care Dentist 1982;2:116–20.
58. de Vries IA, Breugem CC, van der Heul AM, et al. Prevalence of feeding disorders in children with cleft palate only: a retrospective study. Clin Oral Investig 2014;18(5):1507–15.
59. Cu SR, Sidman JD. Rates and risks of gastrostomy tubes in infants with cleft palate. Arch Otolaryngol Head Neck Surg 2011;137:275–81.
60. Redford-Badwal DA, Mabry K, Frassinelli JD. Impact of cleft lip and/or palate on nutritional health and oral-motor development. Dent Clin North Am 2003;47:305–17.
61. Pandya AN, Boorman JG. Failure to thrive in babies with cleft lip and palate. Br J Plast Surg 2001;54:471–5.
62. Eipe N, Alexander M, Alexander R, et al. Failure to thrive in children with cleft lips and palates. Paediatr Anaesth 2006;16:897–8 [author reply: 898–90].
63. Hayes D. State programs for universal newborn hearing screening. Pediatr Clin North Am 1999;46:89–94.

64. Chen JL, Messner AH, Curtin G. Newborn hearing screening in infants with cleft palates. Otol Neurotol 2008;29:812–5.
65. Barker SE, Lesperance MM, Kileny PR. Outcome of newborn hearing screening by ABR compared with four different DPOAE pass criteria. Am J Audiol 2000;9: 142–8.
66. Vohr BR, Oh W, Stewart EJ, et al. Comparison of costs and referral rates of 3 universal newborn hearing screening protocols. J Pediatr 2001;139:238–44.
67. Paradise JL, Bluestone CD, Felder H. The universality of otitis media in 50 infants with cleft palate. Pediatrics 1969;44:35–42.
68. Paradise JL, Bluestone CD. Early treatment of the universal otitis media of infants with cleft palate. Pediatrics 1974;53:48–54.
69. Anteunis LJ, Brienesse P, Schrander JJ. Otoacoustic emissions in screening cleft lip and/or palate children for hearing loss–a feasibility study. Int J Pediatr Otorhinolaryngol 1998;44:259–66.
70. Goudy S, Lott D, Canady J, et al. Conductive hearing loss and otopathology in cleft palate patients. Otolaryngol Head Neck Surg 2006;134:946–8.
71. Joint Committee on Infant Hearing, American Academy of Audiology, American Academy of Pediatrics, et al. Year 2000 position statement: principles and guidelines for early hearing detection and intervention programs. Joint Committee on Infant Hearing, American Academy of Audiology, American Academy of Pediatrics, American Speech-Language-Hearing Association, and Directors of Speech and Hearing Programs in State Health and Welfare Agencies. Pediatrics 2000;106:798–817.
72. Jugessur A, Farlie PG, Kilpatrick N. The genetics of isolated orofacial clefts: from genotypes to subphenotypes. Oral Dis 2009;15:437–53.
73. Andrews-Casal M, Johnston D, Fletcher J, et al. Cleft lip with or without cleft palate: effect of family history on reproductive planning, surgical timing, and parental stress. Cleft Palate Craniofac J 1998;35:52–7.
74. Starr P, Zirpoli E. Cleft palate patients–the social work approach. Health Soc Work 1976;1:104–12.
75. Perkins JA, Sie KC, Milczuk H, et al. Airway management in children with craniofacial anomalies. Cleft Palate Craniofac J 1997;34:135–40.
76. Muntz H, Wilson M, Park A, et al. Sleep disordered breathing and obstructive sleep apnea in the cleft population. Laryngoscope 2008;118:348–53.
77. Muntz HR. Management of sleep apnea in the cleft population. Curr Opin Otolaryngol Head Neck Surg 2012;20:518–21.
78. Tweedie DJ, Skilbeck CJ, Wyatt ME, et al. Partial adenoidectomy by suction diathermy in children with cleft palate, to avoid velopharyngeal insufficiency. Int J Pediatr Otorhinolaryngol 2009;73:1594–7.
79. Abdel-Aziz M. The effectiveness of tonsillectomy and partial adenoidectomy on obstructive sleep apnea in cleft palate patients. Laryngoscope 2012;122:2563–7.
80. Ahn JH, Kang WS, Kim JH, et al. Clinical manifestation and risk factors of children with cleft palate receiving repeated ventilating tube insertions for treatment of recurrent otitis media with effusion. Acta Otolaryngol 2012;132:702–7.
81. Gordon AS, Jean-Louis F, Morton RP. Late ear sequelae in cleft palate patients. Int J Pediatr Otorhinolaryngol 1988;15:149–56.
82. Drake AF, Rosenthal LH. Otolaryngologic challenges in cleft/craniofacial care. Cleft Palate Craniofac J 2013;50(6):734–43.
83. Mildinhall S. Speech and language in the patient with cleft palate. Front Oral Biol 2012;16:137–46.

84. Hardin-Jones M, Chapman KL. Cognitive and language issues associated with cleft lip and palate. Semin Speech Lang 2011;32:127–40.
85. Kummer AW. Communication disorders related to cleft palate, craniofacial anomalies, and velopharyngeal dysfunction. Semin Speech Lang 2011;32:81–2.
86. Kummer AW, Clark SL, Redle EE, et al. Current practice in assessing and reporting speech outcomes of cleft palate and velopharyngeal surgery: a survey of cleft palate/craniofacial professionals. Cleft Palate Craniofac J 2012;49:146–52.
87. Kummer AW. Disorders of resonance and airflow secondary to cleft palate and/or velopharyngeal dysfunction. Semin Speech Lang 2011;32:141–9.
88. Rullo R, Di Maggio D, Festa VM, et al. Speech assessment in cleft palate patients: a descriptive study. Int J Pediatr Otorhinolaryngol 2009;73:641–4.
89. Schuster T, Rustemeyer J, Bremerich A, et al. Analysis of patients with a cleft of the soft palate with special consideration to the problem of velopharyngeal insufficiency. J Craniomaxillofac Surg 2013;41:245–8.
90. McDonagh S, Pinson R, Shaw AJ. Provision of general dental care for children with cleft lip and palate–parental attitudes and experiences. Br Dent J 2000;189: 432–4.
91. Becker DB, Lee F, Hill S, et al. A survey of cleft team patient experience in obtaining dental care. Cleft Palate Craniofac J 2009;46:444–7.
92. Rivkin CJ, Keith O, Crawford PJ, et al. Dental care for the patient with a cleft lip and palate. Part 1: from birth to the mixed dentition stage. Br Dent J 2000;188: 78–83.
93. Rivkin CJ, Keith O, Crawford PJ, et al. Dental care for the patient with a cleft lip and palate. Part 2: the mixed dentition stage through to adolescence and young adulthood. Br Dent J 2000;188:131–4.
94. Dungy AF. General dental care of the cleft palate patient. Dent J 1976;42:356–7.
95. Noble J, Karaiskos N, Wiltshire WA. Future provision of orthodontic care for patients with craniofacial anomalies and cleft lip and palate. World J Orthod 2010; 11:269–72.
96. McWilliams BJ. Speech and language problems in children with cleft palate. J Am Med Womens Assoc 1966;21:1005–15.
97. Nelson PA, Kirk SA, Caress AL, et al. Parents' emotional and social experiences of caring for a child through cleft treatment. Qual Health Res 2012;22:346–59.
98. Baker SR, Owens J, Stern M, et al. Coping strategies and social support in the family impact of cleft lip and palate and parents' adjustment and psychological distress. Cleft Palate Craniofac J 2009;46:229–36.
99. Schneiderman CR, Harding JB. Social ratings of children with cleft lip by school peers. Cleft Palate J 1984;21:219–23.
100. Richman LC. Self-reported social, speech, and facial concerns and personality adjustment of adolescents with cleft lip and palate. Cleft Palate J 1983;20:108–12.
101. Starr P, Oppenheimer ME. Social factors in the patients in a cleft palate clinic. Plast Reconstr Surg 1979;64:253.
102. Evans KN, Sie KC, Hopper RA, et al. Robin sequence: from diagnosis to development of an effective management plan. Pediatrics 2011;127:936–48.
103. Meyer AC, Lidsky ME, Sampson DE, et al. Airway interventions in children with Pierre Robin sequence. Otolaryngol Head Neck Surg 2008;138:782–7.
104. Evans AK, Rahbar R, Rogers GF, et al. Robin sequence: a retrospective review of 115 patients. Int J Pediatr Otorhinolaryngol 2006;70:973–80.
105. Caouette-Laberge L, Bayet B, Larocque Y. The Pierre Robin sequence: review of 125 cases and evolution of treatment modalities. Plast Reconstr Surg 1994; 93:934–42.

106. Chang AB, Masters IB, Williams GR, et al. A modified nasopharyngeal tube to relieve high upper airway obstruction. Pediatr Pulmonol 2000;29:299–306.
107. Parhizkar N, Saltzman B, Grote K, et al. Nasopharyngeal airway for management of airway obstruction in infants with micrognathia. Cleft Palate Craniofac J 2011;48:478–82.
108. Schaefer RB, Stadler JA 3rd, Gosain AK. To distract or not to distract: an algorithm for airway management in isolated Pierre Robin sequence. Plast Reconstr Surg 2004;113:1113–25.
109. Papoff P, Guelfi G, Cicchetti R, et al. Outcomes after tongue-lip adhesion or mandibular distraction osteogenesis in infants with Pierre Robin sequence and severe airway obstruction. Int J Oral Maxillofac Surg 2013;42:1418–23.
110. Kochel J, Meyer-Marcotty P, Wirbelauer J, et al. Treatment modalities of infants with upper airway obstruction-review of the literature and presentation of novel orthopedic appliances. Cleft Palate Craniofac J 2011;48:44–55.
111. Mackay DR. Controversies in the diagnosis and management of the Robin sequence. J Craniofac Surg 2011;22:415–20.
112. Collins B, Powitzky R, Robledo C, et al. Airway management in Pierre Robin sequence: patterns of practice. Cleft Palate Craniofac J 2013;51(3):283–9.
113. Bijnen CL, Don Griot PJ, Mulder WJ, et al. Tongue-lip adhesion in the treatment of Pierre Robin sequence. J Craniofac Surg 2009;20:315–20.
114. Huang F, Lo LJ, Chen YR, et al. Tongue-lip adhesion in the management of Pierre Robin sequence with airway obstruction: technique and outcome. Chang Gung Med J 2005;28:90–6.
115. Denny AD, Amm CA, Schaefer RB. Outcomes of tongue-lip adhesion for neonatal respiratory distress caused by Pierre Robin sequence. J Craniofac Surg 2004;15:819–23.
116. Kirschner RE, Low DW, Randall P, et al. Surgical airway management in Pierre Robin sequence: is there a role for tongue-lip adhesion? Cleft Palate Craniofac J 2003;40:13–8.
117. Parsons RW, Smith DJ. A modified tongue-lip adhesion for Pierre Robin anomalad. Cleft Palate J 1980;17:144–7.
118. Dauria D, Marsh JL. Mandibular distraction osteogenesis for Pierre Robin sequence: what percentage of neonates need it? J Craniofac Surg 2008;19:1237–43.
119. Ow AT, Cheung LK. Meta-analysis of mandibular distraction osteogenesis: clinical applications and functional outcomes. Plast Reconstr Surg 2008;121:54e–69e.
120. Chowchuen B, Jenwitheesuk K, Chowchuen P, et al. Pierre Robin sequence: challenges in the evaluation, management and the role of early distraction osteogenesis. J Med Assoc Thai 2011;94(Suppl 6):S91–9.
121. Roy S, Patel PK. Mandibular lengthening in micrognathic infants with the internal distraction device. Arch Facial Plast Surg 2006;8:60–4.
122. Marston AP, Lander TA, Tibesar RJ, et al. Airway management for intubation in newborns with Pierre Robin sequence. Laryngoscope 2012;122:1401–4.
123. Rosenfeld RM, Schwartz SR, Pynnonen MA, et al. Clinical practice guideline: tympanostomy tubes in children. Otolaryngol Head Neck Surg 2013;149:S1–35.
124. Paradise JL. Management of middle ear effusions in infants with cleft palate. Ann Otol Rhinol Laryngol 1976;85:285–8.
125. Gravel JS, Wallace IF, Ruben RJ. Auditory consequences of early mild hearing loss associated with otitis media. Acta Otolaryngol 1996;116:219–21.
126. Gravel JS, Roberts JE, Roush J, et al. Early otitis media with effusion, hearing loss, and auditory processes at school age. Ear Hear 2006;27:353–68.

127. Valtonen H, Dietz A, Qvarnberg Y. Long-term clinical, audiologic, and radiologic outcomes in palate cleft children treated with early tympanostomy for otitis media with effusion: a controlled prospective study. Laryngoscope 2005;115: 1512–6.

128. Gould HJ. Hearing loss and cleft palate: the perspective of time. Cleft Palate J 1990;27:36–9.

129. Fria TJ, Paradise JL, Sabo DL, et al. Conductive hearing loss in infants and young children with cleft palate. J Pediatr 1987;111:84–7.

130. Sheahan P, Blayney AW. Cleft palate and otitis media with effusion: a review. Rev Laryngol Otol Rhinol (Bord) 2003;124:171–7.

131. Sheahan P, Miller I, Sheahan JN, et al. Incidence and outcome of middle ear disease in cleft lip and/or cleft palate. Int J Pediatr Otorhinolaryngol 2003;67: 785–93.

132. Phua YS, Salkeld LJ, de Chalain TM. Middle ear disease in children with cleft palate: protocols for management. Int J Pediatr Otorhinolaryngol 2009;73: 307–13.

133. Maw R, Wilks J, Harvey I, et al. Early surgery compared with watchful waiting for glue ear and effect on language development in preschool children: a randomised trial. Lancet 1999;353:960–3.

134. Paradise JL, Feldman HM, Campbell TF, et al. Effect of early or delayed insertion of tympanostomy tubes for persistent otitis media on developmental outcomes at the age of three years. N Engl J Med 2001;344:1179–87.

135. Paradise JL, Feldman HM, Campbell TF, et al. Tympanostomy tubes and developmental outcomes at 9 to 11 years of age. N Engl J Med 2007;356:248–61.

136. Ponduri S, Bradley R, Ellis PE, et al. The management of otitis media with early routine insertion of grommets in children with cleft palate – a systematic review. Cleft Palate Craniofac J 2009;46:30–8.

137. Pool R, Farnworth TK. Preoperative lip taping in the cleft lip. Ann Plast Surg 1994;32:243–9.

138. Ahmed MM, Brecht LE, Cutting CB, et al. 2012 American Board of Pediatric Dentistry College of Diplomates annual meeting: the role of pediatric dentists in the presurgical treatment of infants with cleft lip/cleft palate utilizing nasoalveolar molding. Pediatr Dent 2012;34:e209–14.

139. Suri S, Disthaporn S, Atenafu EG, et al. Presurgical presentation of columellar features, nostril anatomy, and alveolar alignment in bilateral cleft lip and palate after infant orthopedics with and without nasoalveolar molding. Cleft Palate Craniofac J 2012;49:314–24.

140. Grayson BH, Maull D. Nasoalveolar molding for infants born with clefts of the lip, alveolus, and palate. Clin Plast Surg 2004;31:149–58, vii.

141. Seibert RW. The role of lip adhesion in cleft lip repair. J Ark Med Soc 1980;77: 139–41.

142. Seibert RW. Lip adhesion in bilateral cleft lip. Arch Otolaryngol 1983;109:434–6.

143. Wakami S, Fujikawa H, Ozawa T, et al. Nostril suspension and lip adhesion improve nasal symmetry in patients with complete unilateral cleft lip and palate. J Plast Reconstr Aesthet Surg 2011;64:201–8.

144. van der Heijden P, Dijkstra PU, Stellingsma C, et al. Limited evidence for the effect of presurgical nasoalveolar molding in unilateral cleft on nasal symmetry: a call for unified research. Plast Reconstr Surg 2013;131:62e–71e.

145. Uzel A, Alparslan ZN. Long-term effects of presurgical infant orthopedics in patients with cleft lip and palate: a systematic review. Cleft Palate Craniofac J 2011;48:587–95.

146. van der Woude DL, Mulliken JB. Effect of lip adhesion on labial height in two-stage repair of unilateral complete cleft lip. Plast Reconstr Surg 1997;100:567–72.
147. Millard D, editor. Cleft craft: the evolution of its surgery. Boston: Little; 1976. p. 165–73.
148. Sitzman TJ, Girotto JA, Marcus JR. Current surgical practices in cleft care: unilateral cleft lip repair. Plast Reconstr Surg 2008;121:261–70.
149. Mohler L. Unilateral cleft lip repair. Plast Reconstr Surg 1987;80:511.
150. Noordhoff M. Reconstruction of vermilion in unilateral and bilateral cleft lips. Plast Reconstr Surg 1984;73:52.
151. Tennison C. The repair of the unilateral cleft lip by the stencil method. Plast Reconstr Surg 1952;9:115.
152. Randall P. A triangular flap operation for the primary repair of unilateral clefts of the lip. Plast Reconstr Surg 1959;23:331.
153. Millard D. Closure of bilateral cleft lip and elongation of columella by two operations in infancy. Plast Reconstr Surg 1971;47:324.
154. Noordhoff M. Bilateral cleft lip reconstruction. Plast Reconstr Surg 1986; 78:45–54.
155. Mulliken J. Principles and techniques of bilateral complete cleft lip repair. Plast Reconstr Surg 1985;75:477–87.
156. Manchester W. The repair of the bilateral cleft lip and palate. Br J Surg 1965;52: 878.
157. Dorf DS, Curtin JW. Early cleft palate repair and speech outcome. Plast Reconstr Surg 1982;70:75.
158. Gundlach KK, Bardach J, Filippow D, et al. Two-stage palatoplasty, is it still a valuable treatment protocol for patients with a cleft of lip, alveolus, and palate? J Craniomaxillofac Surg 2013;41:62–70.
159. Bardach J, editor. Unilateral cleft palate repair. Philadephia: Decker; 1985. p. 350.
160. Furlow LJ. Cleft palate repair by double opposing Z-plasty. Plast Reconstr Surg 1986;78:724–38.
161. Katzel EB, Basile P, Koltz PF, et al. Current surgical practices in cleft care: cleft palate repair techniques and postoperative care. Plast Reconstr Surg 2009;124: 899–906.
162. Aboul-Wafa AM. Islandized mucoperiosteal flaps: a versatile technique for closure of a wide palatal cleft. Can J Plast Surg 2012;20:173–7.
163. Wilhelmi BJ, Appelt EA, Hill L, et al. Palatal fistulas: rare with the two-flap palatoplasty repair. Plast Reconstr Surg 2001;107:315–8.
164. Losken HW, van Aalst JA, Teotia SS, et al. Achieving low cleft palate fistula rates: surgical results and techniques. Cleft Palate Craniofac J 2011;48:312–20.
165. Furlow LT. Cleft palate repair by double opposing Z-plasty. Plast Reconstr Surg 1986;78:724–38.
166. Millard D. Columella lengthening by a forked flap. Plast Reconstr Surg 1958;22: 454–7.
167. McComb H. Primary repair of the bilateral cleft lip nose: a 15-year review and a new treatment plan. Plast Reconstr Surg 1990;86:882–9.
168. Witt PD, D'Antonio LL. Velopharyngeal insufficiency and secondary palatal management: a new look at an old problem. Clin Plast Surg 1993;20: 707–21.
169. Sipp JA, Ashland J, Hartnick CJ. Injection pharyngoplasty with calcium hydroxyapatite for treatment of velopalatal insufficiency. Arch Otolaryngol Head Neck Surg 2008;134:268–71.

170. Brigger MT, Ashland JE, Hartnick CJ. Injection pharyngoplasty with calcium hydroxylapatite for velopharyngeal insufficiency: patient selection and technique. Arch Otolaryngol Head Neck Surg 2010;136:666–70.
171. Sie KC, Tampakopoulou DA, Sorom J, et al. Results with Furlow palatoplasty in management of velpharyngeal insufficiency. Plast Reconstr Surg 2001;108:17.
172. Cable BB, Canady JW, Karnell MP, et al. Pharyngeal flap surgery: long-term outcomes at the University of Iowa. Plast Reconstr Surg 2004;113:475–8.
173. Sloan G. Posterior pharyngeal flap and sphincter pharyngoplasty: the state of the art. Cleft Palate Craniofac J 2000;37:112–22.
174. Seagle MB, Mazaheri MK, Dixon-Wood VL, et al. Evaluation and treatment of velopharyngeal insufficiency: the University of Florida experience. Ann Plast Surg 2002;48:464–70.
175. Jackson I. Sphincter pharyngoplasty. Clin Plast Surg 1985;12:711.
176. Sie KC, Tampakopoulou DA, De Serres LM, et al. Sphincter pharyngoplasty: speech outcome and complications. Laryngoscope 1998;108:1211–7.
177. Lesavoy MA, Borud LJ, Thorson T, et al. Upper airway obstruction after pharyngeal flap surgery. Ann Plast Surg 1996;36:26–30.
178. Abyholm FE, Bergland O, Semb G. Secondary bone grafting of alveolar clefts. Scand J Plast Reconstr Surg 1981;15:127–40.
179. Turvey TA, Vig K, Moriarty J, et al. Delayed bone grafting in the cleft maxilla and palate: a retrospective multidisciplinary analysis. Am J Orthod 1984;86:244.
180. Hopper RA, Birgfeld CB, editors. Gingivoperiosteoplasty. New York: McGraw-Hill; 2009.
181. Wang YC, Liao YF, Chen PK. Outcome of gingivoperiosteoplasty for the treatment of alveolar clefts in patients with unilateral cleft lip and palate. Br J Oral Maxillofac Surg 2013;51:650–5.
182. Goudy S, Lott D, Burton R, et al. Secondary alveolar bone grafting: outcomes, revision, and new applications. Cleft Palate Craniofac J 2009;46:610–2.
183. Herber SC, Lehman JA Jr. Orthognathic surgery in the cleft lip and palate patient. Clin Plast Surg 1993;20:755.
184. Weinzweig J, Panter KE, Seki J, et al. The fetal cleft palate: IV. Midfacial growth and bony palatal development following in utero and neonatal repair of the congenital caprine model. Plast Reconstr Surg 2006;118:81–93.
185. Association ACP. Parameters for evaluation and treatment of patients with cleft lip/palate or other craniofacial anomalies. ACPA Publication; 2000.

Index

Note: Page numbers of article titles are in **boldface** type.

A

Airway, abnormalities of, syndromes associated with, 807
    and breathing, assessment of, in cleft lip and/or cleft palate, 835–836
    disorders of, endoscopy in, 809–810
        gastroesophageal reflux disease and, 809
        pulmonary health and, 809
    lesions of, diagnosis and management of, 797
Analgesia, in acute otitis media management in children, 655
Antibiotic therapy, in acute otitis media management in children, 655–659
Attention deficit hyperactivity disorder, 784–785
    symptoms of, 784
Autism, diagnosis of, 785
    examination procedures in, 787
    in children with hearing issues, 785–786
    treatment of, 786–787
    warning signs of, 787

B

Balloon catheter dilation, in chronic rhinosinusitis, 740
Bernoulli principle, 798
Bone grafting, alveolar ridge, in cleft lip and/or cleft palate, 842–843

C

Cheiloplasty, in cleft lip and/or cleft palate, 838–839
Cleft lip and/or cleft palate, 782–783
    bilateral incomplete, 827, 828
    by cleft team, 831
    classification of, 824–827
    complete, 826
    disorders with, 821
    early interventions in, assessment of airway and breathing, 835–836
        assessment of feeding in, 836
        assessment of hearing in, 836–837
        presurgical orthopedics in, 837
    embryology of, 822
    epidemiology of, 822–824
    evaluation of new childhood/adolescent with, 833–835
    follow-up care in, interdisciplinary teams in, 843
        surgical management of, orthognathic surgery in, 843
    incidence of, 822

Otolaryngol Clin N Am 47 (2014) 853–858
http://dx.doi.org/10.1016/S0030-6665(14)00105-4
0030-6665/14/$ – see front matter © 2014 Elsevier Inc. All rights reserved.

Printed and bound by CPI Group (UK) Ltd, Croydon, CR0 4YY

18/10/2024

01775920-0002